THE MILLON CLINICAL MULTIAXIAL INVENTORY:

A Clinical Research Information Synthesis

THE MILLON CLINICAL MULTIAXIAL INVENTORY:

A Clinical Research Information Synthesis

Edited by

ROBERT J. CRAIG

Illinois School of Professional Psychology
Chicago, Illinois

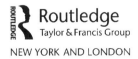

Routledge
Taylor & Francis Group

NEW YORK AND LONDON

First Published by
Lawrence Erlbaum Associates, Inc., Publishers
10 Industrial Avenue
Mahwah, New Jersey 07430

Transferred to Digital Printing 2009 by Routledge
270 Madison Ave, New York NY 10016
27 Church Road, Hove, East Sussex, BN3 2FA

Library of Congress Cataloging-in-Publication Data

The Millon Clinical Multiaxial Inventory : A clinical research
  information synthesis / edited by Robert J. Craig.
      p.   cm.
    Includes bibliographical references and index.
    ISBN 0-8058-1145-1
    1. Millon Clinical Multiaxial Inventory.   I. Craig, Robert J.,
  1941–   .
    [DNLM: 1. Personality Inventory.   WM 141 M656]
    RC473.M47M55   1992
    616.89′075—dc20
    DNLM/DLC
    for Library of Congress   92-23350
                                                                  CIP

Publisher's Note
The publisher has gone to great lengths to ensure the quality of this reprint
but points out that some imperfections in the original may be apparent.

Contents

Foreword

Theodore Millon
University of Miami

It was most gratifying to read the following chapters on the MCMI by Craig and his coauthors. Together, these authors comprise an impressive group of active researchers who have made major contributions to the MCMI, and from whom I have learned much. Their straightforward examination of the strengths and weaknesses of the inventory reflects their careful scholarship. No punches are pulled but they do give the MCMI its fair due. What they record here deserves close reading. Few fail to find features that may be faulted in the instrument, but almost all conclude that, despite these limits, the MCMI may well be the most diagnostically useful self-report inventory to appear in recent years, especially since the advent of DSM-III and the central role it assigns the personality disorders of Axis II.

Let me presume a measure of objectivity and orient the reader to what I view to be the major virtues and limitations of the MCMI (which is currently undergoing a second major revision, to be known as MCMI-III, a step I have decided to take owing to my desire to further refine the instrument's accuracy and utility). I turn first to what I judge to be the instrument's primary strengths.

With but a few notable exceptions (e.g., the TAT), assessment techniques and personality theories have developed almost independently. The MCMI is different. Each of its clinical scales was designed to be an operational measure of a syndrome derived from its author's theory of personality and psychopathology. As such, MCMI scales and profiles measure theory-anchored variables directly, hence providing specific patient diagnoses and clinical dynamics, as well as testable hypotheses.

No less important than its link to theory is whether the scales comprising a clinically oriented instrument are coordinated with the official diagnostic system and its syndromal categories. Despite a number of divergences, few self-report instruments are as fully consonant as is the MCMI with the nosological format and conceptual terminology of the official DSM system.

Separate scales have been constructed for the MCMI to help distinguish the enduring personality characteristics of patients (Axis II) from the more acute clinical disorders they display (Axis I). As such, profiles based on all MCMI scales should assist clinicians in understanding the interplay between longstanding characterological patterns and the distinctive clinical symptomatology a patient manifests under stress. Similarly, scales were constructed to distinguish syndromes in terms of their levels of psychopathologic severity. Thus, the characteriological *pattern* of a patient is assessed independently of its *degree* of pathology.

Scales designed for differential diagnosis were not developed by selecting items that discriminated clinical groups from normals; normals are no longer judged an appropriate comparison group. All item selections for the MCMI were based on data in which target diagnostic groups were contrasted with a population of representative but undifferentiated psychiatric patients. Moreover, item selection and scale development progressed through a sequence of *three* validation steps: (a) theoretical-substantive; (b) internal-structural; and (c) external-criterion. By using different validation strategies, the MCMI sought to uphold the standards of test developers committed to diverse methods of construction and validation.

There are limitations to the MCMI that also should be kept in mind by the reader. First, it is important to note that the MCMI is not a general personality instrument to be used for "normal" populations or for purposes other than diagnostic screening or clinical assessment. Hence, it contrasts with other, more broadly applied, inventories whose presumed utility for diverse populations has been encouraged by their developers. Normative data for the MCMI are based entirely on clinical samples and are applicable only to persons who evidence psychological symptoms or are engaged in a program of professional psychotherapy or psychodiagnostic evaluation. To administer the MCMI to a wider range of problems or class of subjects is to apply the instrument to settings and samples for which it is neither intended nor appropriate.

Along the same lines, the MCMI's scale cutoffs and profile interpretations are oriented to the majority of patients who take the inventory, that is, to those displaying psychic disturbances in the midranges of severity, rather than those whose difficulties are either close to "normal" (e.g., workers compensation litigants, spouses of patients) or of marked clinical severity (e.g., acute psychotics, chronic schizophrenics).

Important in evaluating the MCMI for purposes of differential diagnoses is the fact that certain personality disorder scales are sensitive to the patient's current affective state. All self-report inventory scales, be they personality- (Axis II) or syndrome-oriented (Axis I), reflect in varying degrees both "traits" and "states."

Despite methodologic and psychometric procedures to tease the enduring characteristics of personality apart from clinical features of a more transient quality, every scale reflects a mix of predisposing and generalizing attributes, as well as those of a more situational or acute nature. Noteworthy are the partial blurring effects of current depressive and anxiety states upon specific personality disorder scales. These results stem in part from shared scale items, but the level of covariation is appreciably greater than can be accounted for by item overlap alone.

As most sophisticated readers of this text will recognize, the mysterious and seemingly mythic powers of computer technologies have imbued its associated tests and reports with an undue measure of scientific merit and clinical acumen. Users of diagnostic characterizations provided via computer systems should be wary lest they find themselves lulled over time into an uncritical acceptance of its results.

There are distinct boundaries to the accuracy of the self-report method of clinical data collection. The inherent psychometric limits of the tool, the tendency of similar patients to interpret questions differently, the effect of current affective states on trait measures, the effort of patients to effect certain false appearances and impressions, all narrow the upper boundaries of this method's potential accuracy. However, by constructing self-report instruments in line with accepted techniques of validation, an inventory should begin to approach these upper boundaries. Given that it has progressed through a developmental sequence of this nature, we find that MCMI reports prove on the mark in about 55–65% of patients to whom it is administered; it is appraised useful and generally valid, although with partial misjudgments, in about another 25–30% of cases; and it appears off target, that is, appreciably in error, about 10–15% of the time. These positive figures are in the quantitative range of five to six times greater than chance or random diagnostic assignments.

As I have tried to note, the MCMI remains a less than perfect diagnostic tool. It neither reflects its theoretical foundation of clinical constructs precisely nor mirrors all facets of the syndromal disorders fashioned for the DSM, to which it has sought to be coordinated. Within the restrictions on validity set by the limits of the self-report mode, the frontiers of psychometric technology, as well as the slender range of consensually shared diagnostic knowledge, all steps were taken to maximize the MCMI's concordance with its generative theory and the official classification system. Pragmatic and philosophical compromises were made where valued objectives could not be simultaneously achieved (e.g., instrument brevity versus item independence; representative national patient norms versus local base rate specificity; theoretical considerations versus empirical data).

The MCMI is not cast in stone. It is and will continue to be an evolving assessment instrument, upgraded and refined to reflect substantive advances in knowledge, be it from theory, research, or clinical experience. Modifications have been introduced since the original MCMI publication 14 years ago; these fine-tunings continue regularly as our understanding of the MCMI's strengths, limits, and potentials develop further. For this reason, and to reflect theoretical advances and DSM-IV changes, work is currently underway on the forthcoming MCMI-III, likely to be published in 1993. We intend to address many of the concerns raised in the following chapters, and thereby improve the instrument's validity and clinical efficacy.

In closing, I express again my appreciation to this book's editor and contributors. Although I might take exception to some points raised in one or another chapter, I am pleased to record my estimation of their generally high quality and scholarly character.

Preface

"One man alone ain't got no . . . chance" (Ernest Hemingway, *To Have and Have Not,* 1937).

Hemingway was correct. Without the help of a large number of people, this project never would have happened. First, Ted Millon's brilliant theorizing about personality pathology, clinical syndromes, and the relationship between them, and his subsequent development of an instrument that provides us with a state-of-the-art psychometric application with which to assess mainstream personality styles and clinical syndromes, forms the basis of this work. Without the heuristics of his writings and his ideas shared at many workshops, the research and clinical studies that comprise this volume would not exist. However, his influence on this project is far greater than mere inspiration. Without his support and encouragement, the contributing authors would have been more reluctant to participate in this project and I would not have been able to attain a major publisher, such as Lawrence Erlbaum Associates. Thus, Dr. Millon played a very instrumental role throughout this project.

Second, I deeply appreciate the contributing authors, who wrote original chapters for this volume. I thank them for the quality of their work and for meeting deadline requirements amidst their busy schedules. Assembled here are the researchers and clinicians who have significantly contributed to the advance of knowledge in their specialty area, as it applies to the MCMI/MCMI-II. I was particularly impressed by the fact that no author contacted refused to participate. All were very excited about this volume and were enthusiastic towards their own contributions. I think the results are self-evident.

Finally, I thank the staff at Lawrence Erlbaum Associates, especially Larry Erlbaum, who put his faith and name towards this endeavor, my editor, Hollis

Heimbouch, who allowed me "space" to provide the kind of document of which I could be proud, Kathleen Dolan, editorial assistant, who managed a number of small yet major details that facilitated this publication, and Sondra Guideman, for her expeditious handling of copy editing and production of this volume.

The Millon Clinical Multiaxial Inventory (MCMI/MCMI-II) now occupies a central place in Objective Personality tests, and it is in use in a number of agencies, hospitals, medical centers, counseling centers, and clinical private practices. With this prolific use comes the opportunity to provide its users and its researchers with a compendium of current knowledge concerning this test. Also, the book provides teachers and students with "hands on" information that is useful for a primary or supplementary text in graduate schools in the areas of personality assessment, personality testing, and objective personality tests, psychopathology, and assessment. I hope this is the kind of book that will not sit on a shelf but one that will be used in the routine activities of those who use this instrument. The reader is invited to communicate with me about any aspects of this volume or about similar or related projects, by writing to me at the Illinois School of Professional Psychology, 220 So. State St., 5th Floor, Chicago, Illinois 60604.

Robert J. Craig

Contributors

Michael Antoni, Ph.D.
University of Miami
Coral Gables, Florida

Linda Bresolin, Ph.D.
Lakeside Veterans Administration
    Medical Center and
Northwestern Medical School
Chicago, Illinois

James Choca, Ph.D.
Lakeside Veterans Administration
    Medical Center and
Northwestern Medical School
Chicago, Illinois

Elizabeth M. Corbitt, M.A.
University of Kentucky
Lexington, Kentucky

Robert J. Craig, Ph.D.
Illinois School of Professional
    Psychology
Chicago, Illinois

William E. Davis, Ph.D.
Hines Veterans Administration Hospital
Hines, Illinois

Robert C. McMahon, Ph.D.
University of Miami
Coral Gables, Florida

Mary Melton, Ph.D.
Augusta Veterans Administration Medical
    Center
Augusta, Georgia

Ted Millon, Ph.D.
University of Miami
Coral Gables, Florida

Kevin Moreland, Ph.D.
Fordham University
Bronx, New York

Linda Pendleton, Ph.D.
MetroHealth Medical Center
Cleveland, Ohio

Harry Piersma, Ph.D.
Pine Rest Christian Hospital and
Michigan State University
Grand Rapids, Michigan

James Reich, M.D., M.Ph.
Harvard Medical School
Brookline, Massachusetts

Michael Gibertini, Ph.D.
Moffitt Cancer Center and Research
    Institute
Tampa, Florida

Cheryl Gratton, Ph.D.
Augusta Veterans Administration Medical
    Center
Augusta, Georgia

Richard L. Greenblatt, Ph.D.
Hines Veterans Administration Hospital
Hines, Illinois

Leon Hyer, Ed.D.
Veterans Administration Medical Center
    and
Medical College of Georgia
Augusta, Georgia

Maurice Lorr, Ph.D.
Catholic University of America
Washington, D.C.

Paul Retzlaff, Ph.D.
University of Northern Colorado
Greeley, Colorado

Stephen Strack, Ph.D.
Veterans Administration Outpatient Clinic
Los Angeles, California

Martha Tisdale, Ph.D.
MetroHealth Medical Center
Cleveland, Ohio

To Jo Ann
28 Years and Counting

INTRODUCTION

1

The Millon Clinical Multiaxial Inventory: An Introduction to Theory, Development, and Interpretation

Robert C. McMahon, Ph.D.

The Millon Clinical Multiaxial Inventory (MCMI) is increasingly recognized as a major differential diagnostic instrument. It is now widely used in clinical practice and increasingly used in research settings. The popularity of the MCMI apparently derives from a number of factors including its anchorage to Millon's (1969, 1981) comprehensive theory of personality and psychopathology and its coordination with DSM-III and DSM-III-R personality disorder and clinical symptom syndrome categories. Approximately 200 papers have been published which deal with the various aspects of the reliability, validity, and clinical utility of the MCMI. These studies have been exceedingly useful in clarifying the strengths and limitations of this popular inventory and, together with the careful development and validation effort documented in the MCMI manual, provided the foundation upon which its clinical usefulness should be judged.

The following chapter: (a) presents an overview of Millon's (1969, 1981) model which served as the theoretical framework upon which the MCMI was constructed, (b) summarizes development and standardization efforts connected with the original and revised versions of the MCMI, (c) describes clinical characteristics associated with MCMI-II scale elevations and the use of validity scales, and (d) provides a brief overview of recommended clinical interpretive procedures. Much of what is presented was drawn from several of Millon's major published works including *Modern Psychopathology* (Millon, 1969), *Disorders of Personality* (Millon, 1981), *A Theoretical Derivation of Pathological Personalities* (Millon, 1986a), *Personality Prototypes and Their Diagnostic Criteria* (Millon, 1986b), *Toward a New Personology: An Evolutionary Model* (Millon, 1990), and the *Manual for the MCMI-II* (Millon, 1987). The interested reader should consult these sources which provide in-depth presentations of Millon's theoretical model, and in the case of the Manual, a carefully detailed presentation of MCMI I and MCMI-II development and standardization procedures.

NORMAL AND PATHOLOGICAL PERSONALITIES

Millon (1981) conceives of personality as an organized pattern of deeply embedded, largely unconscious, psychological characteristics that are revealed in most significant aspects of life functioning. These characteristics develop as a result of interacting biological dispositions and social learning experiences and ultimately form a well organized psychic system of stable structures and coordinated functions (Millon, 1981, 1986a). This system of interconnected perceptions, regulatory mechanisms, feelings, thoughts, and behaviors provides a framework for structuring how the individual interacts with his environment and relates to himself (Millon, 1986a; Millon & Everly, 1985).

Millon (1981, 1986a) argues that normal and pathological personality styles derive from the same developmental influences. It is assumed to be "differences in the character, timing, and intensity of these influences which lead some individuals to acquire pathological traits and others to acquire adaptive traits" (Millon, 1981, p.9). Although no clear discontinuity exists between normal and pathological personality styles, several features are argued to be useful as differentiating criteria (Millon, 1969, 1981, 1986a). First, normal personalities are capable of meeting social responsibilities, achieving goals, and coping with inevitable stressors in a manner that is flexible and which leads to personal satisfaction and goal attainment. Pathological personalties, in contrast, tend to have few developed capacities for coping with the demands of life. What skills they do have tend to be applied inflexibly and in situations in which they are inappropriate. Second, normal personalities are relatively free from dysfunctional cognitions, defense mechanisms, and behaviors that foster vicious circles and intensify preexisting difficulties. In contrast, pathological personalities have habitually distorted cognitions and maladaptive behaviors that provoke punishing reactions from others, reactivate earlier conflicts, perpetuate and intensify ongoing difficulties, and severely limit opportunities for new learning. Finally, normal personalities demonstrate reasonable stability and resilience when subject to stressful life experiences. Pathological personalities demonstrate pronounced fragility and lack of resilience associated with the ease with which conflicts connected with troublesome past events are activated and with the meager mechanisms available to cope with both unresolved conflicts and with the impact of new difficulties (Millon, 1969, 1981, 1986a).

PERSONALITY PROTOTYPES

Millon (1986b) identifies the construct "prototype" as potentially useful for incorporating the diverse features that comprise personality as well as the elements that differentiate personality pathology from other forms of psycho-pathology. A prototype refers to the most typically found characteristics of members of a category and represents a theoretical ideal against which potential members of that category can be evaluated. Horowitz, Post, French, Wallis, and Siegelman (1981) point out that all the elements that make up the prototype are assumed to represent at least some members of the category. However, no single element is either necessary or sufficient for membership. One consequence of this conceptual flexibility is that individuals may vary widely in the degree to which they may be considered to approximate the prototype. Individuals who possess more of the correlated features that represent the concept are considered more typical instances and are thus more readily classified. This approach to matching people with personality prototypes contrasts with the classical approach to diagnosis which involves the specification of one or more necessary or sufficient features (Millon, 1986b; Cantor, Smith, French, & Mezzich, 1980).

Millon (1986b) suggests that the prototype model is particularly appropriate to represent the "typical, pervasive, durable, and holistic features that distinguish personality categories from the more symptomatic, less widespread, frequently transient, and narrowly circumscribed clinical syndromes" (p.674). Although it is true that the prototype model allows for categorical diversity and overlap, Millon argues that it is highly desirable to clarify distinctions around the boundaries so as to reduce the number of unclassifiable and borderline cases. In an effort to accomplish this goal of enhancing diagnostic discrimination, Millon (1986b) has developed distinctive criteria for all diagnostically pertinent clinical attributes associated with each prototypical category.

THEORETICAL CLASSIFICATIONS BASED ON THREE POLAR DIMENSIONS

Millon (1969, 1981) using a biosocial learning model, drew upon three classic polar dimensions (pain–pleasure, self–other, active–passive) in constructing a classification system that yields recognized pathological personality categories and articulates their relationships with other mental disorders. In Millon's (1986a) view, personality reflects of an organized pattern of structures and functions that operate to enhance pleasure and reduce pain, reveal whether the individual pursues these objectives primarily in self or others, and illuminate whether the individual utilizes an active or passive approach to goal attainment. Various interacting constitutional vulnerabilities and maladaptive social learning experiences result in deficiencies or imbalances in an individual's orientation to one or more of these polarities. In Millon's (1986a) model, these diverse dysfunctional developmental processes result in any of a number of basic maladaptive or more severely pathological personality patterns.

Millon (1981) uses reinforcement as the central construct around which his classification system is built. It incorporates the pleasure–pain dimension and

TABLE 1.1
Theory-Based Framework for Personality Pathology

Pathology Domain	Self-Other			Pain–Pleasure	
	Other + Self -	Self+ Other -	Self ↶ Other ↴	Pain ↔ Pleasure	Pleasure - Pain ±
Reinforcement source					
Interpersonal pattern/ Instrumental coping style	Dependent	Independent	Ambivalent	Discordant	Detached
Passive variant	Dependent	Narcissistic	Compulsive	Self-Defeating (masochistic)	Schizoid
Active variant	Histrionic	Antisocial	Passive-Aggressive	Aggressive (sadistic)	Avoidant
Dysfunctional variant	Borderline	Paranoid	Borderline or Paranoid		Schizotypal

From Millon (1987) Manual for the MCMI-II. Reproduced by permission of National Computer Systems, Inc.

reflects that drives, motivations, and emotions are ultimately aimed toward events which are attractive, pleasurable, or positively reinforcing, and away from those that are unattractive, aversive, or negatively reinforcing. Millon (1986a) argues that there are three primary ways in which pathology may exist in the nature of pain-pleasure systems. First, it is hypothesized that certain individuals experience significantly diminished capacity to experience pain or pleasure in association with life experiences. That is, both reward and punishment systems are deficient. Second, one motivational system may be abnormally prominent. That is, some individuals may show abnormal pain-responsivity while others may reveal unusual pleasure reactivity. Obviously, the more clinically relevant are those who experience many life events as aversive and few as pleasurable (Millon, 1986a). Finally, there are some individuals in whom there is a significant reversal of the pain–pleasure polarity. These individuals seek out what might be objectively negative or aversive events and experience them as rewarding.

Also central to the framework upon which the classification scheme is built is the assumption that major dimensions of personality pathology may result from disruptions or imbalances in the degree to which, or the manner in which, reinforcement is sought from self and others. Millon (1986a) emphasizes the fundamental importance of this dimension and systematically describes personality styles that involve seeking pleasure or avoiding pain by focusing excessively on self or on others. Other pathological personality patterns involve lack of ability to experience pain and/or pleasure from self or others. Finally, several personalities experience a fundamental conflict about whether to turn to self or others in efforts to seek pleasure and avoid pain.

Millon (1986a) also utilizes the active–passive dimension to define pathological aspects of personality styles. A distinction is drawn between those who are active, engaged, persistent, and initiating in their efforts to seek the rewards and avoid the punishments of life and those who are passive, detached, and acquiescent in such endeavors.

From the three polar dimensions just described, Millon (1986a) has extended his classification to 10 basic pathological personality styles defined in accordance with a 5-by-2 matrix. The classification scheme also includes three more severely dysfunctional personality variants which reflect significantly lower levels of structural cohesion and functional integrity. Each of these 13 maladaptive personality styles is represented in Table 1.1 and basic clinical features are outlined later in this chapter in association with MCMI-II scale descriptions.

THE MILLON CLINICAL MULTIAXIAL INVENTORY:
AN OVERVIEW

The original and revised versions of the MCMI were developed as measures of the basic constructs outlined in Millon's (1969, 1981, 1986a, 1986b) theory of personality and psychopathology. Ongoing efforts have been made to refine the instrument to enhance its correspondence both with the author's evolving theory and with various Axis I and Axis II syndromes in the DSM-III and the DSM-III-R (American Psychiatric Association, 1980, 1987; Millon, 1987). This self-report instrument has 175 items structured in a *true* or *false* response format. Thirteen of the 22 clinical scales in the current version are designed as measures of the basic and pathological personality styles outlined in Millon's (1981, 1986a, 1986b) theory and are designed to be coordinated with DSM-III-R Axis II personality disorder categories. The remaining 9 clinical scales are designed to measure a number of the more common Axis I clinical symptom syndromes.

This separation of pathological personality from symptom scales reflects a central feature of Millon's theory emphasizing the distinction between features of psychopathology that are pervasive and enduring from those that are circumscribed and transient (Millon, 1987). Indeed, interpretation of the 22 clinical scales that make up the MCMI-II profile is designed to "illuminate the interplay between long-standing characterological patterns and the distinctive clinical symptomatology a patient manifests under psychic stress" (Millon, 1987, p.4).

The first 10 scales (Scales 1–8B) are used to gauge basic maladaptive personality styles, while the next three assess personality disorders reflecting greater pathology in structure and function (Scales SS, CC, and PP). Similarly, the next 6 scales (Scales A, H, N, D, B, and T) are designed to tap the less severe clinical symptom syndromes; the final 3 (Scales SS, CC, and PP) are constructed to measure more severe symptom disorders (Millon, 1987). These scales are arranged to reflect categories which are assumed to be interrelated in such a way that each may serve as a precursor, extension, or modification of another. Severe personality disorders are assumed to be extensions of basic maladaptive personality styles. Clinical symptom syndromes are conceived as disturbances in the patient's basic personality style that emerge under conditions of perceived stress (Millon, 1987).

DEVELOPMENT OF THE MCMI-I

The MCMI was developed in accordance with a sequential 3-step validation process. The first step has been labeled "theoretical-substantive" and focuses on the selection of items that reflect the content of formal theory-derived personality disorder and clinical symptom prototypes. Careful efforts were made to include items that reflect the most salient or essential characteristics relevant to each clinical prototype in the classification system. In addition, items were examined to determine their "lack of fit" with conceptually dissimilar or opposing clinical categories. An initially large item pool was further reduced on the basis of patient's judgments regarding ease of self-rating and expert's blind sorting of items into theory relevant categories. Surviving items were further sorted on the basis of their second and third "best fit," as well as on the basis of their "negative fit," with various theory-relevant categories. These sorts were used to guide subsequent decisions regarding differential scoring of items on several scales (Millon, 1987).

The internal–structural validation of the MCMI was approached in accordance with a "polythetic" structural model which emphasizes interrelationships among the basic and pathological personality scales and the clinical symptom syndrome scales. This approach contrasts with models of personality that focus on the identification of factorially pure traits. It recognizes the need for the development of scales that are internally consistent, but which include selective item overlap and moderate to high correlation with theoretically similar and contrasting scales. Millon (1987) indicates that the multiple keying of items and the pattern of correlation among scales was both anticipated by the underlying theory and guided by the polythetic structural model. Point-biserial correlations were calculated between each item and each of the scales on provisional forms of the MCMI. Only those items that were correlated highest with the scale to which they were originally assigned in the theoretical-substantive phase were considered further. Following item reduction on this basis, the median item-scale correlation was .58.

Subsequently, surviving items were examined for meaningful (greater than .3 or −.3) point-biserial correlations with scales other than the ones to which they were originally assigned. Results of this analysis were considered, together with results from the "second-best-fit" and "negative-fit" studies conducted during the previous substantive validation phase, in the development of a scoring system that includes the multiple-scale keying of items. Finally, items showing excessively high or low endorsement frequencies were eliminated because of their typically poor discriminative efficiency (Millon, 1987). Further item reduction resulted from efforts to retain those items that most accurately reflected each scale's personality or syndrome diversity and from the elimination of items that showed a pattern of empirical association with various clinical scales which was inconsistent with the undergirding theoretical model (Millon, 1987).

The external–criterion validation phase of the MCMI-I was designed to ensure its usefulness as a descriptive-interpretive and differential diagnostic tool. One hundred and sixty-seven clinicians participated in this effort by rating a total of 682 patients using a uniform and detailed instruction booklet that included clinical descriptions of each of the theory based personality prototypes and clinical symptom syndromes. Twenty criterion groups were formed that corresponded to each of the MCMI scale related syndromes. Each patient was placed into several of these criterion groups reflecting the assignment of multiple diagnoses. Each of the primary diagnostic groups was further divided on the basis of the degree of diagnostic fit within that group. The endorsement frequency for every MCMI item in relation to each diagnostic group was compared with its average endorsement frequency for the entire clinical population. Items assigned to particular scales on the basis of earlier theoretical-substantive and structural validation procedures were retained only if they demonstrated a significantly higher or lower endorsement frequency for expected criterion groups than the average endorsement frequency for the patient group as a whole (Millon, 1987, p. 48).

Information from all three validation phases was used to eliminate redundant and inefficient discriminating items. After completion of the first criterion validation phase, a decision was made to eliminate the Hypochondriasis, Obsession-Compulsion, and Sociopathy scales due to various factors such as low prevalence and conceptual overlap with other more relevant categories. These scales were replaced with newly constructed Hypomania, Alcohol Abuse, and Drug Abuse scales. Similar substantive, structural, and external validation procedures were followed in the construction of these new scales (Millon, 1987). The addition of these three scales added 25 items to the prior refined list of 150 and created the final 175 item version of the MCMI-I.

DEVELOPMENT OF THE MCMI-II

A revised version of the MCMI was published in 1987. The primary purposes of the revision were to incorporate into the structure of the instrument changes that had taken place in the underlying theory and to enhance the item content and criterion related validity of MCMI scales in relation to DSM-III and DSM-III-R diagnoses. Specifically, scales were developed to measure the aggressive–sadistic and self-defeating personalities. In addition, modifications were made in the item content of the Borderline, Antisocial, and Major Depression scales to reflect changes in the conceptualization of these disorders. Efforts were made to reduce excessive scale overlap and to enhance the criterion related validity of scales in relation to both DSM-III and theory based criteria.

A series of studies were undertaken which examined the correspondence between MCMI items and DSM-III clinical diagnoses. The procedures used to evaluate MCMI items corresponded to those described earlier in the external validity phase of the original MCMI except that criterion groups were constituted based on formal DSM-III criteria rather than on Millon's (1987) theory-based clinical descriptions. Each MCMI item's endorsement frequency for scale relevant diagnostic groups was contrasted with that of all other psychiatric patients under study. Items that did not reflect a pattern of endorsement frequency that enhanced discrimination between relevant criterion groups and the undifferentiated patient groups were considered for possible elimination from the MCMI-II.

Other factors that influenced decisions regarding the retention or deletion of items included the need to retain items that reflected the breadth of underlying personality or symptom dimensions, which reduced content redundancy, which adequately contributed to internal consistency and incremental validity, and which did not contribute to biased estimates in minority groups (Millon, 1987).

One interesting aspect of this analysis was that items varied widely in terms of their efficiency in discriminating between different diagnostic groups. This information was important in the establishment of an a system of weighing items 3, 2, or 1 on scales in a manner that reflected their importance in relation to the prototype. The item weighing procedure was adopted to increase diagnostic efficiency and to reduce correlations among scales (Millon, 1987).

Item replacement studies were designed primarily to identify theoretically, structurally, and criterion valid items for the newly formulated Aggressive–Sadistic and Self-Defeating scales. In addition, modifications of items contributing to existing MCMI scales were required to accommodate changes in Millon's theory and to enhance their association with Axis 1 and Axis II categories of the DSM-II and DSM-III-R (Millon, 1986a, 1986b, 1987). Over 350 items were written to represent criteria for all personality disorders and clinical symptom syndromes associated with the MCMI-I scales. As in the case of the original MCMI validation effort, items were retained on the basis of theoretical and DSM-III-R based content validity, ease of self-rating, and experts fitting of items to theory relevant diagnostic categories.

An internal-structural validation effort was also undertaken. Items were retained only when they demonstrated acceptable endorsement frequencies and correlated highest with the primary scale for which they were identified. Millon (1987) reports that many items that were written to reflect DSM-III or DSM-III-R criteria were eliminated during these item validation procedures. Finally, in the criterion validation phase, 184 patients were administered the provisional form of the MCMI-II. Clinicians used DSM-III-R criteria and, in the case of the aggressive-sadistic personality, a theory-based description in assigning these patients up to three diagnoses. The next step involved the formation of MCMI-II scale relevant diagnostic criterion groups. The primary determinant of item selection at this stage involved whether each item usefully discriminated scale relevant criterion groups from the remaining group of undifferentiated psychiatric patients. The validation procedures described earlier, as well as other pragmatic considerations, led to the replacement of a total of 45 items leaving the MCMI-II with the same total number of items as had been used in the original version.

Millon (1987) developed an item weighing system that was designed to reflect the polythetic structure of his model of clinical prototypes. As discussed earlier, a clinical prototype reflects characteristics that are typically found among members of a category and represents an ideal with reference to which individuals can be evaluated. Members may vary considerably in the degree to which they may resemble the prototype. In addition, members of one prototypical category often manifest some of the features of other prototypes. The elements that define one prototype are often found to blend or overlap with those that define other prototypes that are theoretically congruent. However, particular elements may be much more central to the definition of one clinical prototype than to others with which they are associated. Millon (1987) suggests that it is this polythetic character of clinical prototypes that justifies both the multiple-scoring and differential weighing of items on various scales.

The system for assigning item weights on the MCMI-II was based on the three phase validation system described earlier. Items that were specifically selected on the basis of their correspondence with both theory and DSM based criteria and which were judged valid in theoretical, structural, and criterion validation studies were assigned 3 unit weights. Two unit weights were assigned to items that met two of the following three criteria: (a) items judged to be meaningfully associated with various MCMI-II scale relevant disorders as suggested by theory; (b) items demonstrated meaningful item-scale correlations with one or several secondary scales; (c) items demonstrated a significant endorsement frequency with one or more secondary scales when compared with such frequencies established for primary scale items. A single unit weight was assigned to items that met criteria associated with either b or c above. Items were not given weights on scales which were incompatible with theoretically expected associations (Millon, 1987).

Base-Rate Scores

Both the MCMI-I and MCMI-II make use of Base-Rate scores which involve the transformation of raw scores in such a way that the proportion of patients who score above each scale's cutoff point corresponds to the actual prevalence of scale-related disorders in a representative national population of patients. Millon argues that the use of standard scores is inappropriate in a context in which the clinical disorders being measured are not normally distributed and are not of equal prevalence in patient populations. Further, scores based on actual prevalence data are considered more appropriate when the basic purpose of an instrument is to determine whether an individual is or is not a member of a specific diagnostic group (Millon, 1987).

For the MCMI-I, base-rate (BR) scores were derived primarily from a population of 1,591 patients selected from over 100 hospitals and outpatient centers and from nearly 40 private practices in 27 states and Great Britain (Millon, 1987). A cross-validation population consisting of 256 patients was also utilized. In the selection of these populations, an effort was made to ensure representativeness and diversity of patient characteristics. The centers from which patients were drawn included VA inpatient and outpatient units, general and psychiatric hospitals, college counseling centers, family service agencies, community mental health centers, alcohol and drug treatment programs, and private practices (Millon, 1987). In 1981, MCMI records on more than 40,000 patients were analyzed for the purpose of adjusting BR scores and evaluating adjustment and correction indices. Eighty-four percent of this population was drawn from outpatient settings and 54% were males.

For the MCMI-II, base-rate scores were derived from studies involving two patient populations. In the first, a randomly selected group of 519 clinicians from the United States and Canada administered both the MCMI-I and MCMI-II to between one and three patients. They also completed Axis I and Axis II diagnoses on these patients using DSM-III-R criteria. This study contributed 825 cases to the normative population. In the second study, 93 experienced MCMI-I users, who had some formal training in the application of the author's theory, contributed a total of 467 cases. These samples were combined after a determination was made that prevalence figures on Axis I and Axis II diagnoses were highly similar. This combined normative group included essentially equal numbers of males and females, however over 80% were drawn from outpatient settings and minority groups were underrepresented. Separated norms are provided for Whites, Blacks, and Hispanics. A more detailed description of the characteristics of the normative population is provided in the MCMI-II manual (Millon, 1987).

Base-rate scores of 74 and 84 for all MCMI-I scales were established as the cutting points in which the proportion of patients who score higher would equal the prevalence base rates for the presence (BR = 74) of, or prominence (BR = 84) of, personality or clinical symptom syndrome characteristics which are associated with such scales (Millon, 1987). Although BR scores are used in the MCMI-II in a somewhat similar fashion, several significant changes were made particularly with respect to the meaning of such scores on the 10 basic personality disorder scales.

In light of Millon's (1986a, 1986b) current emphasis on the polythetic structure of personality and the frequency of mixed personality profiles which emerged in studies of the MCMI-II, BR scores on MCMI-II scales 1–8B are no longer to be used to make distinct personality disorder diagnoses. Instead, BR scores on these scales should be considered to represent the highest, second highest, etc., basic personality score in an MCMI-II profile which reflects information about the prominence and mix of various personality features. The most prominent element in the MCMI-II profile will now be represented by the highest BR score whether or not it exceeds BR = 84 (Millon, 1987).

Descriptions of MCMI Scales

The following are brief narrative descriptions of personality prototype and symptom syndrome characteristics associated with each MCMI-II clinical scale. As mentioned previously, Scales 1–8B reflect basic maladaptive personality styles, while Scales S, C, and P tap personality disorders that reflect greater pathology in structure and function. The next 6 scales (Scales A, H, N, D, B, and T) assess clinical symptom syndromes of moderate severity, while the remaining 3 (Scales SS, CC and PP) are designed to gauge symptom disorders of marked severity. These descriptions are based on disorder characterizations found in several of Millon's (1969, 1981, 1986a, 1986b, 1987, 1990) published works. These works should be studied carefully by experienced clinicians prior to attempting interpretive work with the MCMI-II.

Personality Scales

Schizoid (Scale 1).   Passively-detached or schizoid personalities are characterized by limited capacity to experience painful or pleasurable emotional responses. Activation deficits are associated with impoverished cognitive processes, detached interpersonal behavior, and meager emotional responsivity. They are described as experiencing minimal interest in social interactions and limited social participation ultimately leads to broad deficits in the development of interpersonal coping skills. When social demands become intense or inescapable, such patients may display stress-related responses including anxiety reactions, dissociative disorders, somatoform disorders, or brief reactive psychotic episodes.

Avoidant (Scale 2).   Like the schizoid, the avoidant or actively detached personality has limited capacity to derive positive reinforcement from himself or others. However, unlike the schizoid, the avoidant is acutely sensitive to punishing social encounters. These individuals are fundamentally motivated by a desire to avoid social situations that may duplicate painful past rejections. Such patients may constantly survey their social environments for potential dangers and may interpret benign social events as threatening. They desperately desire social approval but chronic social anxiety, frequent disruptive and disturbing cognitions, and meager interpersonal coping skills, make goal attainment unlikely. When subjected to inescapable social demands or conflicts, avoidant patients are considered particularly vulnerable to the development of one or several of the symptom disorders described in connection with the schizoid pattern.

Dependent (Scale 3).   Passively dependent personalities are marked by their need for affection and approval from the significant others upon whom they depend for feelings of worth and adequacy. Avoidance of conflict and efforts to appease mark their interpersonal behavior. They readily subordinate their own wishes and interests to those of supportive others and display limited initiative, competence, and adult responsibility. Dependent personalities may experience a wide range of life demands as stressful because of self-perceptions of weakness and inadequacy. Their primary coping strategy entails efforts to develop secure relationships with caretakers viewed as more competent than themselves. When such support is unavailable, dependent personalities are considered vulnerable to the development of a variety of anxiety, phobic, somatic, dissociative, and depressive disorders.

Histrionic (Scale 4).   Actively-dependent or histrionic personalities are akin to the passive-dependent types in their reliance upon attention and nurturance from others to sustain feelings of self-esteem and adequacy. However, in marked contrast to the passive-dependent's acquiescent interpersonal style, the histrionic personality assertively manipulates events in order to ensure a steady supply of attention and approval and to minimize disinterest and rejection from others. Due to their persistent focus on external social events, they fail to develop flexible and balanced intrapsychic skills and rely excessively on repression to handle troublesome cognitions and emotions. However, they may be keenly sensitive to the thoughts and emotions of others and are often skillful in soliciting support and approval. They avoid meaningful introspection and depth in relationships with others, and although highly reactive emotionally, their responses tend to be dramatic, transient, and superficial. Because of the histrionic's insatiable need for external approval, they are particularly vulnerable to events that interrupt the flow of attention and affection from others. During such stressful periods, they are considered likely to display one or more anxiety, phobic, somatic, dissociative, or affective disorders. Because such reactions do not result from the operation of substantial internal processes or from disruptions in deep external attachments, they are often transient.

Narcissistic: (Scale 5).   Passively-independent or narcissistic personalities derive primary need satisfaction from their overvalued sense of themselves. They have been led to acquire a pretentious self-assurance and sense of entitlement that contributes to exploitive and nonreciprocal interpersonal relationships. Particular difficulty is experienced by those in whom there is a large gap between self-estimated and actual abilities and accomplishments. Personal failures tend to be rationalized and a characteristic retreat to fantasy allows redemption of self-esteem and the characteristic sense of superiority. The efficiency with which they often defend against disappointments, and the ease with which they reward themselves, typically leaves them imperturbably optimistic. However, when circumstances of repeated failure and humiliation lead to an inability to sustain the grandiose sense of self, the narcissist may develop any of various affective, anxiety, somatoform, or paranoid disorders.

Antisocial: Scale 6A.   Actively independent or antisocial personalities focus on themselves as sources of need fulfillment, not because of the excessive self-evaluation that characterizes the narcissist, but because of pervasive mistrust of others. Their security derives from countering anticipated domination and humiliation at the hands of others by means of manipulative, irresponsible, and self-serving behaviors. Although they may view themselves as tough-minded realists, others tend to see them as argumentative and contentious and as displaying minimal human compassion. They have relatively few mechanisms to rework revengeful attitudes and angry feelings which are often expressed directly and forcefully. Although some antisocial personalities display manifestly criminal behavior, most adapt in more socially sanctioned roles in a competitive society in which hard-headed realism is rewarded. Self-perceptions of strength and autonomy lead these individuals to appraise relatively few life events as stressful. However, transient anxiety reactions and paranoid episodes may be associated with feelings of being controlled or betrayed by others.

Aggressive (Sadistic): Scale 6B.   Actively discordant or aggressive–sadistic personalities experience a reversal in the pain–pleasure polarity. They experience pleasure in association with "objectively" aversive behaviors which inflict stress, pain, and humiliation on others. Such individuals derive satisfaction from relationships in which they are dominating, abusive, and even brutal. They tend to be unbendingly dogmatic, intolerant, and argumentative, and readily display hostile affect. They may view themselves as ruggedly independent, realistically toughminded, and vigorously competitive. Depending on social class, and on the vocational roles they assume, they may be viewed as overtly sadistic or as aggressive "type A" personalities. In either case, they experience few tender emotions and little guilt or shame in connection with their abusive social behavior. Because aggressive personalities view themselves as powerful and capable of controlling life circumstances, they tend to deny the significance of "objectively" negative life events and display few stress-related symptoms such as anxiety or depression. However, potent threats to their sense of autonomy may overwhelm typically adequate regulatory controls and lead to explosively aggressive outbursts.

Compulsive (Scale 7).   The passive-ambivalent or compulsive personality experiences intense conflict regarding whether to orient primarily to self or to others as a means of need satisfaction. Consistent exposure to parental over-control, in which narrowly defined patterns of acceptable behavior were imposed, leads to a pattern of constricted, "rule-oriented" attitudes and behavior which are routinely imposed on self and others. Although they have been trained to be compliant, respectful, and conscientious, outward conformity to others' expectations belies a strong wish to assert their own rigidly controlled desires and impulses. Deep ambivalence, conflict, and feelings of hostility are typically controlled through the use of such defensive maneuvers as reaction formation. These individuals have difficulty expressing warm feelings and are often described as serious, tense, or joyless. Compulsive personalities may find indirect expression of their hidden feelings of anger in socially approved careers such as law enforcement. In addition to the ongoing task of coping with deeply repressed contrary impulses, compulsive personalities may be particularly vulnerable to life events that lead them to evaluate their own behavior as having failed to conform to self-imposed standards of propriety or which subject them to the negative evaluations of those upon whom they depend for approval. Under conditions of excessive internal or external stress, they may be expected to manifest any of a variety of reactions including anxiety, depression, and psychosomatic disorders.

Passive-Aggressive Personality: (Scale 8A).   Like the compulsive, the passive-ambivalent or passive-aggressive personality experiences profound conflict over whether to rely on self or others as a means of seeking pleasure and avoiding pain. Unlike the compulsive, however, the conflicts of the passive-aggressive are routinely manifested in sulking, fretful moodiness, feelings of being misunderstood and unappreciated, and interpersonal behavior vacillating between passive-dependence and assertive-independence. The conflict over whether to seek gratification from self or others leads these ambivalent personalities on an erratic course which involves fluctuation between an angry, demanding, resentful posture and a retreat to periods of guilt and compliant acquiescence. They experience persistently conflicted relationships because their labile moods and erratic behavior provoke irritation and resentment in others. Although they may experience an intense need for acceptance, mistrust leads to negative expectancies regarding outcomes in important relationships. The passive-aggressive personality has developed few regulatory mechanisms to control troublesome impulses and emotions which tend to be expressed directly. Thus, they are highly vulnerable both to internally stressful stimuli and to the consequences of their fractious and derogatory interpersonal behavior and frequently suffer from anxiety, depression, and somatic disorders.

Self-Defeating (Masochistic) Personality: Scale 8B.   The passive-discordant or self-defeating personality, like the aggressive–sadistic, experiences a significant reversal in the typical orientation to pleasure and pain. They view themselves as inadequate, as typically having failed to live up to their own and others' expectations, and as deserving of shame, humiliation, and punishment. They relate to others in an unusually self-depreciating and obsequious fashion which allows, if not encourages, exploitation. Their tendency to concentrate on past failures, their negative future expectancies, and their self-sabotaging interpersonal behaviors are hypothesized to serve to raise the experience of suffering to homeostatic levels. Ordinary avenues of need fulfillment are transformed in a manner which leads to frustration and disappointment. The self-defeating personality is not only vulnerable to stressful life events, but seeks out or creates these events which may increase the likelihood of various specific symptom reactions.

Schizotypal Personality: Scale S.   The schizotypal personality represents a more severely dysfunctional variant of either the schizoid or avoidant personality. They tend to have limited social attachments and typically display deficient school and work histories. They often appear self-absorbed and ruminative and their thinking may be obscure involving a mixture of fantasy and reality. Idiosyncratic thoughts and peculiar behaviors are associated with meager and poorly integrated regulatory mechanisms. The active variant is characteristically apprehensive and anxious, whereas the passive subtype is generally deficient emotionally. Schizotypal personalities are highly vulnerable to varied life stressors because of poorly developed coping resources. They are particularly likely to appraise social demands as threatening and react with various anxiety, somatoform, or dissociative disorders. They are also assumed to be vulnerable to schizophrenic disturbances (Millon, 1981).

Borderline Personality: Scale C. The borderline personality experiences broad ranging ambivalence and instability regarding their orientation to pain versus pleasure, activity versus passivity, and self versus other. The tend to fluctuate erratically within these polar dimensions leading to their characterization as inherently unstable. What most clearly distinguishes this severely pathological personality from the diverse basic personality patterns with which it may be associated is intensely labile emotionality. They experience intense endogenous moods which may fluctuate among anxious agitation, anger, euphoria, apathy, and dejection. Vacillating and contradictory self-perceptions contribute to an unstable personal identity. This uncertainty about self leaves them preoccupied with obtaining affection and approval from others. Despite this, they may experience intense ambivalence regarding dependence–independence issues. Their contradictory, manipulative, and erratic interpersonal behavior often leads to rejection rather than approval and, as a consequence, intense dissatisfaction with those upon whom they desperately depend. Borderline personalities have wide-ranging stress vulnerabilities and coping deficiencies. As such, they are likely to experience exacerbations of the fundamental affective instability and periodically display a number of Axis I disorders.

Paranoid Personality: Scale P. Paranoid personalities exhibit a pervasive mistrust of others and display a fiercely independent orientation. They strive to project an image of strength and invulnerability to defend against real or imagined threats of betrayal and humiliation. Their hostile, abrasive, and controlling interpersonal behavior often leads to anger and retaliation from others which only reinforces their distorted social expectancies. Pervasive feelings of mistrust and suspicion lead them to see signs of deception and duplicity in ordinary social transactions and their tendency to distance themselves from people further limits opportunities for corrective social feedback. They have limited appreciation for their own weaknesses and inadequacies and tend to project these qualities onto others. Paranoid personalities are intensely sensitive to threats to their sense of self-determination. When challenged or provoked by an external force perceived as overwhelming, rigid defenses and restricted coping responses leave them vulnerable to acute anxiety, manic disorder, or in more extreme cases, psychotic reactions.

Clinical Symptom Syndrome Scales

Anxiety: Scale A. A generalized state of tension, fatigue, and restlessness is often reported by these patients. Physical complaints may include muscular tightness, sweating, and nausea. They tend to report being worried, apprehensive, or jumpy. Such symptoms may be experienced in a generalized fashion or may be reported in association with specific situations.

Somatoform: Scale H. These patients express psychological difficulties through a variety of physical manifestations which may include multiple somatic complaints involving unrelated parts of the body, weakness, fatigue, or tension. Those with legitimate physical ailments may exaggerate symptoms to gain attention and reassurance.

Bipolar-Manic: Scale N. Periods of overactivity, distractibility, impulsivity, and irritability are commonly seen in these patients. Inflated self-esteem and episodes of manic excitement may lead to unrealistic planning, unselective commitments, and pressured and demanding interpersonal relations. Psychotic processes including delusions or hallucinations may be observed in patients in the very elevated score range.

Dysthymic: Scale D. These patients may be preoccupied with feelings of loneliness, discouragement, failure, and guilt. They tend to experience self-depreciatory cognitions, a pessimistic outlook, and low self-esteem. There may be suicidal ideation, appetite disturbance, fatigue, loss of pleasure associated with formerly reinforcing activities, and generally decreased efficiency in carrying out life responsibilities. An examination of specific items which suggest that such symptoms have been troublesome for two or more years may be of value in determining whether a diagnosis of dysthymic disorder should be considered.

Alcohol Dependence: Scale B. The high scoring patient likely has a history of alcoholism or alcohol abuse, although difficulties associated with current consumption may or may not be indicated. These patients typically report diverse problems frequently related to alcoholism including disrupted interpersonal relationships and family conflict, unstable work histories, and irritability, moodiness, and various other symptoms which may be connected to excessive consumption or withdrawal.

Drug Dependence: Scale T. A history of drug addiction or abuse is typically revealed by high scoring patients. They are often characterized as fearless, impulsive, sensation seeking, or erratic. They may be described as aggressively independent and self-centered and interpersonal relationships are often conflicted or insubstantial. Drug abuse related family and work problems are likely to be reported. This scale emphasizes a sensation seeking rather than a stress-coping pattern of drug abuse.

Thought Disorder: Scale SS. The thinking of these patients tends to be ruminative, fragmented, or bizarre and their behavior may be disorganized and regressive. Social isolation and alienation are common and emotional responses may be blunted, labile, or peculiar. High scoring patients may be diagnosed as having schizophrenic, schizophreniform, or brief reactive psychotic disorders.

Major Depression: Scale CC. These severely depressed patients tend to experience intense feelings of failure, guilt, dread, worthlessness, and hopelessness. Suicidal ideation is common. During acute episodes, most are incapable of independent functioning. Some display a pattern which includes fatigue, motor retardation, social withdrawal, and passive resignation, while others reveal a tense, agitated, irritable, and complaining style. Other manifestations may include significant appetite disturbance, weight loss or gain, insomnia or hypersomnia, and concentration problems.

Delusional Disorder: Scale PP. Interrelated delusions of an often paranoid nature are of central importance in the disturbed thinking, hostile mood, and irrational behavior of these patients. They frequently have suspicions that others intend to mistreat, betray, or disparage them, or fail to recognize their special talents. Delusions of a persecutory or grandiose character may lead to hostile, belligerent, or presumptuous interpersonal behavior.

Validity and Correction Indices

A variety of scales or indices have been introduced into the MCMI-II in an effort to reduce factors that may lead to distortions in results and interpretations. Specifically, the Validity Index was constructed to identify patients who were so confused or uncooperative at the time of testing that they responded in a random fashion. The endorsement of highly improbable items (i.e., I have not seen a car in the last 10 years.) leads to a determination of profile invalidity.

The Disclosure Level Index (Scale X) was designed to identify patients who might be either unusually self-revealing of information of a personally sensitive nature or particularly reticent and secretive in this regard. This index reflects the degree of positive or negative deviation from the midrange of adjusted raw scores on the 10 basic personality scales. The derived BR score transformation is used to identify apparent excesses in either secretiveness or self-disclosure and to adjust BR scores on all MCMI clinical scales up or down accordingly.

The Desirability (Scale Y) and the Debasement (Scale Z) indices are used to reveal the extent to which MCMI-II results may have been influenced by a patient's efforts to appear unrealistically free from psychological difficulties (Scale Y) or to appear more troubled by emotional and interpersonal problems (Scale Z) than might have been objectively evaluated. Adjustments are made on the Schizotypal, Borderline, Anxiety, Hypomanic, and Dysthymic scales to reflect the degree and direction of difference between Scales Y and Z.

The development of Denial-Complaint Adjustments reflected the need to further modify the BR scores of those patients with particular basic personality features. In patients who scored highest on either the Histrionic or Narcissistic scales, or first or second highest on the Compulsive scale, BR increases are made on the Schizotypal, Borderline, Paranoid, Anxiety, Dysthymic, and Hypomanic scales to adjust for denial tendencies. When the Avoidant scale is first or second highest, or when the Self-Defeating scale is the highest among the basic 10 personality scales, BR scores on the Borderline, Paranoid, Schizotypal, Anxiety, Hypomanic, and Dysthymic scales are decreased to adjust for complaint tendencies.

Finally, the Depression-Anxiety Adjustment was adopted to counter the effects of a tendency for patients to distort their responses to personality measures when they are experiencing intense emotional turmoil. Scores on the Avoidant, Self-Defeating, and Borderline scales are reduced when BR scores on the Anxiety and Dysthymic scales are >85 or when admission to inpatient status has been recent. In addition, combinations of elevated Anxiety and Dysthymic scale BR scores, outpatient versus inpatient status, and amount of time in inpatient treatment are used to determine the extent of BR score reductions on the Avoidant, Self-Defeating, and Borderline scales.

MCMI Profile Interpretation

The overall purpose of MCMI-II profile interpretation is to integrate characteristics measured by various MCMI personality and symptom scales with other relevant demographic, psychosocial, and health related information in order to achieve a meaningful clinical synthesis. Millon (1987) suggests dividing the MCMI-II profile into four sections and thoroughly analyzing relevant scale elevations within each before attempting an interpretation based upon the entire profile configuration. In the initial interpretive phase, a distinction should be drawn between scales that tap basic personality features and those that reflect severe personality pathology. Similarly, scales that assess clinical symptom syndromes of moderate severity should be considered separately from those that are designed to reveal more seriously pathological symptom disorders.

After clinically relevant basic and pathological personality features and clinical symptom syndrome characteristics are specified, the task of developing a meaningful clinical synthesis should be undertaken. This is accomplished by interweaving characteristics associated with clinically elevated basic and pathological personality and clinical symptom syndrome scales. As indicated previously, scales arranged in such categories are assumed to be interrelated in such a way that each may function as a precursor, extension, or adaptation of another. Basic personality styles may be seen as precursors to severe personality disorders. Clinical symptom syndromes reflect disturbances in the underlying personality pattern which emerge under conditions of stress. Symptom features should be described in a way that reflects their distinctiveness in relation to the undergirding personality configuration. The MCMI-II manual provides a more complete description, as well as illustrations, of the clinical interpretive process summarized here (Millon, 1987).

Conclusion

This chapter provides an introduction to the theoretical model underlying the development of the MCMI-I and II, summarizes development and standardization procedures, describes clinical characteristics associated with MCMI-II scale elevations, and includes an overview of recommended clinical interpretive procedures. Competent professional use of this increasingly popular diagnostic instrument requires a thorough familiarity with the underlying theory of personality and psychopathology and with the expanding literature examining its usefulness in diverse clinical settings.

REFERENCES

Cantor, N., Smith, E. E., French, R. D., & Mezzich, J. (1980). Psychiatric diagnoses as prototype categorization. *Journal of Abnormal Psychology, 89,* 181–193.

Horowitz, L. M., Post, D. L., French, R. D., Wallis, K. D., & Siegelman, E. Y. (1981). The prototype as a construct in abnormal psychology. 2. Classifying disagreement in psychiatric judgment. *Journal of Abnormal Psychology, 90,* 575–585.

Millon, T. (1969). *Modern psychopathology.* Philadelphia: Saunders.

Millon, T. (1981). *Disorders of personality, DSM-III: Axis II.* New York: Wiley.

Millon, T. (1986a). Personality prototypes and their diagnostic criteria. In T. Millon & G. Klerman (Eds.), *Contemporary directions in psychopathology: Toward the DSM-IV* (pp. 639–669). New York: Guilford Press.

Millon, T. (1986b). A theoretical derivation of pathological personalities. In T. Millon & G. Klerman (Eds.), *Contemporary directions in psychopathology: Toward the DSM-IV* (pp. 671–712). New York: Guilford Press.

Millon, T. (1987). *Millon Clinical Multiaxial Inventory-II: Manual for the MCMI-II.* Minneapolis: National Computer Systems.

Millon, T. (1990). *Toward a new personology: An evolutionary model.* New York: Wiley-Interscience.

Millon, T., & Everly, G. (1985). *Personality and its disorders: A biosocial learning approach.* New York: Wiley.

2 MCMI: Review of the Literature

Robert J. Craig, Ph.D.
Donna Weinberg, M.S.

The *Million Clinical Multiaxial Inventory* (MCMI) (Millon, 1981, 1987) has become a popular instrument for clinical diagnosis. Upon the test's introduction, there were favorable expectations for the MCMI from professionally reputable sources (Butcher & Owen, 1978; Korchin & Schuldberg, 1981), and a recent survey of training directors at diagnostic practicum sites found that 50% believe the test should be taught in graduate psychology programs (Craig & Horowitz, 1990). The instrument is now widely used in clinical settings and increasingly used in research settings.

The test consists of Personality Disorder (PD) scales that were derived from Millon's biopsychosocial theory of personality pathology (Millon, 1981, 1984a, 1986a, 1986b), and symptom scales that emanate from Millon's belief that AXIS I disorders are extensions of the person's basic personality style (see Everly et al., 1987; and Walton, 1986 for further elaboration and evidence). Although the symptom scales are congruent with AXIS I syndromes of the *Diagnostic and Statistical Manual of Mental Disorders* (DSM-III-R) (American Psychiatric Association, 1987), the Personality Disorder scales were not originally designed to be congruent with the diagnostic criteria for AXIS II disorders (Reich, 1985). Nevertheless, recent research has increasingly compared MCMI PD scales to DSM-III-R Axis II disorders.

The MCMI [its precursors were the *Millon Illinois Self-Report Inventory,* and the *Millon Multiaxial Clinical Inventory*], as revised, the MCMI-II (Millon, 1987) has been received favorably by many clinicians. Although critical reviews have been both laudatory and damaging (Dana & Cantrell, 1988; Greer, 1984,1985; Hess, 1985; Lanyon, 1984; McCabe, 1984; Wetzler, 1990; Widiger, 1985; Widiger & Francis, 1987; and Widiger, Williams, Spitzer, & Frances, 1985;) Millon did not find these criticisms compelling (Millon, 1985a, 1985b).

Many of these reviews were published early in the history of the test and some of the criticism are no longer relevant. Our review differs from previous reviews in its comprehensive nature, in the presentation of the most current information and conclusions available from this large body of knowledge, and in the amount of information that may be more useful to practicing clinicians. Our findings may also be used as a benchmark against which subsequent research with the MCMI-II may be judged.

In view of the increasing popularity of this clinical instrument and the increasing number of research publications, it is now time to review the instrument in the light of the first 10 years of its existence. First, we briefly describe the test and its underlying theoretical assumptions.

The MCMI-II[1] is a 175-item self-report inventory with items written at the 8th grade reading level. It consists of 22 clinical scales which were constructed as an operational measure of those syndromes derived from Millon's theory of personality and psychopathology (Millon, 1981, 1986a, 1986b). This theory is presented in Chapter 1, and the classification scheme results in a 5-by-2 matrix that produces ten basic personality styles. The theory also includes a severity dimension that results in three dysfunctional variants, which reflect the decomposition of a basic personality style when stressed, for a total of 13 theory-derived personality styles (see Table 1.1, Chapter 1).

Millon theorizes that these various personality types, when confronted with stressful life events, would decompensate into particular forms of psychopathology or clinical syndromes. This division between clinical symptoms and personality disorders was influential in the DSM-II's change to a multiaxial approach to diagnosis, although DSM-III did not precisely use Millon's typology.

DSM-III and the MCMI were both revised in 1987. Table 2.1 presents the MCMI and MCMI-II Scale designations. For brevity sake, scale designations are used throughout the remainder of this chapter rather than using scale names. Also, the original MCMI had clinical syndrome names that, in some cases, were different than the names specified in the MCMI-II. For example, Scale CC was originally called Psychotic Depression but is now called Major Depression. Throughout this chapter, names of the MCMI-II scales are used when discussing research findings, and earlier MCMI scale names have been converted to their new designations for ease of communication. This is permissible because the dimensions assessed by the scale are purported to be identical, despite a few item changes and a revised name for improved description.

This chapter presents a comprehensive review of the MCMI.[2] We believe that

---

[1]By convention we used MCMI(II) when we address points that apply to the test *qua* test. Distinctions are made between the MCMI and the MCMI-II when necessary for clarification.

[2]We found only two studies that used the earlier versions of the MCMI. Foster (1977) used the MISRI, and Gilbride and Hebert (1980) used the MMCI. They are not included in this review but appear in the References.

TABLE 2.1
MCMI-I and MCMI-II Scale Designations

MCMI-I Scales	*MCMI-II Scales*
Basic Personality Patterns	*Clinical Personality Patterns*
1 Schizoid (Asocial)	1 Schizoid
2 Avoidant	2 Avoidant
3 Dependent (Submissive)	3 Dependent
4 Histrionic (Gregarious)	4 Histrionic
5 Narcissistic	5 Narcissistic
6 Antisocial (Aggressive)	6A Antisocial
	6B Aggressive
7 Compulsive (conforming)	7 Compulsive
8 Passive Aggressive (Negative)	8A Passive Aggressive
	8B Self-Defeating
Pathological Personality Disorders	*Severe Personality Pathology*
S Schizotypal	S Schizotypal
C Borderline (Cycloid)	C Borderline
P Paranoid	P Paranoid
Clinical Syndromes	*Clinical Syndromes*
A Anxiety	A Anxiety
H Somatoform	H Somatoform disorder
N Hypomania	N Bipolar: Manic disorder
D Dysthymia	D Dysthymic disorder
B Alcohol abuse	B Alcohol dependence
T Drug abuse	T Drug dependence
	Severe Syndromes
SS Thought disorder	SS Thought disorder
CC Psychotic depression	CC Major depression
PP Delusional disorder	PP Delusional disorder
	Modifier Indices
	X Disclosure
	Y Desirability
	Z Debasement

our review may help provide researchers with directions for future research with the MCMI-II. We hope to provide clinicians with information about this test that may be useful in their clinical practice as well.

We address both the psychometric and clinical aspects of the MCMI. First, we review research on the test's psychometric properties, including factor structure, reliability, validity, the detection of faking, and the influence of moderator variables on test scores. Second, we review clinical studies conducted with psychiatric populations, including the disorders of psychosis and schizophrenia, affective disorders, anxiety disorders, alcohol and drug abuse, eating disorders, and with criminal offenders. Third, we review the test's use with medical patients and special populations, including geriatric patients, sexual disorders, victims of sexual abuse, elective abortion, military personnel, and normals. Finally, we review the validity of the MCMI computer-generated narrative report. Because much of the research is presented in other chapters in this book, we have eliminated some details to avoid redundancy. However, the research on which the conclusions are presented have been retained in the References, so that that reader would have a relatively complete listing of MCMI/MCMI-II studies.

METHOD

A conscientious search was conducted for all published literature on the MCMI(II) between January, 1980 and June, 1990. Then three independent computer searches were conducted to provide a comprehensive listing of all MCMI(II) references. Excluded from this review were dissertation abstracts and unpublished papers from conferences. Papers delivered at the First Annual Conference on the Millon Inventories (Green, 1987) were excluded if they did not present empirical data. A few references published subsequent to June, 1990 have been added when such research adds clarification to the issue in question. We believe these procedures resulted in the acquisition of a comprehensive listing of relevant MCMI(II) papers. From this body of knowledge we provide a clinical information synthesis.

PSYCHOMETRIC STUDIES

Base Rate Scores

Raw scores are converted to Base Rate (BR) scores, a transformed score which ensures that the "proportion of patients who will score above each scale's cutoff point matches the actual prevalence among a representative national population of patients who possess each scale's corresponding disorder and completed the test." (Millon, 1987, p. 95) A BR score of 85 and above signifies the "most prominent" disorder whereas a BR of 75 and over reflects the "presence of characteristics" of the disorder. MCMI-II diagnostic assignments begin when the BR exceeds 70.

Millon has been criticized by several reviewers for not providing the raw data from which these BR scores were developed and for failing to provide the base rate or prevalence percentages of the populations used in his normative samples. This means that using identical raw scores with patient groups who have prevalence rates different from Millon's standardization group yield BR scores that are not equivalent to the test norms and therefore could lead to faulty diagnoses (see Duthie & Vincent, 1986; and Gibertini, Brandenburg, & Retzlaff (1986). Millon (1987) has responded to this criticism by providing considerable information about the derivations of BR scores in the MCMI-II manual. The manual also advises reserchers and clinicians to take into account local base artes when making interpretive descisions.

Factor Analysis.   Millon (1983) reported a 4-factor structure of the MCMI consisting of General Maladjustment, Paranoid Behavior and Thinking, Schizoid Behavior and Detachment, and Social Restraint/Aggression. For the MCMI-II (1987), he found an 8-factor matrix that is presented in Table 2.3, which also includes studies that have investigated the internal structure of the MCMI(II). Millon did not label the factors for the MCMI-II, and the labels presented in this table reflect nominal categories that seem to reflect the meaning of those factors as discussed in the test manual.

There has been a remarkable amount of interest in studying the factor structure of the MCMI. At the time this chapter was completed, no study had published the results of an MCMI-II factor structure, (besides Millon) but this will surely be done soon, if not already.

The 20 studies presented in Table 2.2 all used large sample sizes, consisting of a variety of clinical populations (psychiatric inpatients and outpatients, substance abusers, and criminal offenders.) They also conducted a principle components analysis with varimax rotation, using BR scores, so that method variance is not a confounding issue in comparing results. Furthermore, many of these studies reported that they used oblique rotations or a different factor method with no change in findings.

Researchers have used different cutoff scores to identify factor loadings. Some have used a score of .30 and above, while others have used scores at .5 or .6. Despite these differences, which might account for the variations in number and order of factors found and the labels attached to them, and despite varying populations used with the factor studies, there is a remarkable similarity across these studies. From three to six factors have been found for the MCMI. In reviewing these findings, there seems to be general agreement on the following dimensions: General Maladjustment, Schizoid/Asocial, Paranoid Behavior and Thinking, and Submission/Aggression. These factors emerge when all the scales are factored and essentially conform to Millon's (1983) original report on the MCMI factors. Also, these same factors appear among the factors reported for the MCMI-II (Millon, 1987).

When the personality scales and symptom scales were factored separately, three factors were found that were similar to the four factors identified above (Hamberger & Hastings, 1986; Retzlaff, & Gibertini, 1987a). We can conclude that the MCMI factor structure is remarkably robust across a wide variety of different psychopathologies.

There are three problematic issues: (a) the choice of scores, (b) the influence of acquiescent response bias on scale intercorrelations, and (c) the problem of item-overlap.

The MCMI(II) provides raw scores that are converted to BR scores. BR

TABLE 2.2
Factor Analytic Studies With the Millon Clinical Multiaxial Inventory (MCMI)

Author / Year	Population	Sample Size	Findings		
Millon (1983)	General psychiatric	744	MCMI: General maladjustment Paranoid behavior and thinking Schizoid detachment Restraint/Aggression		
Millon (1987)	General psychiatric	769	MCMI-II: General maladjustment Acting out/Self-indulgence Neurotic symptoms Emotional control Submissing/Intimidating Addiction Confused thinking Interpersonal ambivalence		
Flynn and McMahon (1984b)	Drug abusers	139	Negativistic-Avoidant (50%) Paranoid (6%) Emotional detachment/Social isolation (25%) Passive/Submissive (18%)		
Butters, Retzlaff, and Gibertini (1986)	Trainees referred to base MHC	175	General distress (44%) High social anxiety (18%) Social submissiveness (18%) Suspiciousness (10%)		
Choca, Peterson, and Shanley (1986)	Psychiatric inpatients	478	Maladjustment (61%) Extroverted acting out (27%) Psychoticism (7%)		
Hamberger and Hastings (1986)	Spouse abusers	99	Personality Scale Factors: Schizoidal/Borderline (44%) Narcissistic/Antisocial (25%) Passive-Dependent/Compulsive (11%)		
Piersma (1986)	Psychiatric inpatients	151	Withdrawal/Avoidance (50%) Emotional distress (24%) Impulsive/Negativistic (13%) Paranoid distrust/Delusions (7%) Dependency/Submission (6%)		
Everal et al. (1987)	General psychiatric	301	(Three factors accounted for over 80%) Ambivalence/Unstable Detached Independent/Vigilant		
Choca, Peterson, and Shanley (1987)	Psychiatric inpatients	155 (blacks) 155 (whites)	Maladjustment Acting out Psychoticism	Blacks (65%) (28%) (07%)	Whites (59%) (28%) (08%)
Montag and Comrey (1987)	Drivers License applicants in Israel	527	Anxiety-Depression Paranoia Histrionic vs. Compulsive Schizoid Antisocial		
Retzlaff and Gibertini (1987a)	Five different samples of psychiatric patients and drug abusers	175 250 249 478 not cited	Personality Scale Factors: Aloof-Asocial (21%) Aggressive-Submissive (22%) Lability-Restraint (19%)		

TABLE 2.2
(*Continued*)

Author / Year	Population	Sample Size	Findings
Retzlaff and Gibertini (1987)	Psychiatric inpatients	136	(Four factors accounted for 78% of the variance) Schizotypal Paranoid Aggression Polyneuroticism Social deviancy
Langevein et al. (1988)	Offenders in jail	419	General psychopathology (58%) Psychotic tendencies (20%) Extroversion (6%) Dependent-Submissive/ Antisocial-Aggressive (5%)
Gibertini and Retzlaff (1988)	Air Force Recruits in MHC Cadets in alcohol rehab	175 250	(Factor analysis performed on the matrix of item-overlap coefficients (62%)) General distress Social/Acting out Suspiciousness Submissive/Aggressive Psychotic-Detached
Marsh et al. (1988)	Addicts on Methadone	159	Passive-Aggressive with Anxiety and Depression (39%) Somatization (22%) Schizoid Avoidant (12%) Paranoid (6%)

Lorr, Retzlaff, and Tarr (1989)	Psychiatric outpatients
	Alcoholic inpatients
		253
		185
			(Factored MCMI at the item level)
			Personality Scales:
			  Social Introversion
			  Dependency on others
			  Verbal hostility
			  Orderliness
			Symptom Scales (44%)
			  Depression & Tension
			  Drug abuse
			  Drinking problem
			  Manic excitement
			  Suicidal ideation

McCormack, Barnett, and Wallbrown (1989)	Offenders in Jail	1200	Social isolation (35%) Agitated impulsivity (24%) Anxious/Ambivalent (25%) Paranoid/Psychoticism (25%)
Retzlaff and Gibertini (1990)	Psychiatric outpatients Alcoholic inpatients Air Force recruits at base MHC	253 185 184	(Three factors found across all populations) Aloof-Asocial (21%) Aggressive/Submission (22%) Liability/Restraint (19%)
Ownby et al. (1990)	Criminal offenders	2245	Withdrawn behavior Affective symptomology Neurotic anxiety Exploitive interpersonal attitude Passivity vs. Activity

Percent of variance accounted for by the factors appear in parenthesis, if reported. If no values indicated, than author(s) did not provide this information.

scores are used for statistical purposes throughout the test manual, and these are the scores clinicians use for diagnostic purposes. All research on MCMI factor structure has used BR scores, which are nonlinear transformations of weighted scores and correlate well with them. No study has compared differences between raw scores and BR scores, and the correlations between weighted and un-weighted scores approach unity (Retzlaff, Sheehan, & Lorr, 1990). Until studies demonstrate the superiority of one set of scores over another, it is likely that researchers will continue to use and report BR scores.

Theoretically, the number of items endorsed "True" can adversely affect the factor structure, which is likely to reduce the number of factors within the matrix due to the issue of item-overlap. No study has addressed this problem to date.

The major issue pertains to the problem of item-overlap within the MCMI(II). This introduces a forced similarity between the scores which artificially elevates the correlations between the scales, thus leading to factor loadings that are also artificially elevated. Gibertini and Retzlaff (1988) have succinctly described this problem:

> The similarity indices indicate a high degree of parallelism between the structure of the subject response patterns and that of the item-overlap coefficient matrix . . . the factor invariance reported in the literature is a function of the built-in structure created by the partial linear dependency of the scales. The artifact created by item-overlap among the scales represents a powerful source of variance relative to the subject response patterns. (p 71)

This suggests item-overlap is the controlling aspect of the factor structure.

To avoid the problem of item overlap, Lorr, Retzlaff, and Tarr (1989) conducted a factor analysis at the item level, by taking the 175 items of the test and separating them into 100 personality descriptions and 75 clinical symptom descriptions. The latent variables that underlie the items themselves can then be determined without the problem of scale keys. Their results found six factors for the personality scales, five of which matched up with Millon's "types," and five symptom dimensions among the nine MCMI symptom groupings.

Millon's theory does not predict a factor structure that would reflect the test's 3-part division because basic, pathological dimensions, and symptom configurations are assumed to be interrelated in theory. For example, Millon's theory would predict that the MCMI Schizoid, Avoidant, Schizotypal, and Dysthymic scales would all load on a single factor. In fact, this has often been found to be true due, in part, both to item overlap among the scales and to the conceptual similarity of the underlying dimensions.

Although the factors inherent in the MCMI(II) are of psychometric interest, they probably are of little clinical importance. In reflecting on the history of the MMPI, various factor analytic studies of the MMPI item pool have been conducted, as illustrated by the Comrey factor studies of the MMPI individual scales, but they have had no clinical utility. Conversely, Factor scales of randomly selected MMPI items, such as Welsh's Scales A and R, Wiggins Content Scales, and the rationally derived Harris-Lingoes subscales have tremendous clinical utility.

We argue that similar efforts need to be developed for the MCMI-II. There has been a start in this direction. Retzlaff and Gibertini (1990) recently presented factor-based special scales for the MCMI that include the dimensions of Aloof/ Asocial, Submissive/Aggressive and Labile/Restrained for the personality scales, and factor scales labeled Detached, Submissive, Suspicious, High Social Energy, and General Distress, for the symptom scales. They further presented clinical descriptors for elevated scores on these scales. Early research with these scales appears promising. This material is elaborated on in Chapter 14. Adams and Clopton (1990) found that dissonant missionaries (e.g., those who were more willing to question and challenge Church missionary policies) scored lower on the Special Content Scales of Compulsive and Submissive/Aggressive. The clinical usefulness of these scales remains to be demonstrated, but we argue that this is an important direction for future research. We believe that researchers should stop wasting their time and journal space by factor analyzing the MCMI-II scales.

Also, no one has conducted a factor analysis on a scale by scale basis. This has been done for the MMPI by Comrey and by Serkownek, and should also be done for the MCMI-II. In addition to ascertaining which dimensions are salient within an individual domain labeled by the scale, such research would contribute to the debate concerning the MCMI items and their correspondence to DSM-III-R categorizations (Millon, 1985a; Streiner & Miller, 1989; Widiger et al., 1985, 1986).

Test-Retest Reliability.   Table 2.3 presents the results of studies that assessed the MCMI test-retest reliability.[3] Only studies that presented the individual scale stability coefficients are shown. Also presented are Millon's (1983, 1987) stability coefficients reported in the test manuals.

Reliability data with clinical samples is somewhat confounded by the effects of treatment and by fluctuating changes in clinical states. Inasmuch as Millon (1983, 1987) reported stability coefficients using these same kinds of patients, published research should be directly comparable to the data presented in the test manuals.

---

[3]Besides these studies, Malec et al., (1988) reported that MCMI stability coefficients in cancer patients (N = 68) ranged from .52 to .79 between admission and four or eight months of chemo/radio therapy, but they did not present individual scale data. Flynn and McMahon (1983a) studied 161 drug addicts in treatment tested at different intervals but reported data only for Scale T. After 1 month post intake, this stability coefficient ranged from .45 to .55; from admission to 3 months it was .56 and from 1 month to 3 months it was .74.

TABLE 2.3

MCMI Stability Coefficients for Different Populations and Retest Intervals

Population		Heterogeneous Psychiatric Patients*		Hetergeneous Drug Abusers**	Inpatient Psychiatric***	
Retest Interval		5-9 days	4-6 Weeks	Intake to 1 Month	Intake to 3 Mos	Intake to Discharge
MCMI Scale	Scale Code	(N = 59)	(N = 86)	(N = 33)	(n = 33)	(N = 151)
Schizoid	1	.85	.82	.65	.82	.56
Avoidant	2	.90	.84	.70	.80	.56
Dependent	3	.83	.79	.61	.79	.65
Histrionic	4	.91	.85	.87	.82	.75
Narcissistic	5	.85	.81	.71	.88	.61
Antisocial	6A	.90	.83	.72	.79	.55
Aggressive/Sadistic	6B	X	X	X	X	X
Compulsive	7	.81	.77	.70	.77	.56
Passive-Aggressive	8A	.89	.81	.54	.69	.48
Self-Defeating	8B	X	X	X	X	X
Schizotypal	S	.86	.78	.74	.76	.57
Borderline	C	.84	.77	.42	.70	.27
Paranoid	P	.85	.77	.32	.38	.46
Anxiety Disorder	A	.80	.68	.61	.72	.31
Somatoform Disorder	H	.81	.62	.45	.62	.21
Bipolar: Manic Disorder	N	.79	.65	.62	.78	.75
Dysthymic Disorder	D	.78	.66	.57	.70	.32
Alcohol Dependence	B	.83	.76	.22	.74	.54
Drug Dependence	T	.83	.74	.41	.74	.75
Thought Disorder	SS	.80	.68	.51	.72	.40
Major Depression	CC	.79	.61	.61	.61	.52
Delusional Disorder	PP	.82	.66	.44	.61	.58

Population		Inpatient Alcoholic****		Heterogeneous Psychiatric Outpatients****		Heterogeneous Psychiatric Inpatients****	
Retest Interval		Intake to 4-6 Weeks	Intake to Midphase	Midphase to Midphase	Intake to Midphase	Intake to Discharge	Midphase to Midphase
MCMI Scale	Scale Code	(N = 96)	(N = 37)	(n = 35)	(N = 23)	(N = 47)	(N = 26)
Schizoid	1	.69	.76	.79	.72	.74	.78
Avoidant	2	.70	.77	.83	.76	.71	.74
Dependent	3	.58	.71	.85	.67	.73	.70
Histrionic	4	.83	.80	.81	.83	.74	.75
Narcissistic	5	.61	.79	.78	.73	.70	.77
Antisocial	6A	.63	.73	.83	.69	.64	.69
Aggressive/Sadistic	6B	X	.75	.80	.70	.73	.78
Compulsive	7	.70	.78	.85	.73	.70	.73
Passive-Aggressive	8A	.61	.69	.77	.62	.59	.68
Self-Defeating	8B	X	.80	.82	.76	.72	.75
Schizotypal	S	.65	.73	.84	.67	.64	.69
Borderline	C	.50	.63	.78	.51	.49	.60
Paranoid	P	.66	.59	.83	.64	.59	.62
Anxiety Disorder	A	.44	.60	.77	.58	.47	.59
Somatoform Disorder	H	.40	.59	.72	.55	.43	.46
Bipolar: Manic Disorder	N	.67	.71	.64	.64	.61	.64
Dysthymic Disorder	D	.44	.62	.75	.57	.43	.51
Alcohol Dependence	B	.57	.73	.83	.70	.59	.66
Drug Dependence	T	.70	.72	.80	.73	.66	.71
Thought Disorder	SS	.63	.65	.72	.44	.49	.53
Major Depression	CC	.55	.59	.71	.59	.57	.58
Delusional Disorder	PP	.69	.65	.79	.62	.60	.62

(continued)

33

TABLE 2.3
(Continued)

Population		Psychiatric Inpatients****	Psychiatric Inpatients*****	Impatients with Major Depression*****	Depressed Outpatients******
Retest Interval		3 Weeks	12 Months	6 Weeks	3 Months
MCMI Scale	Scale Code	(N = 98)	(n = 25)	(N = 15)	(N = 28)
Schizoid	1	.60	.71	.86	.77
Avoidant	2	.51	.76	.80	.65
Dependent	3	.67	.67	.45	.48
Histrionic	4	.74	.80	.86	.81
Narcissistic	5	.68	.87	.80	.51
Antisocial	6A	.84	.85	.79	.62
Aggressive/Sadistic	6B	.69	NR	NR	NR
Compulsive	7	.62	.44	.66	.35
Passive-Aggressive	8A	.69	.61	.55	.19
Self-Defeating	8B	.49	NR	NR	NR
Schizotypal	S	.47	.75	.83	.40
Borderline	C	.66	.64	.54	.27
Paranoid	P	.63	.51	.91	.66
Anxiety Disorder	A	.36	NR	NR	NR
Somatoform Disorder	H	.44	NR	NR	NR
Bipolar: Manic Disorder	N	.77	NR	NR	NR
Dysthymic Disorder	D	.53	NR	NR	NR
Alcohol Dependence	B	.66	NR	NR	NR
Drug Dependence	T	.78	NR	NR	NR
Thought Disorder	SS	.47	NR	NR	NR
Major Depression	CC	.50	NR	NR	NR
Delusional Disorder	PP	.49	NR	NR	NR

MCMI Scale	Scale Code	Median Correlations	Nonclinical Population**** (N = 91)
Schizoid	1	.76	.84
Avoidant	2	.76	.86
Dependent	3	.71	.85
Histrionic	4	.82	.80
Narcissistic	5	.77	.83
Antisocial	6A	.73	.88
Aggressive/Sadistic	6B	.75	.81
Compulsive	7	.70	.89
Passive-Aggressive	8A	.62	.85
Self-Defeating	8B	.76	.86
Schizotypal	S	.73	.89
Borderline	C	.63	.79
Paranoid	P	.64	.87
Anxiety Disorder	A	.59	.80
Somatoform Disorder	H	.55	.85
Bipolar: Manic Disorder	N	.67	.79
Dysthymic Disorder	D	.57	.78
Alcohol Dependence	B	.70	.88
Drug Dependence	T	.73	.85
Thought Disorder	SS	.63	.80
Major Depression	CC	.59	.78
Delusional Disorder	PP	.62	.91

*Millon (1983)
**McMahon, Flynn, and Davidson (1985b)
***Piersma (1986b)
****Millon (1987)
*****Piersma (1989b)
NR = Not reported.

35

A review of the data from these studies suggests the following conclusions:

1. Stability coefficients across all scales are generally lower than presented in the test manual for the MCMI (Millon, 1983) and for the MCMI-II (Millon, 1987).

2. Consistent with Millon's theory, stability coefficients are higher for the personality scales, moderately stable for the pathological personality scales, and lowest for the symptom scales.

3. Median stability coefficients for the personality scales range from .62 (8A) to .82 (4); for the pathological personality scales, median coefficients range from .63 (C) to .73 (S); for the symptom scales, median values ranged from .55 (H) to .73 (T). The Alcohol and Drug Dependence Scales appear particularly stable, suggesting they are probably measuring enduring personality traits as well as symptomatic expression of substance abuse.

4. Median stability coefficients are lower for clinical populations compared to nonclinical populations.

5. The stability coefficients for the MCMI-II are consistently higher than for the MCMI. However, preliminary evidence indicates that the pattern of stability estimates reported here for the MCMI are also true for the MCMI-II (Piersma, 1989a, 1989b).

Researchers have tended to rely on short retest intervals, generally ranging from a few weeks to 3 months. This methodology tends to result in spuriously high correlations. Only one study (Overholser, 1990) reported stability coefficients for MCMI scales beyond 3 months. After a 1-year posttesting interval, the average correlation for the personality scales was .69 and . 67 for the clinical scales.

In summary, the published data show the MCMI scales to be generally stable from 3 months. Stability coefficients show median values in the 60s and 70s for a variety of clinical groups. Axis II scales are more stable that Axis I scales, as would be expected. These scales are stable enough for their continued use, both clinically and in research.

Content Validity. The items of the MCMI were created by developing a theoretically based item pool which was then reduced on rational grounds. Millon opted for scale redundancy by arguing that item overlap is required because the constructs themselves overlap, but he attempted to lessen the psychometric problems created from such overlap by requiring that each item have a higher correlation with that scale than it has with any other scale. The result is that approximately 89% of all MCMI items are scored on two or more scales, more so than on any other test. Millon intentionally developed his instrument on the basis of his theory, which posits an association between personality style and the development of particular clinical syndromes. This insures a large amount of item overlap among scales.

Although scale redundancy has created some debate, the existing research indicates this is not much of a problem at the level of content validity. Lumsden (1987) compared the correlational matrix of the MCMI scales with and without the effects of shared items and found few differences. Also, while item overlap affects factor analysis, a nonmetric multidimensional scaling technique, which is not affected by scale redundancy, produced a pattern of the test's internal structure that was a faithful representation of Millon's theory (Greenblatt, 1987).

Widiger et al. (1985, 1986) conducted a content analysis of Scales 4 and 6A and found MCMI items more congruent to Millon's typology than to DSM-III criteria. Millon (1985a, 1986) argued that DSM-III criteria are not sacrosanct and often change, that the test does not require a one-to-one-correspondence with DSM-III to provide a valid assessment of the syndromes, and that content analysis is not necessarily relevant to a test's predictive validity. The issue remains unresolved.

Concurrent/Convergent Validity.   Two main issues that pertain to convergent validity. First, to what extent does the MCMI intercorrelate with similar measures? Second, what is the degree of correspondence between MCMI-derived personality disorders and DSM-III(R) diagnoses?

Intercorrelation with Other Personality Tests.   The MCMI has been correlated with other personality tests (The Minnesota Multiphasic Personality Inventory [MMPI], California Psychological Inventory [CPI], and Eysenck Personality Questionnaire [EPQ]), with symptom scales (The Profile of Mood States [POMS], Derogatis Symptom Checklist [SCL-90], Beck Depression Inventory (BDI), Hamilton Rating Scale for Depression (HRSDI and special rating scales (Robbins & Patton, 1986), with the General Health Questionnaire [GHQ]), with scales measuring perfectionism, narcissism, and interpersonal behaviors, and with personality scales derived from the MMPI.

In samples of heterogeneous psychiatric patients and substance abusers, the intercorrelations between the MCMI and the MMPI scales have been low to moderate, depending on the scales in question, though generally below .50 (Dubro, Wetzler, & Kahn, 1988; Marsh, Stile, Staughton, & Trout-Lauden, 1988; Smith, Carroll, & Fuller 1988). Correlations between MCMI personality scales and those derived from the MMPI have tended to be somewhat higher, ranging from −.31 to .87 (McCann, 1989; Morey & LeVine, 1988). Research suggests that both tests have shared and unique dimensions (Ownby, Wallbrown, Carmin, & Barnett, 1990). Studies have shown that, whether the criterion is symptoms established from chart review (Helmes & Barilko, 1988), concordance with Axis I disorders (Patrick, 1988), or agreement between the MacAndrew Alcoholism Scale (MAC) compared to Scale B (Miller & Streiner, 1990), the concurrent validity of the MMPI has been equal to or better than the MCMI.

Common factorial space has been reported for the MCMI and the MMPI (Ownby et al., 1990), the CPI (Holliman & Guthrie, 1989), and the (EPQ) (Gabrys et al., 1988), with correlations generally in the low to moderate range. Similar findings have been reported between the MCMI and more narrow band instruments, including the POMS (McMahon & Davidson, 1985a; 1986b), the GHQ (Leaf et al., 1987), the interpersonal problem checklist (Morey, 1986), the Burns Perfectionism Scale (Broday, 1988) the Narcissistic Personality Scale (Auerbach, 1984), and the Superiority and Goal Instability scales (Robbins, 1989). Moderate associations have been reported for DSM-III PDs and different measuring instruments of these disorders, including the MCMI (Morey, 1986.) Despite these associations, studies report poor correspondence between instruments purporting to measure DSM-III-R personality disorders (Helmes & Barilko, 1988; Morey, 1986; Reich, Noyes, & Troughton, 1987a; and Widiger & Francis, 1987). These results suggest the MCMI taps dimensions that are both similar yet unique from these instruments.

Correspondence with Axis I & II Disorders.   Although the MCMI was developed to measure Millon's taxonomy of personality styles and associated disorders and although it was developed prior to the appearance of DSM-III(R), it has been often used as a measure of DSM-III(R) Axis I and II disorders. The concordance of MCMI with DSM-III(R) syndromes and PDs has been the subject of much polemics (Widiger et al., 1985, 1986; Millon, 1985a), and a major concern of previous reviews was the extent to which the MCMI(II) corresponds to DSM-III(R) disorders in general. Chapters 11 and 12 provide the reader with an excellent discussion of this issue from both a theoretical and empirical perspective.

Correspondence with Axis I Syndromes

The Chapters in Part II of this book present research that bears substantially on the agreement with MCMI-based diagnosis with DSM-III Axis I syndromes. The reader is referred to those chapters for a more detailed presentation of the results. Evidence so far suggests poor agreement between MCMI computer-generated and clinician-determined diagnoses when the methodology compared MCMI test results with diagnosis established by other procedures on identical patients. When the methodology used statistics to differentiate groups (Choca, Bresolin, Okonek, & Ostrow, 1988) or asked graduate students to rate the accuracy of a real versus "random" MCMI reports of patients, (Moreland & Onstead, 1987), more favorable results were reported. However, these conclusions are based on only a few studies.

Correspondence with Axis II Disorders.   Studies have the following results: (a) The convergent validity is better for DSM-III PDs that are congruent with Millon's typology (e.g., Avoidant, Dependent) than it is for those inconsistent with the typology (Antisocial, Passive-Aggressive) (Morey & LeVine, Widiger & Sanderson, 1987). The MCMI-II subdivides the antisocial style into an Aggressive/Sadistic and Antisocial subtypes and this distinction should make the latter subtype more congruent with DSM-III(R). (b) The rates of diagnostic agreement between MCMI-derived and clinically-derived PDs have generally been disappointingly low (Piersma, 1987a; Reich, Noyes, & Treighton, 1987a; Wetzler & Dubro, 1990). This finding appears whether the clinical diagnosis is based on routine psychiatric examination or from structured clinical interviews designed to be isomorphic with Axis II categories.

It is too early to conclude that the MCMI is a poor instrument to measure DSM III-R Axis II disorders, since there are other interpretations of these research findings. First, clinical diagnosis may be a poor criterion by which to judge the MCMI(II). Some of this research was conducted in private psychiatric hospitals, where more influence might have been given to the diagnosis of Axis I syndromes based on insurance reimbursement considerations rather than on their true diagnoses. Second, even if a clinician is conscientious, a structured instrument that reviews the entire spectrum of disorders will almost always show more disorders than will an evaluation by an individual clinician, thus reflecting poor statistical correspondence. Third, the patients used in these studies have often had a coexisting Axis I syndrome which might have differentially affected the manifestation of PDs and/or inflated scores on a structured inventory. Fourth, studies have relied on computer-generated MCMI diagnoses to compare test results with other criterion measures. This confounds test results with the issue of whether computer-generated MCMI diagnoses themselves are valid. The methodologies used in these studies rarely addressed these issues. Fifth, the clinical popularity of this instrument attests to its clinical utility. Research has not yet tapped this area of inquiry. However, the rather consistent reports that the MCMI tends to overdiagnose PDs in a variety of populations (Cantrell & Dana, 1987; Craig, 1988; Holliman & Guthrie, 1989; Libb et al., 1990; Rebillot, 1985; Repko & Cooper, 1985) is disquieting. The MCMI-II uses more stringent criteria to establish a diagnosis than did the MCMI, and Millon continues to try and reduce the problem.

Predictive Validity.   There is a dearth of MCMI(II) predictive validity research. Two studies found that the MCMI was unable to predict treatment dropout (Cantrell & Dana, 1987; Craig, 1984), and one study found that Scale B successfully predicted polydrug use among college students (Jaffe & Archer, 1987). MCMI scores were able to predict return to duty or discharge from service (Butters, Retzlaff, & Gibertini, 1986) and poorer outcomes to lumbar laminectomy (Uomoto, Turner & Herron, 1988). These studies were all retrospective.

No one has used a prospective design to actual *predict* criterion. The need for future researchers to engage in predictive validity studies with the MCMI-II is all too apparent.

Detection of Faking.   Millon has developed a measure that was designed to detect malingering, a response set that exaggerates psychopathology. He reported that the Index detected 75% of college students who were instructed to take the test under "fake bad" instructions, but only 19% of those instructed to "fake good." Millon (1987) further argued that "deliberate or random misrepresenta-tion on clinical inventories is much less frequent than is commonly thought . . . the role of response styles seems to be a minor factor when com-pared with the substantive content of the scales" (p. 115).

There has been a surprising lack of research that addresses the various MCMI(II) validity indices (i.e., Disclosure Level, Desirability Gauge, Debase-ment). Van Gorp and Meyer (1986) studied the MCMI's ability to detect faking under one of six different instructional sets. A total of 95 psychiatric outpatients and 90 medical/surgical inpatient controls were randomly assigned to one of six instructional conditions. The MCMI was able to detect the faked bad profiles but not the faked good ones, results that substantiate Millon's earlier report. Further-more, the MCMI(II) Validity Scales were not found useful in screening out cases among 419 sex offenders, since the scales were especially influenced by social desirability (Langevein et al., 1988). In settings where a clinician can expect faked good response sets, such as in custody evaluations, the MCMI may not be the instrument of choice.

Demographic Variables

Race.   The MCMI was standardized on a sample that was 81% White. While the MCMI did provide separate norms for Black and White respondents, the MCMI-II manual presents no reports on racial differences, if any, with the inventory. Three studies have now addressed the issue.

Choca, Shanley, Peterson, and Denburg (1990) compared 235 Black with 471 White, male psychiatric inpatients and found significant differences for all diag-noses, except the personality disorders, by race. The patients were then sub-divided into two matched groups, of 209 subjects each, based on psychiatric diagnosis, and the data was analyzed at the item, scale, and structural level. Results showed that 45 of 175 items were answered differently by race, which was higher than chance. At the scale level, Blacks scored higher than Whites on Scales 4, 5, 6, P, N, B, T, and PP, and lower on scale D, though factor analysis indicated the factor structure within each racial group looked identical.

Davis, Greenblatt, and Pochyly, (1990) used a factorial design that analyzed the effects of race (Black/White), education (high school/less than high school) and diagnosis (schizophrenic/nonschizophrenic) on scales 2, 6, SS, and PP, among 310 newly admitted psychiatric patients. These scales were chosen as the ones most likely to differentiate schizophrenics from nonschizophrenics. Blacks scored higher than Whites on all scales studied. The MCMI described Black psychiatric patients as more asocial, avoidant, and psychotic in their thinking than White schizophrenics.

Though the study is praiseworthy for its elegant design and large sample size (N = 310), the results only demonstrated differences between Black and White schizophrenics on the MCMI and did not address the issue of bias. Differences in means do not establish test bias. Perhaps these differences were actual differences between the two populations. Holliman and Guthrie (1989) found no MCMI-based racial differences in a large sample of college students. We conclude that the issue of racial bias in the MCMI has not been demonstrated and remains an open question.

Education.   Holliman and Guthrie (1989) also found no educational differences on the MCMI, although one study reported nine of the scales were moderately influenced by IQ scores and education (Langevein et al., 1988).

Age.   Langevein et al. (1988) found that none of the MCMI scales correlated above .20 with age (N = 313) and 15 of the 20 scales correlated below 0.10, suggesting age does not significantly influence MCMI scales. Holliman and Guthrie (1989) found no age differences on MCMI scales among college students. Craig, Verinis, and Wexler (1985) found age to be correlated with the MCMI scales for alcoholics and opiate addicts but only 5% of the variance could be attributed to the effects of age. The research so far indicates that age is not a substantial variable that affects MCMI scores, but few studies have addressed the question.

Gender.   Millon has developed separate norms on the MCMI(II) for males and females. Piersma (1986a) found that female psychiatric inpatients scored significantly higher than males on scales 3, C, H, CC, and PP. No other scales showed sex differences initially. Cantrell and Dana (1987) found that female psychiatric outpatients scored higher than males on scales 3, C, A, H, D, and CC; males scored higher than females on scales 5 and 6. Gabrys et al., (1988) found that male outpatients (N = 325) scored higher on scales 2, 4, 5, 6, P, N, B, T, SS, and PP; female outpatients (N = 531) scored higher on Scale 7. These differences may correspond to differences in prevalence rates by sex and not imply test bias.

Descriptive Clinical Studies

By "clinical studies" as used here, we mean giving the MCMI to a particular population and then describing the personality style from group data. In a series of studies by Millon and his associates at the University of Miami (Antoni, Levine, Tischer, Green, & Millon, 1986, 1987; Antoni, Tischer, Levine, Green, & Millon, 1985a, 1985b; and Levine, Tischer, Antoni, Green, & Millon, 1985), patients with common MMPI profiles (i.e., 24/42, 27/72, 28/82, 78/87, and 89/98) were also given the MCMI and the high point MCMI codes within each MMPI profile type were then categorized into one of several "types," each representing a specific cluster of personality traits. The attributes of their MCMI correlate groups were then used to describe the subtype within the specific MMPI code.

The determination and interpretation of these MCMI clusters was arbitrary rather than statistical and sample sizes within each cluster were small. Also, the findings were generally based on an MCMI cutoff score of BR 65, which is below the BR score used to define the prevalence of a given disorder (BR 70), and well below the BR score that reflects the most severe manifestations of the disorder (BR 85). The approach is descriptive with some empirical features, but it lays the foundation for more empirically based actuarial diagnostic classification systems. Chapter 16 presents this material in depth and adds new data that has not appeared in the published literature.

Similar types of studies are beginning to appear in the literature. McCann and Suess (1988) studied 35 psychiatric inpatients with a 1238 MCMI codetype and found that patients had clinical diagnoses of affective disorder (44%), Schizophrenia (22%), Severe Personality Disorder (19%), Schizoaffective disorder (11%), or Adjustment Disorder with Depressed Mood (4%). A Previous suicide attempt was reported by 65% of the sample and 85% reported suicidal ideation. Greenblatt, Mozdzierz, Murphy, and Trimakas (1987) studied 53 psychiatric inpatients with a 28/82 codetype and found six subgroups with various symptom pictures, suggesting that patients with the same basic personality style can decompensate into a variety of pathological personality styles and report diverse patterns of symptoms. Benjamin (1987) combined the MCMI with the Structural Analysis of Social Behavior (SASB) INTREX Questionnaire to document change in Axis I symptoms through reconstructive psychotherapy.

These kinds of clinical studies are only just appearing on the individual scales. Auerbach (1987) found that patients who score high on the Scale S endorsed statements on scales that measure social anxiety, withdrawal, cognitive impairment, rage and somatic preoccupation, whereas patients who scored low on Scale 5 did not endorse these items.

These studies are important because they form the initial basis for the development of an MCMI personality "cookbook" of interpretations (Millon, 1984b). Although the clinical utility and validity of such schemata remain to be demonstrated, and though there are some methodological considerations extant in the development of these identified subtypes, such research is critical because it lays the foundation for MCMI-based personality description which would have clinical and heuristic value.

Clinical Populations

The concurrent validity of the MCMI with clinical populations can be determined by (a) comparing the pattern of profile scores on patients with a defined disorder to determine if a reliable profile exists, (b) assessing the validity of MCMI scales that relate specifically to the disorder, and (c) correlating these disorder-related scales with similar measures from other instruments.

In the following section we review the instruments' utility with specific clinical populations. For each disorder we present the modal MCMI profile suggested in the test manual, present the psychometric characteristics of the MCMI scale(s) that most pertain to the assessment of the disorder, and conclude with a review validity studies for that disorder.

Psychosis/Schizophrenia.

Modal Profile.   Scales P, SS, and PP are the three scales that would be most likely elevated in psychotic states. Millon (1987) reported that a combined elevation on Scales 2 and S may be as good a gauge of schizophrenia as is Scale SS. He provided modal profiles for Paranoid Disorder and Delusional disorder but none for psychosis

Paranoid.   Scale P item content pertains to vigilant mistrust, edgy defensiveness, irritability and issues with independence. It has an internal consistency of .90 and a median test-retest correlation of .63.

Scale Intercorrelations.   Millon (1987) reported that Scale P correlates .41 with both MMPI Paranoia (Pa) and Wiggins Psychoticism (PSY). McCann (1989) reported a correlation of .08 with MMPI Personality Disorder Scale "Paranoid."

Thought Disorder.   Scale SS pertains to disorganized and confused thinking, inappropriate affect, delusions and hallucinations. Internal consistency of the scale is .81 and median test-retest correlations is .63.

Scale Intercorrelations.   It correlates .61 with MMPI Schizophrenia (Sc), .39 with Pa, and .62 with PSY. McMahon and Davidson (1986b) reported a .49 correlation with POMS "Confusion/Bewilderment."

Delusional Disorder.   Item content on Scale PP deals with delusions, persecutions, grandiosity, hostile mood, and ideas of reference. It has an internal consistency estimate of .81 and a median test-retest correlation of .62.

Scale Intercorrelations.   Millon (1987) reported correlations of .39 with Pa, .41 with PSY, and .41 with SCL-90 "Anger/Hostility" and .42 with Wiggins

"Hostility (HOS) (Millon, 1983.) The scale shows minimal associations with the POMS "Anger/Hostility" scale (McMahon & Davidson, 1985a, 1986b.)

Validity Studies.   The evidence is mixed with respect to the instrument's ability to diagnose schizophrenia. Chapter 5 provides the reader with detailed information about this research. Studies that have assessed the congruence of the MCMI with DSM-III-R psychotic disorders have often reported poor agreement between test and clinician diagnosis (Bonato et al., 1988; Cantrell & Dana, 1987; DeWolfe, Larson, & Ryan, 1985; Patrick, 1988; and Sexton, McIlwraith, Barnes, & Dunn, 1987.) These results compel caution when using the MCMI to establish a DSM IIIR diagnosis involving psychosis. Millon admits that the instrument does not work as well at the "extremes of the distribution [of psychopathology]" and presumably this applies to severe forms of psychopathology, such as psychosis.

Affective Disorders

Studies have appeared that have assessed the MCMI with the disorders of Dysthymia, Major Depression, and Mania. We present a review of the studies for each of these diagnoses.

Dysthymia

Modal Profile.   Millon reported the modal profile had peak elevations on Scales D and A and mild elevations on 2, 8B, and 3 in that order. These results have not been replicated. McCann and Suess (1988) found that 64% of psychiatric patients with a 1238 codetype had some type of affective disturbance (Affective Disorder, Schizoaffective, Adjustment Disorder with Depressed Mood). Of these patients, 65% reported a previous suicide attempt, while 85% reported suicidal ideation. However, the codetype was not specific to Affective Disorder.

Dysthymia Scale.   Scale D is a 36-item scale that deals with behavioral apathy, self-deprecatory cognitions, guilt, and feelings of discouragement. Millon (1987) reports a stability estimate for the scale of .95, a correlation of .82 between the MCMI and MCMI-2 revisions of the scale, and test-retest correlations ranging from .32 to .78 among six separate samples of psychiatric patients and substance abusers. Our review found a median test-retest correlation of .57.

Scale Intercorrelations.   Millon (1987) reported Scale D correlates .70 with the MMPI Depression (Dep), .06 with Hypomania (Hyp), .74 with Wiggins Depression (DEP), and .12 with Hypomania (HYP), and a correlation of .69 with the SCL-90 Depression scale (Millon, 1983). The scale shows moderate correlations with structured depression rating scales including .62 with the BDI (Goldberg, Shaw, & Segal, 1987), and .62 with the HRSD (Choca et al., 1988), but lower associations (.26) were found with psychiatric ratings of depression (Tamkin, Carson, Nixon, & Hyer, 1987.)

McMahon and Davidson (1986b) found moderate associations between Scale D and the POMS scales of Tension/Anxiety (.46), Depression/Dejection (.47), and Fatigue/Inertia (.46), This data indicates there is convergent validity of Scale D with other measures of depression.

Validity Studies.   Scale D showed limited usefulness in identifying depressive-related symptoms reported on a screening survey among drug abusers (Flynn & McMahon, 1983b), and moderate concurrent validity in identifying depression in alcoholics (Hyer, Carson, Nixon, Tamkin, & Saucer, 1987; Tamkin et al., 1987.) The scale did not discriminate between anxious and depressed states (McMahon & Davidson, 1986b), but Choca et al., (1988) found the scale was able to discriminate between three mood states (depressed, euthymic, and hypomanic.) Among 95 outpatients, 68% of whom were depressed, the mean BR score was 84, suggesting dysthymia (Goldberg, Shaw, & Segal, 1987). Scale D was able to assess Major Depression with an accuracy of about 65%, which was better than chance (Wetzler, Kahn, Strauman, & Dubro, 1989). The scale was able to correctly classify depression-related symptoms with a 72% hit rate among psychiatric inpatients (Helmes & Barilko, 1988). In fact, studies have reported that Scale D is consistently elevated in the moderate to severe range of BR scores among patients with Major Depression (Joffe, Swinson, & Regan, 1988; Piersma, 1989a; and Wetzler et al., 1989.) The research to date suggests that, though the scale may not be able to distinguish between Dysthymia and Major Depression, it appears adequate to suggest a depressive diagnosis, since hit rates for "depression" have indicated a 60%–79% accuracy.

Major Depression

Modal Profile.   Millon (1987) reported the modal MCMI-II profile for Major Depression consisted of peak elevations on Scales CC, D, and A, and moderate elevations on 2, 8A, 8B, and 3, in that order. Three subsequent studies have now been published that provide partial substantiation of Millon's earlier data (Joffe et al., 1988; Piersma, 1989a; and Wetzler et al., 1989.) Scales A and D have consistently appeared as the two most elevated scales among the clinical symptom scales, with Scale CC often ranking third in elevation with mean BR scores at 73. None of these studies found the same pattern of elevations among the personality disorder scales, but Scales 2 and 8A were among the two most elevated scales. The one study that used the MCMI-2 (Piersma, 1989b) found that Scales 2, 8B, and 3 were the most elevated, corroborating Millon's report.

Major Depression.   Scale CC is a 31-item scale with an internal consistency estimate of .90 and a test-retest correlation ranging from .52 to .79 in six separate samples (Millon, 1987). We report a median stability estimate of .59. Scale content deals with suicidal ideation, cognitive signs of depression, crying spells, depressed affect, and withdrawn behavior.

Scale Intercorrelations.   The scale shows moderate associations with similar measures of depression. Millon (1987) reported Scale CC correlated .63 with MMPI Dep, .06 with Ma, .83 with Wiggins DEP, and .29 with HYP, and .83 with the SCL-90 Depression (Millon, 1983.) McMahon and Davidson (1986b) found moderate associations with the POMS Depression/Dejection (.54), Tension/Anxiety (.47) and Confusion/Bewilderment (.56). Also, moderate associations have been reported with depression rating scales, including the BDI (.62) (Goldberg et al., 1987) and the HDI (.56) (Choca et al., 1988.)

Validity Studies.   Despite these moderate associations to other measures of depression, the evidence is quite clear that scale CC is seriously deficient in establishing a diagnosis of Major Depression. The majority of studies have found poor concurrent validity using scale CC on patients with a clinical diagnosis of Major Depression (Choca et al., 1988; Flynn & McMahon, 1983b; Goldberg et al., 1987; Patrick, 1988; Piersma, 1987b; Silverstein & McDonald, 1988; and Wetzler et al., 1989). Patients with a clinical diagnosis of Major Depression often attain average BR scores below the recommended cutoff score (BR > 84), which is inconsistent with their clinical diagnosis, although they often score in the clinically elevated range on Scale D, suggesting some form of depression. Some studies have found that Scale CC is insensitive to true depression but quite good at ruling it out (e.g., true negatives) (Choca et al., 1988; Patrick, 1988; and Wetzler et al., 1989), though support for the scale was found in a drug abuse sample (Flynn & McMahon, 1983b). Helmes and Barilko (1988) found that the test correctly classified 78% of patients with histories of suicide attempts. The reader is referred to Chapter 6 for specific details.

Item content of the scale ignores the vegetative and somatic symptoms (appetite, weight loss, energy, sleep, libido) that constitute a major part of the criteria used to define the disorder. Factor analysis of the scale reflect three primary components consisting of mental disturbance, suicidal ideation and dependency conflicts (Goldberg et al., 1987), confirming the largely cognitive symptoms composed in this scale.

Mania

Modal Profile.   Millon (1987) reported the modal MCMI-II profile for Bipolar Mania showed mild elevations on most clinical symptom scales, a mean BR score of 63 and 76 with two separate samples of manics, and mild elevations of the personality disorder scales, peaking on Scales 8B and 2. There have been no other studies that report similar data.

BiPolar Manic Disorder Scale.   Scale N is a 37-item scale that measures symptoms related to the manic state. Item content deals with labile emotionality, restlessness, overactivity, distractibility and impulsivity. The scale correlated .79 between the MCMI and MCMI-II. Stability estimates for Scale N range from .62 to .79 on six different samples of psychiatric patients and substance abusers for the MCMI and from .61 to .79 for the MCMI-II (Millon, 1987.) We found a median test-retest correlation of .67. The scale has an internal consistency estimate of .84.

Scale Intercorrelations.   Millon (1987) reported correlations between Scale N and MMPI Depression of $-.18$, Hypomania .66, Wiggins Depression $-.12$, and Wiggins Hypomania of .07. Choca et al. (1988) reported a correlations of .36 with the Mania Rating Scale and Scale N. McMahon and Davidson (1986b) found low associations with POMS scales of Depression/Dejection (.10), Anger/Hostility (.25), and Vigor/Action (.26).

Validity Studies.   There have been few studies using the MCMI with Bipolar manic disorder. The reader is referred to Chapter 6 for specific details on these studies.

Comorbidities.   Some investigators have used the MCMI to evaluate depression in patients with comorbidities. The MCMI has been useful in evaluating depression among alcoholics. In a sample of 80 male alcoholics, Scale D was able to accurately detect 73% of the alcoholics who were also depressed. The depression among alcoholics has been rated as mild (Hyer, Carson, Nixon, Tamkin, & Saucer, 1987), a finding that appears when other instruments have been used with this population.

McMahon and Davidson (1986a) compared depressed alcoholics (N = 144) with nondepressed alcoholics (N = 74) and found the depressed group characterized by a detached interpersonal style of avoidant or asocial, with disorganized cognition and mixed emotionality of anxiety and depression.

Alcoholics whose depression did not abate after 6 weeks of inpatient treatment were characterized on the MCMI as having confused and disorganized thinking and an avoidant personality style (McMahon & Davidson, 1985b).

Flynn and McMahon (1983b) studied Scales D and CC among 88 drug abusers in treatment. Low but statistically significant correlations were found between these scales and survey items dealing with suicidal ideation, but these scales showed limited usefulness in identifying depressive-related symptoms among drug abusers.

Several studies have explored the characterization of depression among different psychiatric patients. Joffe, Swinson, and Regan (1988) found that the frequency of personality disorders among depressed patients with obsessive-compulsive disorders was not significantly different from that of patients with Major

Depression. Both groups had their most frequently occurring elevations on Scales 8A, 2, and 3.

Overholser, Kabakoff, and Norman (1989) used the MCMI to operationally classify depressed and dependent groups. Results showed that depression and dependency both affected symptoms directly rather than interactively, suggesting that the determination of personality disorders among depressed or dependent patients should be deferred until their clinical condition stabilizes.

Geriatric psychiatric patients with depression generally had a detached interpersonal style (schizoid, avoidant) and passive-aggressive style, while Millon's independent styles (N, 6A) and actively dependent or histrionic styles were inversely related to depression (Hyer, Harrison, & Jacobsen, 1987).

These studies show that the personality styles associated with affective disorders are characterized mostly by Millon's "detached" and/or "dependent" interpersonal styles, consistent with his theory on the association between personality style and symptom expression as it relates to depression. Clinicians are cautioned to defer diagnosing personality disorders in patients with an affective disorder, until the clinical condition remits, since the clinical state can influence the observed personality style (Overholser et al., 1989) and often change in the remitted state (Joffe & Regan, 1988; Piersma, 1989b).

In summary, there is a paucity of research that replicates Millon's suggested modal profiles for Affective Disorders (Dysthymia, Bipolar: Manic), and there has been partial replication of the modal profile for Major Depression. Scale intercorrelations for the affective disorder scales (D, N, CC) show moderate convergent validity with similar measures. Validity studies suggest that Scale D is sensitive to depression but not specific to Dysthymia vs. Major Depression. Scale CC is deficient in diagnosing Major Depression because item content of the scale omits the vegetative signs that often define the disorder. There have been only a few studies that investigated the MCMI with manic states, but preliminary results are encouraging. Most patients with an affective disorder shows detached or dependent personality styles, which is consistent with Millon's personality disorder typology.

Anxiety Disorders

Modal Profile.   Millon (1987) reported that the modal MCMI profile for patients with Anxiety disorders showed mild elevations on Scales 2, 8A, and 8B and mild-to-moderate elevations on Scales A and D. No research has appeared, as yet, to replicate these results.

Anxiety.   Scale A item content deals with somatic complaints, nervous tension, social apprehension, crying, and indecisiveness. Millon (1987) reported a stability estimate of .94, and we found a median test-retest correlation of .59.

Scale Intercorrelations.   Scale A correlates .57 with MMPI D, .41 with Pt, .67 with Wiggins DEP, .59 with HEA and .57 with ORG, .67 with SCL-90 Anxiety and .47 with SCL-90 Phobic Anxiety (Millon, 1983, 1987). McMahon and Davidson (1986b) reported that Scale A showed moderate correlations (>.35) with the POMS Scales of Tension-Anxiety, Depression-Dejection, Fatigue-Inertia, and Confusion-Bewilderment.

Validity Studies.   Despite the prevalence of anxiety disorders among psychiatric populations, they have been infrequently studied with the MCMI. Chapter 10 provides a review of these studies.

Elevated Scale A scores have been frequently observed in patients with PTSD (Hyer & Boudewyns, 1985; Hyer, O'Leary, Elkins, & Arena, 1985; Hyer, Woods, Boudewyns, Bruno, & O'Leary, 1988; McDermott, 1987; and Robert et al., 1985), substance abuse (Bartsch & Hoffman, 1985; Craig, Verinis, & Wexler, 1985; McMahon & Davidson, 1985b, 1986b; McMahon, Davidson, & Flynn, 1986; and McMahon, Gersh, & Davidson, 1989), and in various medical conditions (Herron, Turner, & Weiner, 1986; Malec, Romsaas, & Trump, 1985; Malec, Wolberg, Romsaas, Trump, & Tanner, 1988; and Snibbe, Peterson, & Sosner, 1980). These results attest to the Scale's construct validity.

Post-Traumatic Stress Disorder

There have been six publications using the MCMI with patients with PTSD. Two were clinical reports that suggest the usefulness of the MCMI as part of an assessment battery for evaluating the syndrome (Dalton, Garte, Lips, & Ryan, 1986; Hyer et al., 1985). The remaining four studies were empirical reports, only two of which used a contrasting control group.

Millon did not report a modal profile for PTSD, and there are no MCMI scales that directly measure the condition. Clinically, it appears that the modal PTSD profile is an 82 pattern, characterized by Passive-Aggressive and Avoidant personality features. Secondarily, Borderline traits are commonly observed, along with elevated scores on A, D, and B (Hyer & Boudewyns, 1985; Hyer et al., 1985, 1988; McDermott, 1987; and Robert et al., 1985.)

PTSD profiles had different mean BR scores, were more significantly elevated, had greater variability and a different shape than comparison groups with diagnoses that often obfuscates a differential diagnosis (Robert et al., 1985.)

This 8A2 modal profile has appeared often enough in these reports that a clinician can feel confident that it is accurate. However, it is based on results of an all-male sample of Vietnam veterans in inpatient PTSD programs at VA Medical Centers. The total sample size across published studies with this population is N = 96. It is unknown if these results will generalize to other PTSD victims (e.g., rape, fire, earthquake survivors,). The relative absence of comparison groups in this area suggests that further research is needed.

In summary, anxiety disorders have been insufficiently researched with the MCMI. Preliminary evidence indicates that Scale A has acceptable convergent and construct validity. Clinical studies have revealed that the 82 codetype is the modal profile for male PTSD inpatients. Chpater 9 provides further information on this area of research.

Obsessive-Compulsive Disorders

Patients (N = 23) who met RDC criteria for a primary diagnosis of obsessive-compulsive disorder showed no differences on personality trait scales compared to depressives. A mixed disorder with avoidant, dependent, and passive-aggressive features was most commonly observed. Scale 7 showed a mean BR score of only 56 in the clinical sample, similar to the mean scores for Millon's normative sample on this scale (Joffe, Swinson, & Regan, 1988).

Substance Abuse

Chapter 7 provides a full account on the use of the MCMI with alcoholics and drug abusers. We will not repeat this information here for brevity sake.

Eating Disorders (anorexia/bulimia)[4]

Seven studies have reported on the use of the MCMI with eating disordered patients. Five have used hospitalized patients, one used an outpatient sample, and one assessed university females. Sample sizes were quite small in three of the studies. This literature is presented in Chapter 8.

Overall, in the published literature, the MCMI has been given to 31 anorexics and to 262 bulimics, and 62 morbidly obese patients. Results can only be suggestive because of low sample sizes, particularly in the anorexics. Based on limited data with MCMI scores, bulimics tend to score higher on the more active interpersonal styles, whereas the anorexics score on the more detached and withdrawn interpersonal styles. It is uncertain if these results reflect basic personality dimensions in these populations or whether they are a reaction to the disorder itself.

Criminal Populations

Sex Offenders. Millon presented no information on the use of the MCMI(−II) with an offender population, but research is beginning to appear that uses the instrument with this population. The MCMI could not differentiate between specific versus anomalous sexual preferences or between sexual offenders (rapists, pedophiles, and perpetrators of incest) with and without these

---

[4]The succeeding material diverges from the original organization because Millon has not presented Modal Profiles or Scales for these disorders.

sexual proclivities (Langevein et al., 1979) and overdiagnosed PDs in this population, although all scales except 6 and T differentiated sex offenders from community controls (Langevein et al., 1988).

The mean profile among 99 rapists and child molesters was 654 characterized by aggression, narcissism, and gregariousness. Cluster analysis found four separate personality "types": (a) a detached type (213), (b) a narcissistic, aggressive, and gregarious type (564), (c) an aggressive, narcissistic type (68), and (d) a "healthy" group with no BR score over 75, but with some elevation on Scale T, and a subclinical 567 profile type (Bard & Knight, 1987).

Hamberger and Hastings (1986) found that 99 males in a domestic violence abatement treatment program had three "types" of personalities, Schizoid/Borderline, Narcissistic/Antisocial, or Passive-dependent/Compulsive. Cluster analysis of MCMI profiles from a similar population (N = 188) revealed two pathological clusters (Passive-Aggressive/Avoidant [N = 66], Antisocial/Narcissistic [N = 74], and a nonpathological group (N = 48). Abusers with personality disorders showed more affective lability and held more irrational beliefs than abusers without these disorders (Lohr, Hamberger, & Bonge, 1988.)

MEDICAL PATIENTS

Though intended for psychiatric populations, the MCMI has been used with medical patients to examine the role psychosocial factors play in the etiology, diagnosis, treatment, and prognosis of medical conditions. Often the differentiation between medical and psychological conditions is unclear, as in the case of obesity or chronic pain, due to the interacting effects which are not conclusively understood. Thus, the question of cause and effect remains unanswered and complicates the process of personality assessment.

We found 10 such studies. The samples include patients with testicular cancer, breast cancer, chronic headache, chronic pain, chronic fatigue syndrome, choreoacanthocytosis. Workman's Compensation claimants, and surgical patients (gastric stapling for morbid obesity, lumbar laminectomy). Once again, the diversity of populations and small number of published studies preclude easy summation.

The first group of studies are essentially descriptive. Medalia, Merriam, and Sandberg (1989) presented a neuropsychological case report of a woman diagnosed with choreoacanthosytosis and used the MCMI to assess the patient's psychopathology and character structure. Malec, Romsaas, and Trump (1985) studied 59 patients with testicular cancer, all of whom had at least one testicle surgically removed, to explore whether severe psychopathology was more prevalent among these patients. Because the patients were also at different phases of postoperative treatment, personality assessment was confounded with reactions to surgery and chemotherapy/radiation therapy. There was no consistently elevated personality scales among these patients, but the most frequent peak elevations on the symptom scales were A and H, which were logically related to their medical treatment and which attested to the construct validity for those particular scales.

Patients with Chronic Fatigue Syndrome (N = 24) scored highest on Scales 1, 3, 4, and 7, but BR scores were generally below 60. On the MCMI-II personality scales these patients scored highest on Scales 4, 2, and 1. They also scored highest on symptom scales measuring distress (A and H), with BR scores around 70 (Millon et al., 1989).

These studies were merely case reports for group data, as no comparison groups were included in the design. The next group of studies were more elegant in design, using more refined clinical groupings, control groups, and/or more elaborate statistical analyses.

Chronic headache (HA) patients (N = 25) differed from nonheadache chronic pain (CP) patients (N = 26) on several MCMI scales, and had a mean group MCMI profile characterized by elevated scores on Scales 7, C, A, H, and D. Results also showed greater overall psychopathology among the CP group (Jay, Grove, & Grove, 1987). These findings are consistent with many other studies that report traits similar to those underlying the scales elevated in the HA group.

Twenty-seven patients with benign breast biopsy were compared with 41 patients with breast cancer. The patients were assessed at the time of the initial evaluation and again at either 4 months (benign group) or 8 months (cancer group) in a test-retest design. Results showed the breast cancer group experienced more distress (Scale A) and somatic concerns (Scale H) following breast surgery and adjunctive therapy. Also, there was poor concordance of MCMI personality scales between pre- and posttesting, suggestive that treatment for breast cancer (and perhaps with other medically stressful procedures) may not provide a reliable occasion for the assessment of personality (Malec et al., 1988).

Two studies have used the MCMI with Worker's Compensation claims. Snibbe, Peterson, and Sosner (1980) studied 47 such claimants, using univariate and multivariate procedures. Subjects were categorized into one of four groups, head injury, psychiatric, low back pain, and a miscellaneous group. No significant differences among groups were found. When the MCMI group mean profile was plotted, peak scores were obtained on Scales 3, C, A, and D. In another study with a similar population, the MCMI suggested a passive-dependent personality style with anxiety and depression. This pattern was also found on the MMPI (Repko & Cooper, 1985).

The next two studies extend the usefulness of the MCMI a step further by attempting to demonstrate or "predict" postsurgical outcomes with various surgical procedures. In the first of these reports, 129 patients who were treated by lumbar laminectomy for discogenic disease were evaluated preoperatively with the MCMI. Patients with good versus fair or poor postsurgical outcomes were compared on their preoperative MCMI scores. Patients with poorer outcomes had scores associated with higher elevations on Scales 1, 2, 3, 8A, D, and A. However, the MCMI was only moderately associated with treatment outcomes, whereas MMPI scales were found to have higher predictive value (Herron, Turner, & Weiner, 1986). In a subsequent report, a discriminant function analysis based on MCMI scale scores correctly classified postsurgical outcomes with 66% accuracy. There was no attempt at cross-validation. Thus the MCMI was only moderately successful in predicting outcome to lumbar laminectomy. However, this may not be the fault of the test. Other variables besides personality factors, such as presence or absence of disc herniation, pending status of workman's compensation claims, etc., may be involved in postsurgical outcomes with this population (Uomoto, Turner, & Herron, 1988).

Chandarana, Holliday, Conlon, and Deslippe (1988) compared 31 morbidly obese patients awaiting gastric stapling with 31 similar patients who had already undergone the procedure. The postsurgical group scored lower on Scales 2 and S, perhaps suggesting an improvement in their satisfaction with interpersonal relationships.

The *Millon Behavioral Health Inventory* was constructed to provide health clinicians with an instrument that would capture the relationships between basic coping style and the relationship to psychosocial stress that can precipitate or exacerbate physical illness. However, the studies reported here indicate the MCMI may also be useful in medical settings as well. The test has now been given to 530 medical patients in the published literature. Its most relevant applications in such settings seems to be as a measure of psychopathology or a predictor of medical and surgical treatment outcomes. The bulk of the research presented normative data for the given population. One consistent finding is that these patients, irrespective of diagnosis, tend to score high on Scales H, A, and D. This would seem to establish the concurrent, if not construct, validity of these MCMI scales. Much more research needs to be done before the MCMI establishes its usefulness with medical patients, but it appears promising. Also, a number of these studies have printed mean MCMI profiles for different medical groups which could be useful in the construction of an MCMI interpretive "cookbook" for these populations.

SPECIAL POPULATIONS

Geriatric Psychiatric Population.   Hyer and Harrison (1986) applied Millon's typology to a later-life personality model and presented BR scores on four case histories. They extended their model to a larger clinical study (N = 60) with male later-life psychiatric patients. Consistent with Millon's theory, the detached (Scales 1 and 2) and the ambivalent (Scale 8A) styles were more prone to depression in later life, whereas independent styles (Scales 5, 6A,) were inversely related to depression (Hyer, Harrison, & Jacobsen, 1987). The most frequent personality style was that of submission, followed by the detached types and the passive aggressive type. The more energetic types, Scales 4, 6, and 7) were less in evidence (Hyer, 1987).

Sexual Disorder.   In a clinical report, Sugrue (1987) reported that 25 males in a treatment program for nonorganic erectile dysfunction generally had MCMI configurations peaking on Scale 7, suggesting an overcontrolled, rigid and ruminative person; Scale 6A suggesting the traits of independence, tough, and competitive superiority; or Scale 3, reflecting a lack of self-confidence and insecurity in relationships. The clinical usefulness of these findings remains to be seen.

Victims of Sexual Abuse.   A high proportion of patients with elevations on Scale C characterized a group of females (N = 14) who were sexually abused and later admitted to a private psychiatric hospital for a variety of disorders unrelated to the abuse (Bryer, Nelson, Miller, & Krol, 1987.) Mothers of incest victims (N = 43) had MCMI profiles characterized by the personality disorders of Dependent, Borderline, or Narcissistic (Myer, 1984–85).

Elective Abortion.   Campbell, Franco, and Jurs (1988) studied women who had abortions during adolescence compared with those who had abortions as adults (N = 66). The women were attending a support group for females who had experienced an abortion. Females who had aborted during adolescence scored higher in Scales 6A, P, T, and PP. The total sample scored high on scales A, H and D, though these scales did not differentiate between groups.

Military Personnel.   Three studies have used the MCMI with military personnel, but they all emanate from the same research group. Two studies identified normative data using the MCMI with 350 Air Force pilots in training. These officers obtained their highest scores on Scales 5 and 4 (Retzlaff & Gibertini, 1988.) Distinct MCMI scales, each with Scales 4, 5, 6, & 7 in varying degrees of saliency, were associated with different Personality Research Form test profiles when cluster analyzed (Retzlaff & Gibertini, 1987b). These scales generally tap more attenuated traits associated with less severe manifestations of or an absence of psychopathology rather than psychopathology per se. For example, pilots who score high on Scale 5 or 3 would be seen as sociable, possessing high self-esteem, arrogant, dramatic, excitable, bold, adventurous, thrill-seeking, and playful. Those who score high on Scale 7 might be described as cautious, conforming, and polite.

In a sample of trainees referred for mental health evaluation, the MCMI was an effective predictor of clinical recommendations of either a return to duty, administrative separation, or immediate discharge for reasons of mental health. Higher MCMI scores were associated with recommendations for immediate discharge. Exceptions were scores on Scales 4 and 5, where higher scores were associated with higher levels of ego strength compared to the other personality scales. The test's predictive ability was enhanced when the sample was dichotomized into "return to duty" vs. "discharge" (Butters et al., 1986).

In summary, the clinical usefulness of the MCMI seems promising but remains to be empirically demonstrated in these special populations.

NORMAL POPULATIONS

Several studies have now reported on the use of the MCMI with nonclinical populations. Studies have found meaningful relationships between MCMI scale scores and vocational interests among community college students (Tango & Dziuban, 1984), chronic absenteeism in large corporations (Beck, 1987), and burnout among family practice residents (Lemkau, Purdy, Refferty, & Rudisill, 1988). The MCMI has also been used to study the personality styles of seminary students (Piersma, 1987c) and Air Force Officers in pilot training (Retzlaff & Gibertini, 1987b, 1988).

These studies do raise a serious ethical question, however. The MCMI is a personality instrument specifically designed and normed for use with clinical populations. Millon 1983, 1987) made it clear that the MCMI should not be used outside of mental health settings. Still, we found numerous studies that violated Millon's injunction (Adams & Clopton, 1990; Bard & Knight, 1987; Beck, 1987; Butters et al., 1986; Campbell et al., 1988; Chandarana et al., 1988; Hamberger & Hastings, 1986; Herron et al., 1986; Jaffe & Archer, 1987; Jay et al., 1987; Langevin et al., 1979, 1988; Lemkau et al., 1988; Lohr et al., 1988; Lundholm, 1989; Malec et al., 1985, 1988; McCormack, Barnett, & Wallbrown, 1989; Medalia et al., 1989; Millon et al., 1989; Myer 1984–85; Piersma, 1987c; Retzlaff & Gibertini, 1987b, 1988; Snibbe et al., 1980; Tango & Dziuban, 1984; and Uomoto et al., 1988). An earlier reviewer of this manuscript thought we should emphasize the fact that these studies were ill-conceived and suggest that no more should be done. We do not take quite as strong a position, but clinicians who use this instrument with nonclinical samples are putting themselves at risk for malpractice. Although research with the MCMI with normal populations may be justified, no clinical decision should be made using this instrument on such populations at this time. Alternative approaches include developing special scales from other tests that tap Millon's basic personality types (Strack, 1987) or using regression equations that estimate these constructs from other test scores (Zarella, Schuerger, & Ritz, 1990.) Millon is presently developing a new instrument that would measure his basic personality types in nonclinical (normal) populations.

The history of the MCMI(II) is likely to follow that of the MMPI. Initially the MMPI was developed to study psychopathology. As the instrument became more popular, gradually a variety of normal populations were studied to the point where reliable extra-test correlates among normals were found to be clinically useful. This may eventually be the fate of the MCMI as well. However, it is still too soon to recommend using this test with normals and ethical caveats cited earlier still apply.

Validity of NCS Computer-Generated Narrative Report

Several previous reviews have lamented about the paucity of research on the validity of the NCS computer-generated narrative report. This report is among the more popular and frequently used methods of obtaining MCMI test results, and computer-generated MCMI diagnoses has often been a criterion measure used to evaluate the diagnostic validity of the instrument in many of the published studies included in this review. Hence, its validity is a central issue that has direct clinical implications.

There now have been published seven studies and two rebuttals that have addressed the validity of these narrative reports, as presented in Table 2.4. The range of patients used to generate an MCMI profile has been broad. These include patients with adjustment disorders to schizophrenia (Green, 1982), Bipolar Affective Disorder (DeWolfe et al., 1985), Affective and Anxiety Disorders (Piersma, 1987b), alcoholics (Gualtieri, Gonzaels, & Baldwin, 1987), substance abusers (Siddall, 1986) and heterogeneous psychiatric outpatients (Moreland & Onstad, 1987). The judges have included mental health clinicians, graduate students in clinical psychology, alcohol rehabilitation counselors, and unspecified clinical staff. Methodology has varied dramatically across these studies. Green (1982) had clinicians rate the MCMI narratives, Roche MMPI reports and Mayo MMPI reports, in terms of adequacy of information, description accuracy in nine areas, and report format and utility. This material is elaborated upon in Chapter 13.

When the MCMI computer-generated report has been compared to discharge clinical diagnosis, the results have shown poor diagnostic agreement. The MCMI underdiagnosed or misdiagnosed Affective Disorders (DeWolfe et al., 1985; Piersma, 1987b) and overdiagnosed anxiety disorders (Piersma, 1987b). However, these conclusions are based on only two studies and relates specifically to the concurrent validity of the MCMI, and does not specifically address the quality or usefulness of the report when the computer-generated diagnosis is valid.

The MCMI report has generally received favorable ratings by clinicians on the adequacy of information presented in the report, its accuracy in describing basic personality and symptoms, and its format and usefulness to clinicians (Green, 1982; Gualtieri et al., 1987; Moreland & Onstad, 1987; Sandberg, 1987; and Siddall, 1986). These ratings were shown not to be influenced by instructional sets (Gualtieri et al., 1987) or "Barnum" type effects (Green, 1982; Sandberg, 1987), but were influenced by clinician experience level (Siddall, 1986).

TABLE 2.4
Research on the MCMI Computer-Generated Narrative Reports

Authors	Judges	Population Tested	Task
Green (1982)	23 psychiatrists, psychologists, and social workers	Adjustment Disorders–Schizophrenics (N = 100)	Rate report on adequacy of information, descriptive accuracy and report utility
DeWolfe, Larsen, and Ryan (1985)	None	Bipolar Affective Disorders (N = 148)	Compared computer diagnosis with clinical diagnosis
Siddall (1986)	Clinical staff	Polydrug abusers involved with the Judicial System	Rate accuracy, format and utility of reports along 13 different categories
Piersma (1987b)	None	Affective and Anxiety Disorders (N = 151)	Compared computer diagnosis with clinical diagnosis
Sandberg (1987)	Psychology graduate students (N = 34)	Simulated patient profiles (N = 34)	Rate narrative reports compared to "fake" reports to determine if "Barnum"statements are the cause of high narrative ratings
Guatlieri, Gonzales, and Baldwin (1987)	Alcohol Rehab. Counselors (N = 24)	Inpatient alcoholics (N = 175)	Rate narrative reports of patients who took the MCMI under different instructional sets
Moreland and Onstead(1987)	Clinical Psychologists (N = 8)	Psychiatric outpatients (N = 99)	Rate accuracy of actual compared to random reports on the same patient

Conclusions

—MCMI report rated more accurate in assessing interpersonal relationships, personality traits and coping styles thant the Roche and Mayo MMPI reports.

—Poor corresponsence of MCMI computer diagnosis with clinical discharge diagnosis.

—MCMI report judged useful with diagnosis and treatment planning. Judges with more clinical experience with the MCMI and more experience in substance abuse rated the test more favorably than judges with less experience.

—MCMI reports underdiagnosed depression and overdiagnosed anxiety disorders.

—Real narrative reports attained higher ratings on information adequacy, diagnostic accuracy, and report utility than faked reports.

—Reports judged accurate; instructional sets did not affect MCMI report.

—MCMI reports rated more accurate in symptoms and trait descriptions than reports selected at random, suggesting Barnum effect not operative in computer satisfaction ratings.

57

When the MCMI narratives have been compared to "real" vs. "faked" reports (Sandberg, 1987) or when actual reports were compared to those chosen at random for the "same" patient (Moreland & Onstad, 1987), the MCMI computer report has been rated as more accurate and useful across a variety of dimensions.

In summary, When the MCMI computer-generated reports have been compared to clinician-derived diagnosis with the same patients, there has been poor diagnostic concordance. When computer reports were subjected to clinician ratings on a variety of dimensions, more favorable results appear.

However, there are methodological problems throughout all the studies that render these findings as only suggestive. Green (1982) found that the National Computer Systems MCMI and the Roche MMPI reports had higher ratings than the Mayo MMPI report. There are several problems with this study. The Mayo Report was based on single scale elevation and used library statements were over 25-years-old. Configural and content scale interpretations have since become more common and clinically useful. Thus, almost any report would receive higher ratings when compared to an outdated and skimpy narrative report. Second, demand characteristics were not accounted for in this study.

DeWolfe et al. (1985) found low diagnostic concordance between MCMI computer diagnoses and clinical diagnoses for patients with Bipolar Affective Disorders. However, MCMI admission test protocols were compared to discharge clinical diagnoses and no information was provided on the length of hospitalization. Thus, comparisons were made at two different points of time.

Siddall (1986) did not control for demand characteristics among judges and merely reported clinician opinions about the narrative reports with little focus on the factors influencing ratings, other than experience level.

Piersma (1987b) controlled for this confound and obtained that the MCMI underdiagnosed affective disorders. It is possible, however, that since it was a private psychiatric hospital, the clinicians might have shown a preference for specifying "Major Depression" over "Dysthymia" because it would more often justify inpatient hospitalization under utilization review, and because insurance may be more likely to reimburse this diagnosis.

Though Sandberg (1987) supported the accuracy and utility of MCMI computer reports, data was not provided about the nature of the comparisons, and the study failed to control for the effects of labeling the reports as either "computer analyzed" or "clinician analyzed" on rater judgments.

Gualtieri et al. (1987) concluded that the MCMI was not influenced by instructional sets, but they included no checks to determine whether the alcoholics actually took the test as instructed. It is likely that alcoholics are not able to discern their behavior under different states of sobriety and drunkenness. This would easily account for the finding of no differences in accuracy ratings across the various instructions.

Moreland and Onstad's (1987) study was criticized by Cash, Mikulka, and Brown (1989) who questioned the representativeness of the selected judges, who numbered 8 from a solicited sample of 600 and argued that perhaps these judges may have been favorably predisposed toward the MCMI interpretive reports. They also criticized the fact that the report chosen at random was labeled "experimental" whereas the actual MCMI report did not contain such a designation. Such a label might have reduced the credibility of the report in the eyes of the judges. However, Moreland and Godfrey (1989) argued that these criticisms do not mitigate their general conclusions that the MCMI computer interpretations are more accurate than randomly generated reports.

In summary, serious problems remain in demonstrating the accuracy of MCMI(II) computer narrative reports, though preliminary evidence suggests they are rated favorably across many dimensions despite many methodological problems. We suggest that if the computer-diagnosis corresponds to the clinical diagnosis, then the narrative report is more likely to be clinically useful.

There are many difficulties with computer-generated personality interpretations (Matarazzo, 1986) and APA guidelines (APA, 1985) stipulate that psychologists limit their use of computerized testing to techniques with which they are otherwise familiar and competent to use. Psychologists would serve their clients best if they follow such guidelines. Meanwhile, research in this area should continue to explore the usefulness and limits of these reports.

DISCUSSION

A critical issue is the question of the degree of knowledge transfer from MCMI research as applied to the MCMI-II. To what extent is the literature on the original scales still relevant to research and clinical practice with the new scales? There is insufficient research to empirically answer this question, but some data exist to suggest that we can expect a great deal of knowledge transfer. First, Millon intended for the MCMI-II to be isomorphic with the MCMI except that the antisocial style was subdivided into antisocial and aggressive/sadistic styles, and the passive-aggressive style was subdivided into passive aggressive and self-defeating styles. Second, although very few papers have been published on the MCMI-II, those that address the degree of correspondence between the MCMI and the MCMI-II generally found few, if any, differences between the two versions. This, however, remains a matter for future investigation. Third, the research data suggest that some of the scales are sufficiently similar such that they could be considered parallel forms of the test.

Some Continuing Problems

Our review leads us to conclude that problems continue to exist with the MCMI. These include poor correspondence to several DSM-III-R syndromes and disorders, problems with item overlap across scales, the absence of a well-articulated prinicples of interpretation, lower scale stability over time than reported in the test manual, and continuing difficulties in demonstrating the validity of the MCMI computer-generated reports. We suspect this is more a research problem than a clinical problem. Clinicians are increasingly using this test and the proof of the test's worth may functionally be in their continued use and faith in the output. Researchers need to determine which aspects of the test provide clinicians with "clinical validity" and then capture this in research designs.

Future Considerations

In keeping with the needed improvements in the methodology identified in this review, we are also able to suggest some needed directions for future research in order to continue the development of the MCMI-II:

1. Future published studies with the test should address both *statistical/empirical* and the *clinical* treatment of the data. *Profile differences* should be reported using (M)ANOVA where possible, to report statistical differences. Comparisons of the MCMI-II *profile shape* should be reported along with commentary on any significant differences or similarities in contrasted groups. *High point MCMI profile codes* should be reported. Results should be cross-validated on independent samples, if possible. This kind of data could add to the MCMI clinical literature and form the basis of an MCMI interpretive "cookbook" for different populations.

2. There has been a paucity of research at the individual scale level. Most research has focused on the test as a whole; yet, configural interpretation and group data ultimately rely on the strength of the individual scales on which such data are based. There has been an initial start in this direction (Prifitera & Ryan, 1984), but much more needs to be done, particularly in the area of basic scale validation research.

3. There is a critical need for the establishment of extra-test correlates associated with the basic scales and with profile elevations. Researchers have accepted that elevations means certain things but there is little research to explicate and substantiate those interpretive meanings.

4. It appears that most studies have used the National Computer Systems computer-generated reports to establish a diagnosis. Given the many problems with such procedures reported throughout this review, if the design requires the MCMI to make the diagnosis then we recommend that the clinician/researcher individually inspect the MCMI-II test protocol and clinically establish the diagnosis, rather than use the computer for this requirement. APA (1985) guidelines specify that psychologists must not use computer-based interpretations of tests unless they are otherwise familiar with and competent to interpret the test without a computer. Extraneous knowledge of the clinician that might methodologically compromise the experiment could be dealt with through effective research designs, such as the use of independent judges.

5. The MCMI-II has been available for over 3 years, yet little research has been conducted using this instrument. Through January, 1990, research continues to be published that is based on the MCMI. Although some of this may be explained by the time lag between conducting research studies and journal publication, it is now time to focus our research on the MCMI-II.

6. More comprehensive research is needed to assess not only personality factors that may predispose people to various clinical syndromes and symptoms and affect the expression of symptoms and/or the course of the syndrome, but also personality factors demonstrated during the acute states that may reflect less severe variants of clinical symptoms and personality changes that may result from having had previous episodes. There is increasing attention within psychiatry to study the association between the development of clinical syndromes and premorbid personality factors. Millon's theory provides clear postulates with which to test these associations and the MCMI-II may be a good instrument with which to advance such knowledge. These findings would also help delineate the exact boundaries of the state vs. trait controversy within the field of psychopathology and personality pathology.

The MCMI-II has made impressive gains in clinical usage in the first 10 years of its existence. Although many of the research findings are preliminary in nature and therefore the conclusions should be viewed as tentative, we have begun to develop a rather substantial knowledge base on this test and have a good sense of its strengths and weaknesses based on empirical research. Future needs include an MCMI-II basic text that can be used for graduate study, an interpretive manual that would help remove what earlier reviewers referred to as the "mysteries of interpretation," greater clinician familiarity and understanding of the concept of "base rate" scores, better research designs that would address the many issues identified in this review, and an instrument that would assess Millon's basic personality types in normal populations.

REFERENCES

Adams, W. E., & Clopton, J. R. (1990). Personality and dissonance among Mormon missionaries. *Journal of Personality Assessment, 54,* 684–693.

Antoni, M., Levine, J., Tischer, P., Green, C., & Millon, T. (1986). Refining personality instruments by combining MCMI high-point profiles and MMPI codes, Part IV: MMPI 89/98. *Journal of Personality Assessment, 50,* 65–72.

Antoni, M., Levine, J., Tischer, P., Green, C., & Millon, T. (1987). Refining personality assessments by combining MCMI high-point profiles and MMPI codes, Part V: MMPI code 78/87. *Journal of Personality Assessment, 51,* 375–387.

Antoni, M., Tischer, P., Levine, J., Green, C., & Millon, T. (1985a). Refining personality assessments by combining MCMI high-point profiles and MMPI codes, Part I: MMPI code 28/82. *Journal of Personality Assessment, 49,* 392–398.

Antoni, M., Tischer, P., Levine, J., Green, C., & Millon, T. (1985b). Refining personality assessments by combining MCMI high-point profiles and MMPI codes, Part III: MMPI code 24/42. *Journal of Personality Assessment, 49,* 508–515.

Auerbach, J. S. (1984). Validation of two scales for Narcissistic Personality Disorder. *Journal of Personality Assessment, 48*, 649–653.

Auerbach, J. S. (1987). Schizotypy, narcissism, and psychopathology: Correlations of psychosis-proneness and MCMI scales. In C. Green (Ed.), *Conference on the Millon clinical inventories (MCMI, MBHI, MAPI)* (pp. 235–241). Minneapolis: National Computer Systems.

Bard, L. A., & Knight, R. A. (1987). Sex offender subtyping and the MCMI. In C. Green (Ed.), *Conference on the Millon clinical inventories (MCMI, MBHI, MAPI)* (pp. 133–137). Minneapolis: National Computer Systems.

Bartsch, T. W., & Hoffman, J. J. (1985). A cluster analysis of Millon Clinical Multiaxial Inventory (MCMI) profiles: More about a taxonomy of alcoholic subtypes. *Journal of Clinical Psychology, 41*, 707–713.

Beck, M. (1987). Absenteeism in industry: A bio-psychosocial profile of the chronic absentee. In C. Green (Ed.), *Conference on the Millon clinical inventories (MCMI, MBHI, MAPI)* (pp. 273–284). Minneapolis: National Computer Systems.

Benjamin, L. S. (1987). Combined use of the MCMI and the SASB Intrex questionnaires to document and facilitate personality change during long-term psychotherapy. In C. Green (Ed.), *Conference on the Millon inventories (MCMI, MBHI, MAPI)* (pp. 305–323). Minneapolis: National Computer Systems.

Bonato, D. P., Cyr, J. J., Kalpin, R. A., Prendergast, P., & Sanhueza, P. (1988). The utility of the MCMI as a DSM-III Axis I diagnostic tool. *Journal of Clinical Psychology, 44*, 867–875.

Broday, S. F. (1988). Perfectionism and Millon basic personality patterns. *Psychological Reports, 63*, 791–794.

Bryer, J. B., Nelson, B. A., Miller, J. B., & Krol, P. A. (1987). Childhood sexual and physical abuse as factors in adult psychiatric illness. *American Journal of Psychiatry, 144*, 1426–1430.

Butters, M., Retzlaff, P., & Gibertini, M. (1986). Non-adaptability to basic training and the Millon Clinical Multiaxial Inventory. *Military Medicine, 151*, 574–576.

Calsyn, D., & Saxon, A. (1988). Identification of personality disorder subtypes among drug abusers using the Millon Clinical Multiaxial Inventory. 49th Annual Scientific Meeting of the Committee on Problems of Drug Dependence, Incorporated: Problems of drug dependence, 1987. *National Institute on Drug Abuse: Research Monograph Series.* Rockville, Md., p. 299.

Calsyn, D. A., & Saxon, A. J. (in press). Personality Disorder subtypes among cocaine and Opiod Addicts using the Millon Clinical Multiaxial Inventory. *The International Journal of the Addictions.*

Calsyn, D. A., Saxon, A. J., & Daisy, F. (1990). Validity of the MCMI drug abuse scale with drug abusing and psychiatric samples. *Journal of Clinical Psychology, 46*, 244–246.

Campbell, N. B., Franco, K., & Jurs, S. (1988). Abortion in adolescence. *Adolescence, 23*, 813–823.

Cantrell, J. D., & Dana, R. H. (1987). Use of the Millon Clinical Multiaxial Inventory (MCMI) as a screening instrument at a community mental health center. *Journal of Clinical Psychology, 43*, 366–375.

Cash, T. F., Mikulka, P. J., & Brown, T. A. (1989). Validity of Millon's computerized interpretation system for the MCMI: Comment on Moreland and Onstad. *Journal of Consulting and Clinical Psychology, 57*, 311–312.

Chandarana, P., Holliday, R., Conlon, P., & Deslippe, T. (1988). Psychosocial considerations in gastric stapling surgery. *Journal of Psychosomatic Research, 32*, 85–92.

Choca, J. P., Bresolin, L., Okonek, A., & Ostrow, D. (1988). Validity of the Millon Clinical Multiaxial Inventory in the assessment of affective disorders. *Journal of Personality Assessment, 52*, 96–105.

Choca, J. P., Peterson, C. A., & Shanley, L. A. (1986). Factor analysis of the Millon Clinical Multiaxial Inventory. *Journal of Consulting and Clinical Psychology, 54*, 253–255.

Choca, J. P., Shanley, L. A., Peterson, C. A., & Van Denburg, E. (1990). Racial bias and the MCMI. *Journal of Personality Assessment, 54*, 479–490.

Craig, R. J. (1984). Can personality tests predict treatment dropouts? *The International Journal of the Addictions, 19,* 665–674.

Craig, R. J. (1988). A psychometric study of the prevalence of DSM-III personality disorders among treated opiate addicts. *The International Journal of the Addictions, 23,* 115–124.

Craig, R. J., & Olson, R. E. (1990). MCMI comparisons of cocaine abusers and heroin addicts. *Journal of Clinical Psychology, 46,* 230–237.

Craig, R. J., Verinis, J. S., & Wexler, S. (1985). Personality characteristics of drug addicts and alcoholics on the Millon Clinical Multiaxial Inventory. *Journal of Personality Assessment, 49,* 156–160.

Dalton, J. E., Garte, S. H., Lips, O. J., & Ryan, J. J. (1986). Psychological assessment instruments in PTSD treatment programs. *VA Practitioner, 3,* 41–51.

Dana, R. H., & Cantrell, J. D. (1988). An update on the Millon Clinical Multiaxial Inventory (MCMI). *Journal of Clinical Psychology, 44,* 760–763.

Davis, W. E., Greenblatt, R. L., & Pochyly, J. M. (1990). Test of MCMI black norms for five scales. *Journal of Clinical Psychology, 46,* 175–178.

DeWolfe, A. S., Larsen, J. K., & Ryan, J. J. (1985). Diagnostic accuracy of the Millon test computer reports for bipolar affective disorder. *Journal of Psychopathology and Behavioral Assessment, 7,* 185–189.

Dougherty, R. J., & Lesswing, N. J. (1989). Inpatient cocaine abusers: An analysis of psychological and demographic variables. *Journal of Substance Abuse Treatment, 6,* 45–47.

Dubro, A. F., Wetzler, S., & Kahn, M. W. (1988). A comparison of 3 self-report inventories for the diagnosis of DSM-III personality disorders. *Journal of Personality Disorders, 2,* 256–266.

Duthie, B., & Vincent, K. R. (1986). Diagnostic hit rates of high point codes for the Diagnostic Inventory of Personality and Symptoms using random assignment, base rates, and probability scales. *Journal of Clinical Psychology, 42,* 612–614.

Everly, G. S., Shapiro, S., Levine, S., Newman, E. C., & Sherman, M. (1987). An investigation into the relationships between personality disorders and clinical syndromes (DSM-III, Axis I). In C. Green (Ed.), *Conference on the Millon clinical inventories (MCMI, MBHI, MAPI)* (pp. 295–303). Minneapolis: National Computer Systems.

Flynn, P. M., & McMahon, R. C. (1983a). Stability of the drug misuse scale of the Millon Clinical Multiaxial Inventory. *Psychological Reports, 52,* 536–538.

Flynn, P. M., & McMahon, R. C. (1983b). Indicators of depression and suicidal ideation among drug abusers. *Psychological Reports, 52,* 784–786.

Flynn, P. M., & McMahon, R. C. (1984a). An examination of the Drug Abuse Scale of the Millon Clinical Multiaxial Inventory. *The International Journal of the Addictions, 19,* 459–468.

Flynn, P. M., & McMahon, R. C. (1984b). An examination of the factor structure of the Millon Clinical Multiaxial Inventory: *Journal of Personality Assessment, 48,* 308–311.

Foster, L. (1977). Group Embedded Figures test performance in different instrumental behavior styles. *Journal of Clinical Psychology, 33,* 571–574.

Gabrys, J. B., Untendale, K. A., Schumph, D., Phillips, K., Robertson, G., Sherwood, G., O'Haire, T., Allard, I., & Clark, M. (1988). Two inventories for the measurement of psychopathology: Dimensions and common factorial space on Millon's clinical and Eysenck's general personality scales. *Psychological Reports, 62,* 591–601.

Gibertini, M., Brandenberg, N. A., & Retzlaff, P. D. (1986). The operating characteristics of the Millon Clinical Multiaxial Inventory. *Journal of Personality Assessment, 50,* 554–567.

Gibertini, M., & Retzlaff, P. D. (1988). Factor invariance of the Millon Clinical Multiaxial Inventory. *Journal of Psychopathology and Behavioral Assessment, 10,* 65–74.

Gilbride, T. V., & Hebert, J. (1980). Pathological characteristics of good and poor interpersonal problem-solvers among psychiatric outpatients. *Journal of Clinical Psychology, 36,* 121–127.

Goldberg, J. O., Shaw, B. F., & Segal, Z. V. (1987). Concurrent validity of the Millon Clinical Multiaxial Inventory depression scales. *Journal of Consulting and Clinical Psychology, 55,* 785–787.

Green, C. (1982). The diagnostic accuracy and utility of MMPI and MCMI computer interpretive reports. *Journal of Personality Assessment, 46,* 359–365.

Green, C. (Ed.). (1987). *Conference on the Millon clinical inventories (MCMI, MBHI, MAPI).* Minneapolis: National Computer Systems.

Greenblatt, R. L. (1987). Nonmetric multidimensional scaling of the MCMI. In C. Green (Ed.), *Conference on the Millon clinical inventories (MCMI, MBHI, MAPI)* (pp. 145–154). Minneapolis: National Computer Systems.

Greenblatt, R. L., Mozdzierz, G. J., Murphy, T. J., & Trimakas, K. (1987). Pathological personality style and symptom diversity of 28/82 psychiatric inpatients. In C. Green (Ed.), *Conference on the Millon clinical inventories (MCMI, MBHI, MAPI)* (pp. 243–247). Minneapolis: National Computer Systems.

Greer, S. E. (1984). Testing the test: A review of the Millon Clinical Multiaxial Inventory. *Journal of Counseling and Development, 63,* 262–263.

Greer, S. E. (1985). A reply to Millon and Moreland. *Journal of Counseling and Development, 63,* 632.

Gualtieri, J., Gonzales, E., & Baldwin, N. (1987). The accuracy of MCMI computerized narratives for alcoholics. In C. Green (Ed.), *Conference on the Millon clinical inventories (MCMI, MBHI, MAPI)* (pp. 263–268). Minneapolis: National Computer Systems.

Hamberger, L. K., & Hastings, J. E. (1986). Personality correlates of men who abuse their partners: A cross-validation study. *Journal of Family Violence, 1,* 323–341.

Helmes, E., & Barilko, O. (1988). Comparison of three multiscale inventories in identifying the presence of psychopathological symptoms. *Journal of Personality Assessment, 52,* 74–80.

Herron, L., Turner, J., & Weiner, P. (1986). A comparison of the Millon Clinical Multiaxial Inventory and the Minnesota Multiphasic Personality Inventory as predictors of successful treatment by lumbar laminectomy. *Clinical Orthopaedics and Related Research, 203,* 232–238.

Hess, A. K. (1985). Review of Millon Clinical Multiaxial Inventory. In J. Mitchell Jr. (Ed.), *Ninth mental measurements yearbook, Vol. 1* (pp. 984–986). Lincoln: University of Nebraska Press.

Holliman, N. B., & Guthrie, P. C. (1989). A comparison of the Millon Clinical Multiaxial Inventory and the California Psychological Inventory in assessment of a nonclinical population. *Journal of Clinical Psychology, 45,* 373–382.

Hyer, L. (1987). "Personologic Primacy" of later-life Patients. In C. Green (Ed.), *Conference on the Millon Inventories (MCMI, MBHI, MAPI)* (pp. 13–19). Minneapolis: National Computer Systems.

Hyer, L., & Boudewyns, P. (1985). The 8–2 MCMI personality profile among Vietnam veterans with PTSD. PTSD *Newsletter, 4,* 2.

Hyer, L., Carson, M., Nixon, D., Tamkin, A., & Saucer, R. T. (1987). Depression among alcoholics. *The International Journal of the Addictions, 22,* 1235–1241.

Hyer, L., & Harrison, W. R. (1986). Later life personality model: Diagnosis and treatment. *Clinical Gerontologist, 5,* 399–416.

Hyer, L., Harrison, W. R., & Jacobsen, R. H. (1987). Later-life depression: Influences of irrational thinking and cognitive impairment. *Journal of Rational-Emotive Therapy, 5,* 43–48.

Hyer, L., O'Leary, W. C., Elkins, R., & Arena, J. (1985). PTSD: Additional criteria for evaluation. *VA Practitioner, 2,* 67–75.

Hyer, L., Woods, M. G., Boudewyns, P. A., Bruno, R., & O'Leary, W. C. (1988). Concurrent validation of the Millon Clinical Multiaxial Inventory among Vietnam veterans with Post-traumatic Stress Disorder. *Psychological Reports, 63,* 271–278.

Jaffe, L. T., & Archer, R. P. (1987). The prediction of drug use among college students from MMPI, MCMI and Sensation Seeking Scales. *Journal of Personality Assessment, 51,* 243–253.

Jay, G. W., Grove, R. N., & Grove, K. S. (1987). Differentiation of chronic headache from nonheadache pain patients using the Millon Clinical Multiaxial Inventory (MCMI). *Headache, 27,* 124–129.

Joffe, R. T., & Regan, J. J. (1988). Personality and depression. *Journal of Psychiatric Research, 22,* 279–286.

Joffe, R. T., Swinson, R. P., & Regan, J. J. (1988). Personality features of obsessive-compulsive disorder. *American Journal of Psychiatry, 145,* 1127–1129.

Josiassen, R. C., Shagass, C., & Roemer, R. A. (1987). Somato-sensory evoked potential correlates of schizophrenic subtypes identified by the Millon Clinical Multiaxial Inventory. In C. Green (Ed.), *Conference on the Millon clinical inventories (MCMI, MBHI, MAPI)* (pp. 41–53). Minneapolis: National Computer Systems.

Korchin, S., & Schuldberg, D. (1981). The future of clinical assessment. *American Psychologist, 36,* 1147–1158.

Langevein, R., Lang, R., Reynolds, R., Wright, P., Garrels, D., Marchese, V., Handy, L., Pugh, G., & Frenzel, R. (1988). Personality and sexual anomalies: An examination of the Millon Clinical Multiaxial Inventory. *Annals of Sex Research, 1,* 13–32.

Langevein, R., Paitich, D., Freeman, R., Mann, K., & Handy, L. (1979). Personality characteristics and sexual anomalies in males. *Canadian Journal of Behavioral Science, 10,* 222–238.

Lanyon, R. (1984). Personality assessment. *Annual Review of Psychology, 35,* 667–701.

Leaf, R., DiGuiseppe, R., Ellis, A., Wolfe, J., Yeager, R., & Alington, D. (1987). Treatment intake status and the MCMI's "Axis II" scale scores. In C. Green (Ed.), *Conference on the Millon clinical inventories (MCMI, MBHI, MAPI)* (pp. 21–29). Minneapolis: National Computer Systems.

Lemkau, J. P., Purdy, R. R., Rafferty, J. P., & Rudisill, J. R. (1988). Correlates of burnout among family practice residents. *Journal of Medical Education, 63,* 682–691.

Lepkowsky, C. M. (1987). Personality pathology in eating disorders. In C. Green (Ed.), *Conference on the Millon clinical inventories (MCMI, MBHI, MAPI)* (pp. 215–220). Minneapolis: National Computer Systems.

Levine, J., Tischer, P., Antoni, M., Green, C., & Millon, T. (1985). Refining personality assessments by combining MCMI high point profiles and MMPI codes. Part II. MMPI code 27/72. *Journal of Personality Assessment, 63,* 501–507.

Libb, J. W., Stankovic, S., Sokol, R., Freeman, A., Houck, C., & Switzer, P. (1990). Stability of the MCMI among depressed psychiatric outpatients. *Journal of Personality Assessment, 63,* 209–218.

Lohr, J. M., Hamberger, L. K., & Bonge, D. (1988). The nature of irrational beliefs in different personality clusters of spouse abusers. *Journal of Rational-Emotive and Cognitive-Behavior Therapy, 6,* 273–285.

Lorr, M., Retzlaff, P. D., & Tarr, H. C. (1989). An analysis of the MCMI-I at the item level. *Journal of Clinical Psychology, 45,* 884–890.

Lumsden, E. A. (1987). The impact of shared items on the internal-structural validity of the MCMI. In C. Green (Ed.), *Conference on the Millon clinical inventories (MCMI, MBHI, MAPI)* (pp. 325–333). Minneapolis: National Computer Systems.

Lundholm, J. K. (1989). Alcohol use among university females: Relationship to eating disordered behavior. *Addictive Behaviors, 14,* 181–185.

Lundholm, J. K., Pellegreno, D. D., Wolins, L., & Graham, S. L. (1989). Predicting eating disorders in women: A preliminary measurement study. *Measurement and Evaluation in Counseling and Development, 22,* 23–30.

Malec, J. F., Romsaas, E., & Trump, D. (1985). Psychological and personality disturbance among patients with testicular cancer. *Journal of Psychosocial Oncology, 3,* 55–64.

Malec, J., Wolberg, W., Romsaas, E., Trump, D., & Tanner, M. (1988). Millon Clinical Multiaxial Inventory (MCMI) findings among breast clinic patients after initial evaluation and at 4- or 8-month follow-up. *Journal of Clinical Psychology, 44,* 175–180.

Marsh, D. T., Stile, S. A., Stoughton, N. L., & Trout-Landen, B. L. (1988). Psychopathology of opiate addiction: Comparative data from the MMPI and MCMI. *American Journal of Drug and Alcohol Abuse, 14,* 17–27.

McCabe, S. (1984). Millon Clinical Multiaxial Inventory. In D. Keyser & R. Sweetland (Eds.), *Test critiques (Vol. 1*, pp. 455–465. Kansas City: Westport.

McCann, J. T. (1989). MMPI personality disorder scales and the MCMI: Concurrent validity. *Journal of Clinical Psychology, 45*, 365–369.

McCann, J. T., & Suess, J. F. (1988). Clinical applications of the MCMI: The 1-2-3-8 codetype. *Journal of Clinical Psychology, 44*, 181–186.

McCormack, J. K., Barnett, R. W., & Wallbrown, F. H. (1989). Factor structure of the Millon Clinical Multiaxial Inventory (MCMI) with an offender sample. *Journal of Personality Assessment, 53*, 442–448.

McDermott, W. F. (1987). The diagnosis of Posttraumatic Stress Disorder using the Millon Clinical Multiaxial Inventory. In C. Green (Ed.), *Conference on the Millon clinical inventories (MCMI, MBHI, MAPI)* (pp. 257–262). Minneapolis: National Computer Systems.

McMahon, R. C., & Davidson, R. S. (1985a). An examination of the relationship between personality patterns and symptom/mood patterns. *Journal of Personality Assessment, 49*, 552–556.

McMahon, R. C., & Davidson, R. S. (1985b). Transient versus enduring depression among alcoholics in inpatient treatment. *Journal of Psychopathology and Behavioral Assessment, 7*, 317–328.

McMahon, R. C., & Davidson, R. S. (1986a). An examination of depressed vs. nondepressed alcoholics in inpatient treatment. *Journal of Clinical Psychology, 42*, 177–184.

McMahon, R., & Davidson, R. S. (1986b). Concurrent validity of the clinical symptom syndrome scales of the Millon Clinical Multiaxial Inventory. *Journal of Clinical Psychology, 42*, 908–912.

McMahon, R. C., Davidson, R. S., & Flynn, P. M. (1986). Psychological correlates and treatment outcomes for high and low social functioning alcoholics. *The International Journal of the Addictions, 21*, 819–835.

McMahon, R. C., Flynn, P. M., & Davidson, R. S. (1985a). The personality and symptom scales of the Millon Clinical Multiaxial Inventory: Sensitivity to posttreatment outcomes. *Journal of Clinical Psychology, 41*, 862–866.

McMahon, R., Flynn, P., & Davidson, R. (1985b). Stability of the personality and symptom scales of the Millon Clinical Multiaxial Inventory. *Journal of Personality Assessment, 49*, 231–234.

McMahon, R. C., Gersh, D., & Davidson, R. S. (1989). Personality and symptom characteristics of continuous vs. episodic drinkers. *Journal of Clinical Psychology, 45*, 161–168.

Medalia, A., Merriam, A., & Sandberg, M. (1989). Neuropsychological deficits in choreoacanthocytosis. *Archives of Neurology, 46*, 573–575.

Miller, H. R., & Streiner, D. L. (1990). Using the Millon Clinical Multiaxial Inventory's Scale B and the MacAndrew Alcoholism Scale to Identify Alcoholics with Concurrent psychiatric diagnoses. *Journal of Personality Assessment, 54*, 736–746.

Millon, T. (1981). *Disorders of personality. DSM-III: Axis II*. New York: Wiley.

Millon, T. (1983). *Millon Clinical Multiaxial Inventory Manual (3rd Ed)*. New York: Holt, Rinehart & Winston.

Millon, T. (1984a). On the renaissance of personality assessment and personality theory. *Journal of Personality Assessment, 48*, 450–466.

Millon, T. (1984b). Interpretive guide to the Millon Clinical Multiaxial Inventory. In P. McReynolds & G. J. Chelune (Eds.), *Advances in personality assessment: Vol. 6* (pp. 1–41). San Francisco: Jossey-Bass.

Millon, T. (1985a). The MCMI provides a good assessment of DSM-III disorders: The MCMI-II will prove even better. *Journal of Personality Assessment, 49*, 379–391.

Millon, T. (1985b). Response to Greer's review of the MCMI. *Journal of Counseling and Development, 63*, 631–632.

Millon, T. (1986a). Personality prototypes and their diagnostic criteria. In T. Millon & G. Klerman (Eds.), *Contemporary directions in psychopathology: Toward the DSM-IV* (pp. 639–669). New York: Guilford Press.

Millon, T. (1986b). A theoretical derivation of pathological personalities. In T. Millon & G. Klerman (Eds.), *Contemporary directions in psychopathology: Toward the DSM-IV* (pp. 671–712). New York: Guilford Press.

Millon, T. (1986). The MCMI and DSM-III: Further commentaries. *Journal of Personality Assessment, 50,* 205–207.

Millon, T. (1987). *Millon Clinical Multiaxial Inventory-II:* Manual for the MCMI-II. Minneapolis: National Computer Systems.

Millon, C., Salvato, F., Blaney, N., Morgan, R., Mantero-Atienza, E., Klimas, N., & Fletcher, M. A. (1989). A psychological assessment of chronic fatigue syndrome/chronic Epstein-Barr virus patients. *Psychology and Health, 3,* 131–141.

Montag, I., & Comrey, A. L. (1987). Millon MCMI scales factor analyzed and correlated with MMPI and CPS scales. *Multivariate Behavioral Research, 22,* 401–413.

Moreland, K. L., & Godfrey, J. O. (1989). Yes, our study could have been better: Reply to Cash, Mikulka, and Brown. *Journal of Consulting and Clinical Psychology, 57,* 313–314.

Moreland, K. L., & Onstead, J. A. (1987). Validity of Millon's computerized interpretation system for the MCMI: A controlled study. *Journal of Consulting and Clinical Psychology, 55,* 113–114.

Morey, L. C. (1985). An empirical comparison of interpersonal and DSM-III approaches to classification of personality disorders. *Psychiatry, 48,* 358–364.

Morey, L. C. (1986). A comparison of three personality disorder assessment approaches. *Journal of Psychopathology and Behavioral Assessment, 8,* 25–30.

Morey, L. C., & LeVine, D. J. (1988). A multitrait-multimethod examination of Minnesota Multiphasic Personality Inventory (MMPI) and Millon Clinical Multiaxial Inventory (MCMI). *Journal of Psychopathology and Behavioral Assessment, 10,* 333–344.

Myer, M. H. (1984–85). A new look at mothers of incest victims. *Journal of Social Work and Human Sexuality, 4,* 47–58.

Overholser, J. C. (1990). Retest reliability of the Millon Clinical Multiaxial Inventory. *Journal of Personality Assessment, 55,* 202–208.

Overholser, J. C., Kabakoff, R., & Norman, W. H. (1989). The assessment of personality characteristics in depressed and dependent psychiatric inpatients. *Journal of Personality Assessment, 53,* 40–50.

Ownby, R. L., Wallbrown, F. H., Carmin, C. N., & Barnett, R. W. (1990). A combined factor analysis of the Millon Clinical Multiaxial Inventory and the MMPI in an offender population. *Journal of Clinical Psychology, 46,* 89–96.

Patrick, J. (1988). Concordance of the MCMI and the MMPI in the diagnosis of three DSM-III Axis I disorders. *Journal of Clinical Psychology, 44,* 186–190.

Piersma, H. L. (1986a). The Millon Clinical Multiaxial Inventory (MCMI) as a treatment outcome measure for psychiatric inpatients. *Journal of Clinical Psychology, 42,* 493–499.

Piersma, H. L. (1986b). The stability of the Millon Clinical Multiaxial Inventory for psychiatric inpatients. *Journal of Personality Assessment, 50,* 193–197.

Piersma, H. L. (1986c). The factor structure of the Millon Clinical Multiaxial Inventory for psychiatric inpatients. *Journal of Personality Assessment, 50,* 578–584.

Piersma, H. L. (1987a). The MCMI as a measure of DSM-III Axis II diagnosis: An empirical comparison. *Journal of Clinical Psychology, 43,* 478–483.

Piersma, H. L. (1987b). Millon Clinical Multiaxial Inventory (MCMI) computer-generated diagnoses: How do they compare to clinical judgment? *Journal of Psychopathology and Behavioral Assessment, 9,* 305–312.

Piersma, H. L. (1987c). The use of the Millon Clinical Multiaxial Inventory in the evaluation of seminary students. *Journal of Psychology and Theology, 15,* 227–233.

Piersma, H. L. (1989a). The MCMI-II as a treatment outcome measure for psychiatric inpatients. *Journal of Clinical Psychology, 45,* 87–93.

Piersma, H. L. (1989b). The stability of the MCMI-II for psychiatric inpatients. *Journal of Clinical Psychology, 45,* 781–785.

Prifitera, A., & Ryan, J. J. (1984). Validity of the Narcissistic Personality Inventory (NPI) in a psychiatric sample. *Journal of Clinical Psychology, 40,* 140–142.

Rebillot, J. (1985). Scoring of the MCMI: Effects on utility. *Journal of Counseling and Development, 63,* 631.

Reich, J. H. (1985). Measurement of DSM-III, Axis II. *Comprehensive Psychiatry, 26,* 352–363.

Reich, J. H., & Noyes, R. (1987). A comparison of DSM-III personality disorders in acutely ill panic and depressed patients. *Journal of Anxiety Disorders, 1,* 123–131.

Reich, J., Noyes, R., & Troughton, E. (1987a). Lack of agreement between instruments assessing DSM III personality disorders In C. Green (Ed.), *Conference on the Millon clinical inventories (MCMI, MBHI, MAPI)* (pp. 223–234). Minneapolis: National Computer Systems.

Reich, J., Noyes, R., & Troughton, E. (1987b). Dependent personality disorder associated with phobic avoidance in patients with panic disorder. *American Journal of Psychiatry, 144,* 323–326.

Reich, J., & Troughton, E. (1988). Frequency of DSM-III personality disorders in patients with panic disorder: Comparison with psychiatric and normal control subjects. *Psychiatry Research, 26,* 89–100.

Repko, G. R., & Cooper, R. (1985). The diagnosis of personality disorder: A comparison of MMPI profile, Millon inventory, and clinical judgment in a Workers' Compensation population. *Journal of Clinical Psychology, 41,* 867–881.

Retzlaff, P. D., & Gibertini, M. (1987a). Factor structure of the MCMI basic personality scales and common-item artifact. *Journal of Personality Assessment, 51,* 588–594.

Retzlaff, P. D., & Gibertini, M. (1987b). Air Force pilot personality: Hard data on "The Right Stuff". *Multivariate Behavioral Research, 22,* 383–399.

Retzlaff, P. D., & Gibertini, M. (1988). Objective psychological testing of U.S. Air Force officers in pilot training. *Aviation, Space, and Environmental Medicine,* July, 661–663.

Retzlaff, P. D., & Gibertini, M. (1990). Factor-based special scales for the MCMI. *Journal of Clinical Psychology, 46,* 47–52.

Retzlaff, P. D., Sheehan, E. P., & Lorr, M. (1990). MCMI-II Scoring: Weighted and unweighted algorithms. *Journal of Personality Assessment, 55,* 219–223.

Robbins, S. B. (1989). Validity of the Superiority and Goal Instability scales as measures of defects in the self. *Journal of Personality Assessment, 53,* 122–132.

Robbins, S. B., & Patton, M. J. (1986). Procedures for construction of scales for rating counselor outcomes. *Measurement and Evaluation in Counseling and Development, 19,* 131–140.

Robert, J. A., Ryan, J. J., McEntyre, W. L., McFarland, R. S., Lips, O. J., & Rosenberg, S. J. (1985). MCMI characteristics of DSM-III Posttraumatic Stress Disorder in Vietnam veterans. *Journal of Personality Assessment, 49,* 226–230.

Sandberg, M. L. (1987). Is the ostensive accuracy of computer interpretive reports a result of the Barnum Effect? A study of the MCMI. In C. Green (Ed.), *Conference on the Millon clinical inventories (MCMI, MBHI, MAPI)* (pp. 155–164). Minneapolis: National Computer Systems.

Sexton, D. L., McIlwraith, R., Barnes, G., & Dunn, R. (1987). Comparison of the MCMI and MMPI–168 as psychiatric inpatient screening inventories. *Journal of Personality Assessment, 51,* 388–398.

Siddall, J. W. (1986). Use of the MCMI with substance abusers. *Noteworthy Responses, 2,* 1–3.

Silverstein, M. L., & McDonald, C. (1988). Personality trait characteristics in relation to neuropsychological dysfunction in schizophrenia and depression. *Journal of Personality Assessment, 52,* 288–296.

Smith, D., Carroll, J. L., & Fuller, G. (1988). The relationship between the Millon Clinical Multiaxial Inventory and the MMPI in a private outpatient mental health clinic population. *Journal of Clinical Psychology, 44,* 165–174.

Snibbe, J. R., Peterson, P. J., & Sosner, B. (1980). Study of psychological characteristics of a Workers' Compensation sample using the MMPI and the Millon Clinical Multiaxial Inventory. *Psychological Reports, 47,* 959–966.

Stark, M. J., & Campbell, B. K. (1988). Personality, drug use, and early attrition from substance abuse treatment. *American Journal of Drug and Alcohol Abuse, 14,* 475–485.

Strack, S. (1987). Development and validation of an adjective check list to assess the Millon personality types in a normal population. *Journal of Personality Assessment, 51,* 572–587.

Streiner, D. L., & Miller, H. R. (1989). The MCMI-II: How much better than the MCMI? *Journal of Personality Assessment, 55,* 81–84.

Sugrue, D. P. (1987). Applications of the MCMI in the evaluation of sexual dysfunctions. In C. Green (Ed.), *Conference on the Millon clinical inventories (MCMI, MBHI, MAPI)* (pp. 287–292). Minneapolis: National Computer Systems.

Tamkin, A. S., Carson, M. F., Nixon, D. H., & Hyer, L. A. (1987). A comparison among some measures of depression in male alcoholics. *Journal of Studies on Alcohol, 48,* 176–178.

Tango, R. A., & Dziuban, C. D. (1984). The use of personality components in the interpretation of career indecision. *Journal of College Student Personnel, 25,* 509–512.

Tisdale, M. J., Pendleton, L., & Marler, M. (1990). MCMI characteristics of DSM-III-R Bulimics. *Journal of Personality Assessment, 55,* 477–483.

Tracy, H. M., Norman, D. K., & Weisberg, L. J. (1987). Anorexia and bulimia: A comparison of MCMI results. In C. Green (Ed.), *Conference on the Millon clinical inventories (MCMI, MBHI, MAPI)* (pp. 195–197). Minneapolis: National Computer Systems.

Uomoto, J. M., Turner, J. A., & Herron, L. D. (1988). Use of the MMPI and MCMI in predicting outcome of lumbar laminectomy. *Journal of Clinical Psychology, 44,* 191–197.

Van Gorp, W. G., & Meyer, R. G. (1986). The detection of faking on the Millon Clinical Multiaxial Inventory (MCMI) *Journal of Clinical Psychology, 42,* 742–747.

Walton, H. J. (1986). The relationship between personality disorder and psychiatric illness. In T. Millon & G. Klerman (Eds.), *Contemporary directions in psychopathology toward DSM-IV.* New York: Guilford Press.

Warner, J. S. (1987). Use of the Millon Clinical Multiaxial Inventory (MCMI) in an alcoholism halfway house program. In C. Green (Ed.), *Conference on the Millon clinical inventories (MCMI, MBHI, MAPI)* (pp. 269–272). Minneapolis: National Computer Systems.

Wetzler, S. (1990). The Millon Clinical Multiaxial Inventory (MCMI): A Review. *Journal of Personality Assessment, 55,* 445–464.

Wetzler, S., & Dubro, A. (1990). Diagnosis of personality disorders by the Millon Clinical Multiaxial Inventory. *Journal of Nervous and Mental Disease, 178,* 261–263.

Wetzler, S., Kahn, R., Strauman, T. J., & Dubro, A. (1989). Diagnosis of major depression by self-report. *Journal of Personality Assessment, 53,* 22–30.

Widiger, T. (1985). Review of Millon Clinical Multiaxial Inventory. In J. Mitchell Jr. (Ed.), *Ninth mental measurements yearbook. Vol. I* (pp. 986–988). Lincoln: University of Nebraska Press.

Widiger, T. A., & Frances, A. (1987). Interviews and inventories for the measurement of personality disorders. *Clinical Psychology Review, 7,* 49–75.

Widiger, T. A., & Sanderson, C. (1987). The convergent and discriminant validity of the MCMI as a measure of the DSM III personality disorders. *Journal of Personality Assessment, 51,* 228–242.

Widiger, T. A., Williams, J. B., Spitzer, R. L., & Frances, A. (1985). The MCMI as a measure of DSM-III. *Journal of Personality Assessment, 49,* 366–380.

Widiger, T. A., Williams, J. B., Spitzer, R. L., & Frances, A. (1986). The MCMI and DSM-III: A brief rejoinder to Millon (1985). *Journal of Personality Assessment, 50,* 198–204.

Zarella, K. L., Schuerger, J. M., & Ritz, G. H. (1990). Estimation of MCMI DSM-III Axis II constructs from MMPI scales and subscales. *Journal of Personality Assessment, 55,* 195–201.

Suggested Reading

American Psychological Association. (1985). *Guidelines for computer-based tests and interpretations.* Washington, D.C.: Author.

American Psychiatric Association. (1987). *Diagnostic and statistical manual of mental disorders (3rd ed.–revised).* Washington, D.C.: Author.

Butcher, J. N., & Owen, P. (1978). Objective personality inventories: Recent research and some contemporary issues. In B. Wolman (Ed.), *Clinical diagnosis of mental disorders* (pp. 475–545). New York: Plenum Press.

Craig, R. J., & Horowitz, M. (1990). Current utilization of psychological tests at diagnostic practicum sites. *The Clinical Psychologist, 43,* 29–36.

Matarazzo, J. D. (1986). Computerized clinical psychological test interpretations: Unvalidated plus all mean and no sigma. *American Psychologist, 41,* 14–24.

3 Factors Affecting the Operating Characteristics of the MCMI-II

Michael Gibertini, Ph.D.

One can place a thermometer into a beaker of water, withdraw it, read the temperature and then place the thermometer into another beaker. Two temperatures can be compared and we know if beaker A is warmer or cooler than beaker B. If we are told that beaker A has a temperature below zero degree centigrade, then we may be relatively certain that the water was in its solid phase (ice) at the time of measurement. Assuming, that is, that the water was relatively pure, that it was at sea level, and that the thermometer was reliable and valid. A test can be used to compare entities on amounts of some attribute, to assign a value to the amount of the attribute the entity displays that has meaning in some reference system, and to make probability statements that the entity is in some category that has distinct properties and behavior. The example of the temperature of water is useful to remind psychologists that these three uses of measurement are general uses and not limited to the interpretation of scores on psychological tests. In the water example, the prediction that the water was in solid phase depends on two conditions. First, the person making the prediction must have a number of facts in hand that are all relevant to a veridical theory of the phases of water. And second, he must have a measuring instrument that is both reliable and valid for the purpose of measuring water temperature. In this trivial example of predicting whether water is solid or liquid from its temperature and pressure and purity, the observer can predict the state of the water with a high degree of confidence because he has a strong theory of the phases of water and a powerful measuring device in the thermometer. Neither the theory nor the instrumentation suffers from large imprecisions.

Applied scientists in the fields of biology and psychology must be especially concerned with the third use of measurement cited before. Assigning people to

categories of disease or behavioral disorder is a task of such great human consequence that imprecision anywhere in the process is difficult to tolerate. Intolerance has driven us to reduce this imprecision through improvements in theory
and measurement devices. Also, this intolerance has caused investigators in the
life sciences to be very concerned that the logic of test use remains defensible and
has spawned the creation of measurement theories and technologies for assessing
the operating characteristics of tests.

In the field of clinical assessment in psychology, imprecisions are the rule in
both the theories underlying the nosological categories and in the instrumentation
designed to measure them. Recognition of this fact has caused leading researchers in psychometrics to insist that the instrumentation be tied to theory
from its inception and that instrument partake in theory refinement (Jackson,
1970; Loevinger, 1957). The MMPI is the most important example of a test that
explicitly ignored the theories underlying the categories it measured. The MCMI-
I and MCMI-II are the two most recent and important inventories where theory is
so integrated with the instrument that obvious and fruitful cross-fertilization is
occuring rapidly. Because of the theory- and empirically-driven construction
procedures of the MCMIs, we are finally in a position to seriously examine the
operating characteristics of a major psychodiagnostic inventory in clinical psychology.

THE MCMIs AND THE DSMs

The MCMI has grown up with the Diagnostic and Statistical Manuals of Mental
Disorders (DSM). Examining the operating characteristics of the MCMI is therefore both necessary and difficult. It is necessary because the DSM nomenclature
is becoming "official" in more circles than just our own. Courts, nonpsychiatric
physicians, third-party payers, and even the media make references to the document and to the categories within it. Psychologists will be called upon with
greater urgency to speak, and ultimately think and see, in terms of the DSM
categories. With long practice, clinicians may begin to forget that the categories
of the DSM are approximations of constructed prototypes and that despite our
use of taxonomic methods to refine our categories, personality disorders will
never have the same ontological status as the flora and fauna of the natural world.
Clinicians forced to find diagnoses and to defend their choices may forget that
the DSM is a political document with constructions that fit individuals only
approximately. They may forget, that is, unless they incorporate the logic underlying the operating characteristics of tests in their interpretations every time they
look at a test score.

Both the MCMI and the DSM are based on rapidly evolving and only partially
overlapping systems. At least two strong forces act on the MCMI/DSM concordance to cloud the normally straightforward calculation and interpretation of the

MCMI operating characteristics. First, experience shapes perception no less for clinicians as anyone else. As clinicians begin to accept the official nomenclature they begin to see the categories in their patients. When categories are shaped by politics, then secular trends in political thinking must alter the empirically derived base rates. And nothing makes operating characteristics more difficult to use than shifting base rates.

A second force that complicates the MCMI/DSM concordance and the use of MCMI operating characteristics is that the MCMI must remain an evolving instrument. Millon himself is both a forceful participant in and an astute observer of the political trends in the DSM nomenclature. His commitment to a comprehensive theory of personality disorders that can shape future DSMs has created great pressure to keep the MCMI current. Several exigencies within the changing nomenclature are apparent. Among these are the need to revise the MCMI to accommodate the inclusion of sadism and masochism into DSM-IV. Another is the need to change items, scales, and response bias correction factors. The new MCMI-II is a very different instrument from its predecessor that includes another two categories of basic personality structure (active and passive discordant types) to account for the new thinking on aggressive (sadistic) and self-defeating (masochistic) personalities. These additions change the meaning of the antisocial, passive-aggressive, dependent, and histrionic scales and thereby cause the clinician to consider substantive as well statistical changes when interpreting the new instrument.

THE OPERATING CHARACTERISTICS OF TESTS

The foregoing discussion should make clear that the ability of the MCMI-II to identify the prototypes that so much work has gone into defining over the last several years is of concern to anyone who attempts to interpret the test, whether configurally or with single scales. It should also be clear that the task is complicated. To assist in the assimilation of these concepts into the working vocabulary of MCMI researchers and clinicians using the test, a recapitulation of our earlier exposition of operating characteristics of tests (Gibertini, Brandenburg, & Retzlaff, 1986) is offered.

Actuarial prediction and decision theory have a long history within psychology (Cronbach & Gleser, 1965; Edwards, Lindman, & Savage, 1968; Meehl & Rosen, 1955; Widiger, Hurt, Frances, Clarkin, & Gilmore, 1984). However, only recently have the classic arguments of Meehl and Rosen (1955) been applied to the problem of deciding for the individual diagnostic case whether test results are truly indicative of the presence of a disorder (e.g., Baldessarini, Finklestein, & Arana, 1983). In part, the reason this type of analysis has not been carried out in the past has been that the mapping of tests to diagnoses could not be reliable until the diagnostic nomenclature itself became less vague. To put it in

TABLE 3.1
Definitions and Formulas for Operating Characteristics of Tests

	Disorder		
Test Result	Present	Absent	
Positive	a	b	a + b
Negative	c	d	c + d
	a + c	b + d	

Index	Definition[a]	Formula
Sensitivity	Pr(Test + | Disorder +)	a/(a + c)
Specificity	Pr(Test - | Disorder -)	d/(b + d)
Positive Predictive Power (PPP)	Pr(Disorder + | Test +)	a/(a + b)
Negative Predictive Power (NPP)	Pr(Disorder - | Test -)	d/(c + d)
Overall Diagnostic Power (DP)	Proportion Correctly Classified	(a + d)/N
Prevalence	Proportion of Patients with Disorder	(a + c)/N

Note. Call values in the 2 X 2 table are number of cases.
[a]Definitions are expressed in terms of conditional probabilities. The definition for sensitivity would read:
"the probability that the test is positive given the disorder is present." Adapted from Gibertini,
Brandenburg, and Retzlaff (1986). Reproduced by permission of Lawrence Erlbaum Associates.

epidemiologic terms, the operating characteristics of psychometric tests could not be known before an explicit diagnostic standard was established. The DSM-II, with its explicit and fixed decision rules, provided a basis for such a standard.

The operating characteristics of a test are probability statements unique to a test and a population. Four measures describe the operation of the test in a population. These indices are usually labeled sensitivity, specificity, positive predictive power (PPP), and negative predictive power (NPP) (Baldessarini, et al., 1983; Griner, Mayewski, Mushlin, & Greenland, 1981; Mausner & Bahn, 1974). These terms are defined in Table 3.1.

Sensitivity and specificity are also known as the proportion of true positives and true negatives. The two predictive power indices are almost never used in clinical test construction despite early suggestions that these indices are more useful to the practitioner making decisions about individual patients than are the sensitivity and specificity of the test (e.g., Dawes, 1962; Meehl & Rosen, 1955). Two other indices are overall diagnostic power (DP) and prevalence. DP is a global index of overall classification accuracy. Prevalence is strictly defined as the number of people with the disorder divided by the number of people at risk for the disorder within a specific time period. For the clinician involved in diagnostic decision-making, prevalence is understood to be the prior probability that a patient has the disorder. Prevalence for the clinician is the "walk-in" probability that a patient has some disorder of interest. We use it interchangeably with the term "base rate."

Operating characteristics of a test are conditional probabilities. Sensitivity is defined as the probability that the test is positive given the disorder is present, whereas specificity is defined as the probability that the test is negative given the disorder is absent. Sensitivity and specificity are usually thought of as characteristics of the test that are independent of the prevalence characteristics of the population. The test should identify the same proportion of disordered cases across populations irrespective of the number of actual disordered cases in each of the populations.

Positive predictive power is defined as the probability that the disorder is present given the test is positive and is calculated as the proportion of test-positive cases with the disorder across all test-positive cases. Clinicians will recognize this index as providing the answer to the question they ask while interpreting a clinically significant test score, namely: What is the likelihood that this patient has the disorder now that I know that the test was positive? Negative predictive power is defined as the probability that the disorder is absent given the test is negative. It is the proportion of test-negative cases without the disorder across all test-negative cases.

The predictive power indices are influenced by both the prevalence of the disorder in the population and the magnitude of the sensitivity and the specificity of the test. In general, the predictive power indices are optimal when the sensitivity and specificity are very high (above 90%). Positive predictive power

TABLE 3.2
Positive Predictive Power at Low Prevalence

Prevalence	PPP
10	68
9	65
8	62
7	59
6	55
5	50
4	44
3	37
2	28
1	16
.5	9
.1	2

Note. Figures are percentages. Sensitivity and specificity are set at 95%. NPP remains at 99%, and DP remains at 95% through all levels of prevalence. Adapted from Gibertini, Brandenburg, and Retzlaff (1986). Reproduced by permission of Lawrence Erlbaum Associates.

decreases as prevalence decreases so that even highly sensitive and specific tests have low positive predictive power when used in populations that have very few disordered patients. This is the inevitable dilemma facing the clinician who attempts to identify rare disorders with fallible indicators. Table 3.2 illustrates this phenomenon. Even a very good test (sensitivity and specificity at 95%) loses substantial positive predictive power when prevalence falls below 10%.

Because they are framed as conditional probability statements about test scores, the predictive power indices are extremely valuable to practitioners who want to know the meaning of a test score for an individual patient. Unfortunately, these indices are not generally presented in test manuals because the data necessary to determine them are rarely collected.

THE OPERATING CHARACTERISTICS OF THE MCMI-II

The operating characteristics of the MCMI-I were calculated directly from prevalence data reported in the manual (Millon, 1983). The operating characteristics for the MCMI-II are included in the MCMI-II manual and, paralleling the enlivened complexity of the new test itself, are replete with subtleties that are sure to discourage all but the most intrepid investigator. In considering the operating characteristics of the MCMI-II, Millon has made full use of a fundamental truth about base rates: They are only as stable as the community's agreement on a diagnostic gold standard. In our MCMI-I paper, (Gibertini et al., 1986) we took as a reason for even considering an analysis of operating characteristics the growing consensus of opinion on personality disorders and the fixed decision rules of DSM-III. A lot has changed since DSM-III. The new DSM-III-R and the DSM-IV contain changes in the number and types of personality disorders as well as the decision rules for diagnosis. Likewise, Millon's theory and the scales of the MCMI have expanded. In the new instrument, for example, there are now three types of aggression to be distinguished: passive (passive-aggressive), active (antisocial), and coercive (aggressive-sadistic). Dependency has a similar configuration: passive (dependent), active (histrionic), and collapsed (self-defeating). The point to note is that once the decision was taken to include the two new extensions (sadistic and self-defeating) to the old MCMI dimensions, clinicians faced six new categories; two new ones and conceptual revisions on four old ones. When theoretical and political thinking gallops ahead of front line clinicians this rapidly, interrater reliability must suffer. Also, the MCMI-II judges had 13 categories to choose from (as opposed to the MCMI-I judges who had only 8) and at least half of these were conceptually new to them. In short, the "improvements" on the DSM and the MCMI have caused a temporary, it is hoped, decrease in our confidence in the reliability of the available gold standard for the MCMI-II.

In the manual to the MCMI-II, Millon has attempted to cope with this new

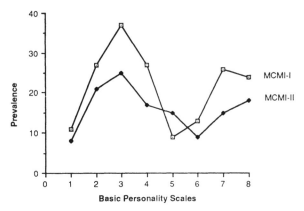

FIG. 3.1. Prevalences of the presence of the eight basic personality disorders for the MCMI-I versus MCMI-II construction samples.

vagueness by using two different definitional schemas for determining whether a particular patient actually had the disorder measured by the MCMI-II scale of interest. In the first table of operating characteristics (Millon, 1987: Table 3-14, p. 173), prevalence is defined as the percentage of cases where the disorder in question was identified by the clinician as either the primary or secondary personality disorder manifested by the patient. In the second table of operating characteristics (Table 3-15, p. 174), prevalence is defined as the percentage of cases where the disorder in question was identified by the clinician as the most prominent personality disorder manifested by the patient. In both cases the criterion was the DSM-III (or DSM-III-R) rather than the scale definitions used on the MCMI-I. The first definition is analogous (but more restrictive) to the MCMI-I definition of the "presence" of the disorder while the second is conceptually identical to the MCMI-I definition of the most prominent disorder.

Figure 3.1 presents the clinician-judged prevalences for the eight basic personality scales that are comparable across the two MCMIs. The effect of having more categories to choose from is apparent in this figure: The prevalences for all the disorders save narcissistic are lower now. Millon has noted a secular trend in his data such that both narcissistic and borderline disorders grew more prevalent between the construction of the MCMI-I and the MCMI-II. Figure 3.2 presents the prevalences for the clinicians' opinions of the most prominent disorder manifested by the patient. Note the MCMI-I and the MCMI-II are much more similar under these more stringent constraints. Base rates, it is apparent, are a final summary statistic reflecting the state of the world (the phenomenon to be observed), the construction of the world (our theories of pathology) and the adequacy of our measuring devices. When all three of these facets are changing, as in the field of psychopathology, then base rates become quite fluid.

Base rates may be genuinely unstable because of unreliability in measures or

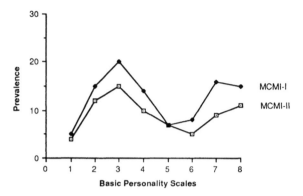

FIG. 3.2. Prevalences of the most prominent of the eight basic personality disorders for the MCMI-I versus MCMI-II construction samples.

changes in theory. Or, they may shift in a more stable manner because of disorder-relevant characteristics of a population. Therefore, the fluidity of base rates is not necessarily a major problem. All prevalence figures are dependent on some aspects of populations. The presence of sickle cell anemia is very low in the United States as whole, it is much higher in the population of African-Americans, and it is extremely high in the population of first degree relatives of people with sickle cell trait (one allele). The problem in these cases is not the fluidity of base rates but the ability of the clinician to identify the relevant population parameters that are associated with large shifts in base rates and then to arrive at a reasonable estimate of the individual's prior probability (i.e., before diagnostic testing) of pathology. Millon has done a great service for clinicians working in mental health clinics, hospitals, and private practice settings by conducting the painstaking research necessary to arrive at the needed "reasonable estimates" of base rates.

As Tables 3.1 and 3.2 above clearly show, consideration of the positive or negative predictive power of the MCMI-II scales can never ignore the prevalence of the disorder under scrutiny. The following formulas make this point forcefully and further articulate that the ability of a test to tell us the truth about the existence of a pathological state in a particular individual at a particular time is always dependent on aspects of the test (sensitivity and specificity) and aspects of the appropriate reference group (prevalence of the pathology in a population).

$$\text{PPP} = \frac{\text{Prev} \times \text{Sens}}{\text{Prev} \times \text{Sens} + (1 - \text{Prev})(1 - \text{Spec})}$$

$$\text{NPP} = \frac{\text{Spec} \times (1 - \text{Prev})}{\text{Spec} \times (1 - \text{Prev}) + \text{Prev} \times (1 - \text{Sens})}$$

When we analyzed the MCMI-I (Gibertini et al., 1986), we found that four (avoidant, dependent, histrionic, and passive-aggressive) of the eight basic personality scales met our criterion for a "good" test (arbitrarily set at PPP>70%). The data provided in the MCMI-II test manual (Millon, 1987; Table 3-14, p. 173) suggest that five (schizoid, avoidant, dependent, antisocial, and aggressive-sadistic) of the 10 MCMI-II basic personality scales meet this criterion. Also, it should be noted that none of the new basic personality scales falls below PPP = 50%. Because the MCMI-II construction procedures used at once a more stringent and a more externally valid "gold standard" (DSM-III criteria met for primary or secondary personality disorder) than did the MCMI-I (mere presence of a category fitting MCMI scale definitions), the prevalences are lower as illustrated in Fig. 3.1. But also true is that by raising the criteria for prevalence, both sensitivity and negative predictive power also decreased. This overall loss of power (lower sensitivity, PPP, and NPP) is a result of fewer cases being identified by the clinicians and some test-positive cases shifting from the true positive cell of Table 3.1 to the false positive cell. In other words, the MCMI-II is over-identifying more cases than was the MCMI-I in a context where a fewer number of true cases are available to be correctly classified.

A few scales on the MCMI-II appear to be much improved over their MCMI-I counterparts. Alcoholism has increased in sensitivity (87% vs. 74%) and PPP (92% vs. 63%) despite more stringent criteria on the gold standard. Major Depression is also greatly improved. These are two important clinical scales that were conspicuously weak on the MCMI-I. A few scales have apparently undergone some post-hoc "adjustments" to improve classification accuracy or to anticipate future trends in diagnostic habits of clinicians. Thus the prevalence figures associated with histrionic, narcissistic, and aggressive-sadistic are apparently less *pure* than those of other scales. Whether they are less accurate is an open question. Overall, however, the diagnostic efficiency of the MCMI-II is very good. The least efficient scale (dysthymia) provides a nearly two-fold increase in predictive power over prevalence alone while the most efficient scale (paranoid) provides a sixteen-fold increase in predictive power over prevalence.

At least two detailed examples (Gibertini et al., 1986; Millon, 1987) of how clinicians may use the definitions of Table 3.1 and the formulas above to aid in the interpretation of the MCMI scale scores exist and interested readers are referred to these sources. Millon (1987) also provides compelling arguments for accepting the prevalences he has arrived at as best estimates for the general case. The call for local base rates is recurrent in the literature since first made by Meehl and Rosen (1955). The logic behind insisting that clinicians make at least a passing effort at estimating base rates of important disorders in the populations they serve is, it should be clear, intimately tied to the problem of knowing the operating characteristics of the tests we use. More to the point, awareness of local base rates is equivalent, in many cases, to a firm knowledge of the risk factors for the disorders the clinician may need to treat. Gender is a risk factor for histrionic (the female to male ratio is on the order of 3:1), borderline, and antisocial personality disorders. Family history of mental illness is a risk factor for schizoid and schizotypal personality disorder. Eating disorders are risk factors for borderline personality disorder. The lists are easily compiled but what are the magnitudes of the risks? This is the question for local base rates. The ease with which we see our base rates shift around because of changes in the nomenclature should encourage us to find the relative risks of these factors so that our reasonable estimates can become precise when we need them.

The MCMI-I gave us the tools and the data we needed to vastly improve our ability to combine empirical actuaries with strong personality theory. The MCMI-II takes us even further. But even Millon's eloquent and sage configural interpretations of the MCMI-II scale scores are no substitute for intimate knowledge of the interconnections among the disorders likely to afflict the people walking into your office.

REFERENCES

American Psychiatric Association. (1980). *Diagnostic and statistical manual of mental disorders (3rd ed.)*. Washington, DC: Author.

Baldessarini, R. J., Finklestein, S., & Arana, G. W. (1983). The predictive power of diagnostic tests and the effect of prevalence of illness. *Archives of General Psychiatry, 40*, 569–573.

Cronbach, L., & Gleser, G. (1965). *Psychological tests and personnel decisions*. Urbana: University of Illinois Press.

Dawes, R. M. (1962). A note on base rates and psychometric efficiency. *Journal of Consulting Psychology, 26*, 422–424.

Edwards, W., Lindman, H., & Savage, L. (1963). Bayesian statistical inference for psychological research. *Psychological Review, 70*, 63–37.

Gibertini, M., Brandenburg, N. A., & Retzlaff, P. D. (1986). The operating characteristics of the Millon Clinical Multiaxial Inventory. *Journal of Personality Assessment, 50*(4), 554–567.

Griner, P. F., Mayewski, R. J., Mushlin, A. I., & Greenland, P. (1981). Selection and interpretation of diagnostic tests and procedures: Principles and applications. *Annals of Internal Medicine, 94*, 557–593.

Jackson, D. (1970). A sequential system for personality scale development. In C. D. Spielberger (Ed.), *Current topics in clinical and community psychology* (Vol. 2, pp. 61–92), New York: Academic Press.

Loevinger, J. (1957). Objective tests as instruments of psychological theory. *Psychological Reports, 3*, 635–694.

Mausner, J. S., & Bahn, A. K. (1974). *Epidemiology: An introductory text*. Philadelphia: Saunders.

Meehl, P. E., & Rosen, A. (1955). Antecedent probability and the efficiency of psychometric signs, patterns, or cutting scores. *Psychological Bulletin, 52*, 194–216.

Millon, T. (1983). *Millon Clinical Multiaxial Inventory*. Minneapolis, MN: Interpretive Scoring Systems.

Millon, T. (1987). *Manual for the MCMI-II, second edition*. Minneapolis, MN: National Computer Systems.

Widiger, T. A., Hurt, S. W., Frances, A., Clarkin, J. F., & Gilmore, M. (1984). Diagnostic efficiency and DSM-III. *Archives of General Psychiatry, 41*, 1005–1012.

4 Dimensional Structure of the Millon Clinical Multiaxial Inventory

Maurice Lorr, Ph.D.

The popular MCMI-II is designed to assess 13 personality disorders and 9 clinical syndromes. An important basic question is what factors or dimensions does the MCMI-II actually measure and how closely do they correspond to the scales? This chapter reviews and evaluates the findings obtained in two recent factor analytic structures of the MCMI-II. One study is by Lorr, Strack, Campbell, and Lamnin (1990); the other was conducted by Retzlaff, Lorr, Hyer, and Ofman (1991).

Both studies involved analyses of the MCMI-II at the item level. The advantage of this approach, as opposed to scale analysis, is that it avoids the problem of item overlap, which characterizes the inventory scales. Item overlap results in spurious scale correlations which in turn impose factor structure that does not result from subject response patterns as Retzlaff and Gibertini (1987) have shown. A second reason for conducting analyses at the item level is that the approach makes possible a comparison of the separate domains of enduring personality disorders and the more transitory symptom syndromes.

Dimensional analyses of inventories are of importance to the clinician for several reasons. Especially if the scale items are numerous, redundant, or complex, the derived factor score measures are fewer in number, more reliable (internally consistent) and more easily conceptualized. Another important advantage is that the factor scores improve profile analysis. The complex correlated scale scores are then transformed into uncorrelated elements. Such elements provide a much sounder basis for assessing the similarity between profiles by means of distance measures or correlations (Cronbach & Gleser, 1953). Then, cluster analysis can be applied to subject samples to identify distinctive profiles or types, or configural patterns such as found in the MMPI (Lorr & Suziedelis,

1982) can be isolated. Such an approach has been discussed by Millon in his *Manual* (1987) in reference to profile development (pp. 106–111).

Another reason for dimensional analysis is that an increasing number of investigators as well as clinicians have adapted the dimensional model for personality disorders (Cloninger, 1987; Widiger & Frances, 1985) instead of the categorical view. Recently, Morey, Waugh, and Blashfield (1985) developed a set of personality disorder scales on the basis of the MMPI. Millon (1987) himself views his personality styles not as types or categories but as continua.

THE FIRST STUDY

Samples and Procedures

The sample in the first study was comprised of 248 psychiatric patients. Of this group, 61 were inpatients and the remainder were outpatients. Diagnostically the sample included Alcoholics, Schizophrenics, Adjustment Reactions, and Major Depressions.

The inventory items are divisible into 120 personality disorder characteristics, 51 clinical symptoms, and 4 validity criteria. Separate correlation matrices were computed for the 120 personality disorder items and the 51 clinical symptoms. Each matrix was subjected to a principal component analysis followed by a "scree" test to determine the number of components to retain. Both the varimax and direct oblimin rotations were applied to solve for simple structure.

The Personality Disorder Factors

The analysis disclosed seven personality disorder factors. Factor interpretations were based on items that loaded ±.35 or more on a factor. The first factor was defined by nine items of which five were keyed for the Schizotypal scale and three for Dependent. Patients report the presence of unseen persons, telepathic influence and strange thoughts. This factor probably represents Millon's Schizotypal disorder.

The second factor, defined by 18 items, is readily interpreted as Social Introversion vs. Extraversion or Schizoid vs. Histrionic. The introversive items are keyed for Schizoid and Avoidant while the extraversive items come from the Histrionic scale.

The third factor, defined by 10 items, corresponds closely to Millon's Compulsive scale but is interpreted as representing Conformity.

A fourth bipolar factor, marked by seven items, is interpreted as Submissive vs. Aggressive. The major items are keyed for Dependent and Antisocial.

The fifth factor is marked by nine items, mostly biographical. All except two items are keyed for the Antisocial scale which was newly introduced in MCMI-

TABLE 4.1
Item-Based MCMI-II Factors in Patients

A. Lorr-Strack et al. (1990)	B. Retzlaff-Lorr et al. (in Press)

Personality Disorders

1. Schizotypal	1. Hostility
2. Social Introversion-Extraversion	2. Histrionic-Schizoid
3. Conformity	3. Dependent
4. Submissive-Aggressive	4. Compulsive
5. Antisocial	5. Sadistic-Narcissistic
6. Narcissism	6. Suspicion
7. Aggressive-Sadistic	

Clinical Syndromes

1. Depressed/Anxious	1. Depression/Fatigue
2. Alcohol dependence	2. Suicide
3. Suicidal ideation	3. Alcohol abuse
4. Hypomania	4. Drug abuse
5. Drug dependence	5. Crying
	6. Manic
	7. Somatization

II. The patient reports changing jobs three or more times, getting in trouble in school, and so on. This factor is confirmatory of Millon's new Antisocial scale.

The sixth factor is defined by four Narcissistic scale items and one from Paranoid. The patient reports himself as creative, with ideas ahead of the times, and as a superior person. Thus the factor is interpreted as Narcissism.

The seventh factor was defined by 15 items. Since all items except one are keyed for the Aggressive (Sadistic) scale, the factor confirms the scale. These factors are presented in Table 4.1.

The Clinical Syndrome Factors

The nine clinical syndrome scales are based on 51 statements. The component analyses of the correlations among these 51 variables yielded five factors that accounted for 44% of the total variance.

The first rotated oblique factor is defined by 18 items keyed mainly for Anxiety Disorder, Dysthymia disorder, and Major Depression. Included here are items indicative of fatigue, depression, and anxiety. The factor was interpreted as Depressed/Anxious.

The second factor items are all keyed for the Alcoholic Dependence scale. These indicate that the patient has an alcohol problem and is unable to stop.

The third dimension appears to represent Suicidal Ideation. The seven defining items are keyed for Major Depression, and Dysthymic Disorder.

The fourth symptom syndrome consists of eight items. Most come from Millon's Bipolar Manic Scale and the remainder from Thought Disorders and Delusional Disorder. The factor is thus interpreted as Hypomania.

The fifth factor, based only on five statements, appears to represent Drug Dependence.

Thus, five of Millon's nine clinical syndromes emerge as factors. The missing dimensions are Somatoform, Thought Disorder, Major Depression, and Delusional Disorder.

THE SECOND STUDY

Sample and Procedure

In the Retzlaff et al. (1991) study, two samples were analyzed. One sample involved 579 male inpatients and outpatients. The second sample consisted of 492 normal college students (35% male and 65% female). As in the Lorr-Retzlaff study, separate analyses were conducted on the personality items and the clinical syndrome items. Use was made of the "scree" test to indicate the number of factors to retain. In both cases the varimax rotational solution was adopted. Six personality factors were isolated in both samples. The variance accounted for was 37% in patients and 25% in normals.

In the patient sample, the first personality factor, labeled Hostility by Retzlaff, was made up of seven items expressive of hostile behaviors. Items were keyed to Borderline, Passive Aggressive, and Aggressive (Sadistic). The content of the second factor was related to sociability and making friends. A Histrionic-Schizoid (or Extraversion-Introversion) dimension is thus implied.

The third factor is a Dependence dimension based on the dependent scale items. The content refers to seeking help, giving in to others, and acting agreeable. Four items define the fourth factor labeled Compulsive; its content reflects respect for authority and morals.

The fifth dimension is shaped by a combination of two sadistic and three narcissistic items. The content reveals a sense of superiority and interpersonal manipulation and use of people. The factor is labeled Sadistic-Narcissistic. The sixth factor items suggest suspicion and grandiosity. Suspicious is the name suggested by Retzlaff.

To what extent do the two personality studies agree on the types of factors isolated? There is good agreement on the Social Introversion-Extraversion factor, on Compulsive and on Hostile Aggression (called Hostility by Retzlaff). However, Lorr and Strack have two well-defined groupings not found by Retzlaff. These are Schizotypal and Antisocial. Also, Retzlaff and his colleagues identify a factor called Dependent and another called Suspicious, not included in Lorr–Strack factors.

Clinical Syndrome Factors

Analysis of the clinical syndrome items disclosed eight patient factors and seven factors for normals as compared to five for the Lorr, Retzlaff, and Tarr study (1989).

The first patient factor was interpreted as Depression/Fatigue. It corresponds fairly well with the Lorr-Retzlaff factor but is much smaller. The second factor was a 3-item Suicidal dimension that is keyed for Major Depression and Dysthymia.

The third factor represents Alcohol Abuse, in that five of the six marker items are from the Alcohol Dependence scale. The fourth factor is defined by four items from the Drug Dependence scale. These refer to need for drugs and arguments about drugs.

The fifth factor may be a residual semantic dimension since the three items use semantically similar terms (crying, tears, and more crying). The sixth factor was labeled Mania since the items refer to over-cheerfulness, excitement, and excessive activity. The last factor, Somatization, refers to reports of losing balance, loss of sensations and lack of awareness of others.

Now the questions are (a) which factors appear to confirm Millon's nine clinical syndromes, and (b) to what extent do the two studies agree with respect to the clinical syndromes? Both studies isolated five dimensions of Depression/Anxiety, Suicidal Ideation, Mania, Alcohol Dependence, and Drug Dependence. The Somatization factor is, however, doubtfully isolated. Thus there is rather good agreement here. Of the nine Millon clinical syndrome scales, Thought Disorder, Major Depression and Delusional Disorder fail to emerge. The Somatoform scale, likewise, needs further confirmation.

THE NORMAL SAMPLE

The first four of the six personality factors isolated in the normal college sample were quite similar to the first four in the Retzlaff patient sample. These factors were Hostile, Histrionic, Dependent, and Compulsive. However, there was only one schizoid item on the Histrionic factor, which is bipolar in the patient sample. The Sadistic-Antisocial scale became more Narcissistic. A sixth Avoidant factor defined by items from Avoidant and Schizotypal also emerged. This factor is not found in other samples.

The clinical syndrome factors agreed quite closely with those for patients. These factors are Depression/Fatigue, Alcohol Dependent, Suicidal, Mania, and Drug Dependent. The remaining factors are Crying and Somatization.

Summary Part 1

A careful comparison of the three samples leads to the conclusion that the patient symptom syndrome factors correspond fairly closely. However, in the normal sample, the Depressed/Anxious factors split into two short factors of Fatigue and Anxiety.

Differences are greater between the personality factors derived in the three samples. Five of the patient and normal factors isolated by Retzlaff et al. (1991) are similar but they differ from three found by Lorr et al. (1990). The Differences are not easily accounted for. The most likely source is patient sample differences. Patients diagnosed as Alcoholic often exhibit antisocial behavior. The alcoholic patients may account for the presence of the Antisocial factor in the Lorr–Strack sample.

Dimensional Structure of the MCMI-I

The first form of the MCMI (Millon, 1982), like MCMI-II, includes 175 items designed to assess eight personality disorders, three chronic personality pathologies and nine symptom syndromes. The personality styles derive from Millon's theory of personality and are intended to evaluate the Axis II disorders listed in DSM-III (American Psychiatric Association, 1981). The eight personality disorder scales are Asocial, Avoidant, Dependent, Histrionic, Narcissistic, Aggressive-Antisocial, Conforming-Compulsive, and Passive-Aggressive. The three pathological disorders were Schizotypic, Cycloid, and Paranoid. The clinical syndrome scales included Anxiety, Hysteria, Hypomania, Neurotic Depression, Alcohol Misuse, Drug Misuse, Psychotic Thinking, Psychotic Depression, and Psychotic Delusion.

A review of the literature discloses that at least 10 factor analytic studies of the MCMI-I have been published. The usual number of factors isolated is four. Retzlaff and Gibertini (1987) pointed out that the scales share items and cause the scales to be linearly dependent; this creates artificial factor structures. The factors formed are interpreted as (a) general distress, (b) high sociability associated with acting out, (c) suspiciousness or paranoia, and (d) Aggressiveness. Retzlaff and Gibertini (1987) also analyzed the MCMI-I basic personality scales in a study of common item overlap. The three factors they isolated were interpreted as Aloof-Social, Aggressive-Submissive and Labile-Restrained.

The Lorr and Retzlaff Study

To avoid the problem of item overlap in scales and the influence of scale keys, Lorr et al. (1989) conducted a study of the MCMI-I at the item level. The 175 items were separated into 100 deemed descriptive of personality and 75 descriptive of clinical symptoms. The item responses analyzed came from a sample of 253 psychiatric outpatients and a second sample of 250 inpatients mainly from

TABLE 4.2
Item-Based MCMI-I Factors in Patients

A. Lorr, Retzlaff, and Tarr (1989)	B. Choca, Greenblatt et al. (1989)
Personality Disorders	
1. Social Introversion-Extraversion	2. Schizoid
2. Dependency on others	4. Dependent
3. Verbal hostility	5. Narcissistic
4. Need to please others (outpatients)	7. Conflictual (hostile)
5. Attention seeking	8. Compulsive
6. Orderliness (conformity)	9. Histrionic
	12. Paranoid

A. Lorr-Strack et al. (1990)	B. Retzlaff-Lorr et al. (1989)
Clinical Syndromes	
1. Depression	1. Depression
2. Drug abuse	3. Hypomania
4. Manic excitement	6. Alcohol abuse
5. Suicidal Ideation	10. Drug abuse
6. Drinking problem	11. Suicidal
3. Infrequent response	15. Somatization
(validity scale)	

alcoholics. The personality and symptom items were intercorrelated separately and analyzed by the method of principal components. The scree test was applied to decide on the number of components to retain. Both varimax and direct oblimin transformations were applied to achieve simple structure. Six factors were isolated to account for the personality items of the alcoholic sample and five were sufficient for the outpatients. The overall results are presented in Table 4.2.

Personality Disorders and Symptom Syndromes

There was close agreement between the outpatients and inpatients on the factors isolated. The main personality disorders were Social Introversion versus Social Extraversion, Dependency on others, Verbal Hostility, Attention Seeking, and Orderliness (Conformity). A Need to Please others appeared only in the outpatient sample.

The solutions for the outpatients and inpatients were also quite similar. Both samples defined symptom syndromes interpretable as Depression plus fatigue, Drug Abuse, Alcohol Abuse, and Manic Excitement. A Suicidal Ideation factor appeared only in the outpatients. A sixth factor for the outpatients was defined by the four validity items such as "I have not seen a car in the last ten years."

The analyses thus indicates that MCMI-I measures five or six personality disorders and five symptom syndromes.

The Choca Study

Choca, Greenblatt, Tobin, Shanley, and Denburg (1989) also sought to avoid the issue of overlapping scales in their analyses of the entire MCMI-I at the item level. Their subjects were 2,129 male psychiatric inpatients. Principal Component Analyses led to 17 factors that accounted for 41% of the total variance. A varimax rotation was applied to the 17 components retained. Of the 17, three factors were defined only by 2 or 3 items and are not considered here. They were interpreted as Tearfulness, Tiredness, and Changeableness. A fourth factor consists of the 4 validity items that were also isolated by Lorr et al. (1989). This leaves 13 factors.

The personality factors isolated were interpreted by Choca, et al. as Schizoid, Dependent, Narcissistic, Conflictual (i.e., hostile and grouchy), Compulsive, Histrionic, and Paranoid. These factors correspond fairly well with Lorr, Retzlaff, and Tarr (1989) findings. If Table 4.2 is examined, it becomes evident that five factors are much the same. These are Social Introversion versus Schizoid, Dependent on others versus Dependent, Verbal Hostility versus Conflictual, Attention Seeking versus Histrionic, Orderliness versus Compulsive. Choca et al. also define Narcissistic and Paranoid factors.

The clinical symptom syndromes identified in the two studies are also listed in Table 4.1. Here agreement is even closer. Five of the factors that correspond are Depression, Manic Excitement, Suicidal, Drug Abuse, and Alcohol Abuse. Analyses of MCMI-II have shown quite similar dimensions. Only Somatization is unique to the Choca et al. study.

Comparison of MCMI-II with MCMI-I

A comparison of the factors that account for individual differences in MCMI-II and MCMI-I is now possible. The personality disorders that are new in the revised form are Antisocial, which Millon had hypothesized. The Self-Defeating scale, however, was not confirmed. The postulated Hostile-Aggressive factor (called Aggressive-Sadistic by Millon) is also confirmed. The Schizotypal factor appears only in the Lorr–Strack study (1990). In general, there are perhaps six personality dimensions assessed by MCMI-II. The nine pathological disorders, Borderline, and Paranoid, were not isolated.

Of the nine clinical syndromes, five or six are confirmed in the analysis. Thought Disorder, Major Depression, and Delusional do not appear in any of the item-level analyses. Anxiety and Dysthymia appear to combine as a single Depression factor. The Somatoform scale is doubtful as it is isolated only by Retzlaff et al. (1991).

Possible Advances

As a result of these dimensional analyses, Millon might consider utilizing the MCMI-II items to establish six Personality Disorder factor scales and perhaps six

Symptom Syndrome factor scales. These could be used, when converted into standard scores, as a basis for profile analyses.

REFERENCES

Choca, J., Greenblatt, R., Tobin, D., Shanley, L., & Denberg, E. (1989, August). *Factor analytic structure of the MCMI items.* Paper presented at the 97th Annual Convention of the American Psychological Association, New Orleans.

Cloninger, C. R. (1987). A systematic method for clinical description and classification of personality variants. *Archives of General Psychiatry, 44,* 573–588.

Cronbach, L. J., & Gleser, G. C. (1953). Assessing similarity between profiles. *Psychological Bulletin, 50,* 456–473.

Lorr, M., Retzlaff, P. D., & Tarr, H. (1989). An analysis of the MCMI-I at the item level. *Journal of Clinical Psychology, 45,* 884–890.

Lorr, M., Strack, S., Campbell, L., & Lamnin, A. (1990). Personality and symptom dimensions of the MCMI-II: An item factor analysis. *Journal of Clinical Psychology, 46,* 749–754.

Lorr, M., & Suziedelis, A. (1982). A cluster analytic approach to MMPI profile types. *Multivariate Behavioral Research, 17,* 285–299.

Millon, T. (1982). *Millon Clinical Multiaxial Inventory Manual* (2nd ed.). Minneapolis, MN: National Computer Systems.

Millon, T. (1987). *Manual for the Millon Clinical Multiaxial Inventory-II.* Minneapolis, MN: National Computer Systems.

Morey, L. C., Waugh, M. H., & Blashfield, R. K. (1985). MMPI scales for the DSM-III personality disorders: Their derivation and correlates. *Journal of Personality Assessment, 49,* 245–251.

Retzlaff, P. D., & Gibertini, M. (1987). Factor structure of the MCMI basic personality scales and common item artifact. *Journal of Personality Assessment, 51,* 588–594.

Retzlaff, P. D., Lorr, M., Hyer, L., & Ofman, P. (1991). An MCMI-II item-level component analysis: Personality and clinical factors. *Journal of Personality Assessment, 57,* 323–334.

Widiger, T. A., & Frances, A. (1985). The DSM-III personality disorder. *Archives of General Psychiatry, 42,* 615–623.

II APPLICATION TO SPECIAL POPULATIONS

5 The MCMI in the Diagnosis and Assessment of Schizophrenia

Richard L. Greenblatt, Ph.D.
William E. Davis, Ph.D.

This chapter evaluates the effectiveness of the MCMI and the MCMI-II in identifying patients afflicted with schizophrenia. The task is complicated because behaviors and experiences associated with schizophrenia are also present in schizophreniform disorder and brief reactive psychosis. Disordered thinking characterizes all three disorders, and the criterion for discriminating among them is duration of illness, a bit of history that is not often reflected in "paper and pencil" tests of personality or psychopathology. To complicate matters further, some nonpsychotic disorders, in their acute phase, inflict on patients experiences similar to those that might be experienced by patients with thought disorders. A prominent example is an acute exacerbation of post traumatic stress disorder, during which the afflicted person may experience constricted affect, social detachment, cognitive-perceptual distortions, and hypervigilance (American Psychiatric Association, 1987)—symptoms that might be shared by acutely disturbed schizophrenics.

Patients suffering from different disorders have the same or similar experiences and, as we discuss shortly, these symptoms are what we ask patients to affirm or deny about themselves when they take paper and pencil tests. As our research suggests, most tests would do better if research hypotheses were broadened. For example, symptom-specific hypotheses such as, "identify patients suffering from confused thinking or problems with impulse control," rather than, "identify the paranoid schizophrenics within a larger group of mixed psychiatric patients," more likely would lead to data supporting the efficacy of a test of psychopathology. The conundrum is that if we broadened our categories to the point that the test might be most accurate, we cease making the diagnostic distinctions that are helpful in good treatment planning and prognostication.

This chapter contains three parts. The first part reviews the use of the MCMI in assessing schizophrenia. Then we discuss empirical studies that evaluate the effectiveness of the MCMI in the diagnosis and assessment of schizophrenia. We conclude with case examples of psychiatric inpatients.

A limitation of this chapter is the exclusion of studies directed at the internal structure of the MCMI, such as factor analytic studies (e.g., Choca, Peterson, & Shanley, 1986). In addition, we exclude studies whose main purpose is to explore relationships between the MCMI and other psychometric measures (e.g., McMahon & Davidson, 1986). We do not link our review to a specific theory of schizophrenia. Instead, we simply propose that assessment should accurately describe a patient's personality and symptomatology. Finally, a note on terminology is necessary. Data that are specific to one version of the MCMI (i.e., either the MCMI-I or MCMI-II) refer to that version. Otherwise, we refer to the MCMI in general.

MCMI SCALES FOR ASSESSING SCHIZOPHRENIA

Directly Relevant Symptom Scales

The MCMI-I and MCMI-II provide two clinical syndrome scales and four personality scales directly relevant to the assessment of schizophrenia. Internal consistency estimates for these six scales are satisfactory, ranging from .81 to .93 (Millon, 1987, p. 129).

To begin with the clinical syndrome scales, the Thought Disorder scale (called Psychotic Thinking on the MCMI-I) most directly addresses the defining features of schizophrenia, including unusual thought processes, inappropriate affect, social withdrawal, and incongruous behavior. All 33 items on the Thought Disorder scale are keyed *True*, and include statements such as:

> Even when I'm awake, I don't notice people who are near me.
> I very often hear things so well that it bothers me.

The Delusional Disorder Scale (called Psychotic Delusions on the MCMI) assesses acute paranoia. Patients with high scores are considered belligerent and harbor persecutory or grandiose delusions. All 22 items on this scale are keyed *True,* and include statements such as:

> I quickly figure out how people are trying to cause me trouble.
> Many people have been spying into my private life for years.

Although the name of this scale is identical with the DSM-III-R disorder of delusional disorder, the DSM describes this disorder as uncommon. Because psychometric instruments are likely ineffectual for diagnosing rare disorders, the Delusional Disorder scale holds more promise in assessing the more common paranoid subtype of schizophrenia.

Personality Scales: Possible Precursors to Schizophrenia

In contrast to the clinical syndrome scales that measure acute dysfunction, the MCMI personality disorder scales measure dysfunctional characteristics that are pervasive and enduring. In addition, these dysfunctional personality characteristics can be mild or more severe.

Two of the severe personality disorders, schizotypal and paranoid, are concomitants or precursors to schizophrenia. The MCMI scales representing these personality disorders are Schizotypal and Paranoid. The 44 items on the Schizotypal scale capture dysfunctional features such as behavioral eccentricity, social detachment, and cognitive autism. Four of the items are keyed *False*. Representative items on the Schizotypal scale include:

I'm so quiet and withdrawn, most people don't even know I exist.
I keep having strange thoughts that I wish I could get rid of.

Millon (1981) suggests that schizotypal personality is the precursor for disorganized, catatonic, and residual schizophrenia, and schizophreniform disorder.

The Paranoid scale captures attributes such as resistance to external control, vigilant mistrust, and abrasiveness. All 44 items are keyed *True,* and include the following statements:

Under no circumstances do I ever let myself be tricked by people who say they need help.
I am ready to fight to the death before I'd let anybody take away my self-determination.

Millon (1981) identifies the catatonic, excited and catatonic, stuporous subtypes of schizophrenia as extensions of the paranoid personality. He does not mention paranoid personality as a possible precursor for paranoid schizophrenia.

The mild to moderately disordered, or basic personality styles, that are most consistent with the diagnosis of schizophrenia are schizoid and avoidant. Both styles are considered detached because of their deficient ability to experience pleasure or reward. They differ in their method of maintaining distance from others. Schizoid personalities are indifferent to human involvement, whereas avoidants actively withdraw from human contact.

The Schizoid (called Asocial on the MCMI-I) scale includes 25 items keyed *True* and 10 items keyed *False*. Items keyed *True* include:

I have little interest in making friends.
I rarely feel anything strongly.

The Avoidant scale includes 35 items keyed *True* and 5 items keyed *False*. Items keyed *True* include:

Talking to other people has almost always been difficult and painful for me. Few people like me.

Other MCMI Scales

Most other MCMI scales might be useful in the assessment of schizophrenia. Of the clinical syndrome scales, the characteristics addressed by the Anxiety, Somatoform, and Dysthymia scales are associated with schizophrenia. Alcohol Dependence and Drug Dependence might be secondary diagnoses of schizophrenics. The Bipolar and Major Depression scales are used for the assessment of schizoaffective disorder. In short, the MCMI holds promise for depicting the diversity of symptoms defining and associated with schizophrenia, and for determining the most salient aspects of the disorder for a given patient.

Of the severely disordered personality styles, only the borderline personality has gone unmentioned. Elevations on the Borderline scale might be associated with schizoaffective disorder. On the basic personality scales, Dependent commonly co-occurs with Avoidant, and thus might be expected as a precursor to schizophrenia. The independent styles (narcissistic and antisocial) can be precursors to paranoid schizophrenia or uncommon variants such as pseudo-psychopathic schizophrenia. The Compulsive scale broaches characteristics found in schizophreniform disorders.

Perhaps the MCMI scales least expected to be elevated in schizophrenic patients are Histrionic and Passive-Aggressive. The active social involvement entailed by these scales seems out of reach for schizophrenics, and more in line with affective disorders. Still, one might find schizoaffective patients with histrionic features, and passive-aggressive behaviors might maintain social withdrawal.

RESEARCH ON THE MCMI AND SCHIZOPHRENIA

This section reviews the empirical evidence evaluating the diagnostic merit of the MCMI for the diagnosis of schizophrenia. The evidence stems from two sources—the validation studies in the MCMI-I (Millon, 1983) and MCMI-II Manuals (Millon, 1987), and studies appearing after the tests were published. All published studies used the MCMI-I.

We begin with a review of the evidence discussed in the manuals. The MCMI-II Manual contains the most up-to-date construction and validity data. Therefore, we refer to the MCMI-I Manual only when information occurs exclusively in that manual.

MCMI Manual Validation for the Assessment of Schizophrenia

The seminal MCMI external validation study (Millon, 1987, pp. 45–50) involved 167 clinicians judging the degree to which patients (well-known to the clinicians) fit detailed descriptions of personality styles and clinical syndromes. These 682 patients had completed a research version of the MCMI. The clinician-supplied diagnoses allowed placement of the patients into 20 criterion groups with sample sizes ranging from 40 to 70. The developers selected items for the final version of the test based on the theoretical model underlying the MCMI and the endorsement frequencies revealed by this data.

Note that this study did not maintain independence among the criterion groups. That is, the investigators assigned subjects to more than one criterion group. A possible confound relevant to the present review would be a patient assigned to the schizoid personality and thought disordered groups. Although the subject might *truly* belong in both groups, this practice forces built-in consistency among the scales. This issue is not identical with the item-overlap controversy that is discussed in the manuals. Rather, this is a matter of test development strategy, and one is clearly in better stead if a subject, regardless of other characteristics, is used in only one criterion group. The implications of subject overlap in the criterion groups are not addressed in the manual.

Another problem is that the manual describes a personality style given to the clinicians, but provides no examples of the clinical syndrome passages used in the study. Thus, we have no examples of the criteria on which the clinicians assigned patients to the thought disordered or delusional disordered groups.

Subsequently, the developers gathered a sample of 1,292 patients from various clinical settings to establish norms and optimal cutting scores for each MCMI-II scale. One study contained 825 patients, and a second study contained 467 patients. In addition, these patients established the frequency of DSM-III diagnoses among patients receiving the MCMI. Millon (1987, pp. 104–107) designated these patients the "MCMI-II Normative Population."

The MCMI-II manual further describes (Millon, 1987, pp. 141–171) the test's "external validation" using clinician-supplied DSM-III diagnoses. These reports directly bear on the topic of the present chapter. The manual describes three studies with samples of 825, 236, and 467 subjects, respectively. The sample of 825 subjects is described as Group A, whereas the samples of 236 and 467 subjects are combined to form a Group B containing 703 subjects. Clinicians assessed Group B patients with attention to the study's specific diagnostic questions.

The manual then displays the median MCMI patient profiles for each diagnosis. For example, Table 3-20 (Millon, 1987, p. 166) displays the median MCMI-II profiles of patients diagnosed as "thought disorder"; from the scale description, these patients primarily carry the diagnosis of schizophrenia. The median profiles of thought-disordered patients attained peaks on the Avoidant, Schizotypal, and Self-Defeating scales. Neither the Thought Disorder nor Delusional Disorder scales attained medians in the clinically interpretable range (i.e., above a BR of 74). The Dysthymic and Anxiety Disorder scales were the only clinical syndrome scales in the interpretable range. The elevations on the Avoidant and Schizotypal scales suggest that the MCMI captures some enduring features of schizophrenia, but fails to capture acute distress.

Yet, a more detailed review of these studies suggests that the results provide little evidence for "external validation" because of the problem of criterion contamination. The patients in Group A are a subgroup of patients included in the MCMI Normative Population that served to establish norms and cutting scores. Two-thirds (467/703) of the patients in Group B were the remainder of the MCMI Normative Population. Millon (1987) does acknowledge that these Group B patients were used in developing item weights, which "inflated scale-diagnosis correspondence" (p. 142). The inflation is more severe: Most of the patients in Groups A and B were used in deriving the norms and cutting scores. These patients were primarily test *construction* subjects who are ineligible to be used as test *validation* subjects. Therefore, the studies of "external validation" in the MCMI-II manual shed no evidence on the test's diagnostic validity.

Similarly, Millon (1987, pp. 171–177) reviews the MCMI-II's validity in terms of classification rates (i.e., true-positive, false-positive, etc.). Millon (1987, p. 172) recognizes that construction samples are unsuitable for validation studies. Still, two-thirds of the subjects used to evaluate the classification efficiency of the MCMI-II cutting scores were members of the Normative Population used to derive the cutting scores. The problem in the classification rates study is equivalent to that of the DSM-III studies described earlier: Test construction subjects cannot be used as validation subjects. The accuracy rates reported in the manual shed little evidence on the validity of the MCMI-II cutting scores.

The validation of the MCMI-I does contain a report on the classification accuracy of 256 patients who were not part of the MCMI-I construction sample (Millon, 1981, p. 58–59). The manual does not include a description of the sample, other than to state that the subjects were comparable (by design) to the MCMI-I construction sample. The results reveal that the valid positive rate for the Psychotic Thinking scale was .46 and for Psychotic Delusion was .40; false positives were minimal for both scales. Valid positive rates for the Schizotypal and Paranoid scales were in the mid .60s, with false positive rates at .06. Schizoid (Asocial) and Avoidant attained valid positive rates of about .80, with false positives less than .10. The correlations between the MCMI-I and MCMI-II versions of these scales range from the .60s to the .70s.

If one supposes that classification accuracy of the MCMI-I and MCMI-II is roughly equivalent, these data provide a gauge for the usefulness of the MCMI-II in assessing schizophrenia. The MCMI is best at identifying mild symptomatology and worst at identifying severe pathology. On the severe clinical syndrome scales, patients scoring above the cut-point more likely than not have the symptoms encompassed by the scale; patients scoring below the cutting score very likely are correctly identified as free of the symptoms.

To summarize, the evidence reported in the MCMI-II Manual regarding the validity of MCMI-II diagnoses, including the diagnosis of schizophrenia, is minimal. Some light could be shed on the test's validity with regard to DSM-III diagnoses and classification accuracy if the manual included separate data from the 236 subjects who were not part of the Normative Population. Evidence inferred from MCMI-I findings suggests more usefulness in assessing milder than more severe disorders. We now turn to studies using nonconstruction subjects that evaluate the assessment of schizophrenia with the MCMI.

The Diagnosis of Schizophrenia with the MCMI

Several studies have evaluated the accuracy of the MCMI (all using the MCMI-I) in the diagnosis of schizophrenia and in the assessment of symptoms relevant to schizophrenia. Some studies attempted to elucidate variables that confound the assessment of schizophrenia.

This section reviews studies directly evaluating the effectiveness of the MCMI in diagnosing schizophrenia. The methods used by these studies include single scale MCMI decisions, MCMI computer-generated diagnoses, and multivariate statistical approaches. Review of the study that apparently used computer-generated diagnoses (Bonato, Cyr, Kalpin, Prendergast, & Sanhueza, 1988) is less than thorough, because the decision rules for generating these diagnoses are not published. The Bonato et al. (1988) study was also the only investigation that used a structured interview as a criterion. All other studies used staff discharge diagnoses.

To begin, Sexton, McIlwraith, Barnes, and Dunn (1987) applied discriminant function analysis to the MCMI to predict the discharge diagnoses of 102 patients diagnosed as unipolar affective, bipolar affective, or schizophrenic disorder. The discriminant function accurately classified 48% of the schizophrenic patients, but misclassified about 19% of the depressed patients. By our calculations, these accuracy rates translate into a positive predictive power of .40 and a negative predictive power of .86. Examination of the significant discriminant function showed that scales relevant to schizophrenia (e.g., Psychotic Thinking and Schizotypal) lacked influence. Scales measuring "neurotic" or "acting-out" behavior (e.g., Dysthymia and Antisocial) most influenced the discriminant function, suggesting that the MCMI might be more useful with these characteristics than psychosis.

Bonato et al. (1988) studied the agreement of diagnoses generated by the MCMI with diagnoses yielded by structured and unstructured interviews. Of the small sample (N = 31), six patients were called schizophrenic according to both the structured and unstructured interviews. The MCMI identified two of these patients as schizoaffective. The authors concluded that "the MCMI provided poor diagnostic agreement" (Bonato et al., 1988, p. 873) with the structured and unstructured interviews.

Patrick (1988) used the discharge diagnoses of 103 inpatients as the criterion to assess single scale MCMI diagnoses. Twenty-six percent of these patients had received a diagnosis of schizophrenia. The positive predictive power for the Psychotic Thinking scale was .33, and the negative predictive power was .74.

Only 2% of the patients were diagnosed as paranoid disorder. The Psychotic Delusions scale attained a positive predictive power of .08 and negative predictive power of .99. The author concluded that the MCMI clinical syndrome scales were "basically invalid" (Patrick, 1988, p. 190) for the diagnosis of psychiatric inpatients.

Davis, Greenblatt, and Pochyly (1990) used the discharge diagnosis of 215 schizophrenic inpatients and 105 inpatients with relatively mild disorders to determine whether the MCMI scales used for schizophrenia would distinguish between these disparate patient groups. Race (White or Black) and education were included with diagnosis as factors in a multivariate analysis. Race was the only significant effect, with Whites scoring lower than Blacks on the Asocial, Avoidant, Psychotic Thinking, and Psychotic Delusions scales. This race effect occurred despite the use of special race-based norms (Millon, 1984). The MCMI was unable to distinguish between schizophrenics and patients with milder disorders.

Limitations of these diagnostic studies include unreliable criteria, small sample sizes, and low base rates. Still, the findings suggest that MCMI correctly identifies, at best, 40% of schizophrenics. When compared with schizophrenics, the MCMI accurately diagnosed about three-quarters of the nonschizophrenics. The studies further showed that the scales most germane to schizophrenia have limited usefulness in distinguishing schizophrenics from other psychopathological groups. A patient's race strongly influences the possibility of being identified as schizophrenic on the MCMI.

Two studies (Patrick, 1988; Sexton et al., 1987) extended their scope by comparing MCMI and MMPI accuracy rates. The results supported no clear superiority of either instrument in diagnosing schizophrenia or paranoid disorders. Comparisons between the instruments in the Patrick (1988) study were difficult to interpret because the way in which the author used the MMPI was unclear.

Patient Characteristics Relevant to Schizophrenia

Rather than evaluate the diagnosis of schizophrenia, a different research approach investigates the MCMI in assessing or describing schizophrenic patients. This section reviews the six studies that take this approach.

Silverstein and McDonald (1988) gathered 27 schizophrenics and 26 major depressives diagnosed according to Research Diagnostic Criteria. These patients were also evaluated for neuropsychological dysfunction. The study investigated selected MCMI scales using analysis of covariance with two factors (diagnosis and neuropsychological status) and two covariates (age and race). Schizophrenics had higher scores than depressives on the Paranoia, Alcohol Abuse, Drug Abuse, Psychotic Thinking, and Psychotic Delusions scales. Significant interactions showed that neuropsychologically impaired schizophrenics attained higher scores on Alcohol Abuse, Drug Abuse, and Psychotic Thinking than nonimpaired schizophrenics. The authors suggested that the results provided limited support for the notion that negative symptoms such as psychotic thinking would be prominent in neuropsychologically impaired schizophrenics. In contrast to expectations, the Paranoid and Psychotic Delusions scales were not elevated in nonimpaired schizophrenics, as compared to impaired schizophrenics. Moreover, subsequent analyses found no effects for the Schizoid, Avoidant, or Dependent scales based on neuropsychological impairment.

In a study using biological and psychometric measures, Josiassen, Shagass, and Roemer (1988) used MCMI computer-generated reports to subtype schizophrenics (diagnosed by DSM-III and RDC criteria) into either "psychotic schizophrenic" or "nonpsychotic schizophrenic" groups; each group had 10 subjects. The investigators then measured evoked potentials using standard procedures. Results showed that the psychotic schizophrenics had larger mean amplitude primary somatosensory potentials. Furthermore, the MCMI Psychotic Delusions scale correlated positively with early somatosensory amplitudes and inversely with later amplitudes. On the personality scales, the psychotic schizophrenics attained elevations on the Paranoid scale, whereas the nonpsychotics attained elevations on the Avoidant and Dependent scales. These findings supported the MCMI's ability to discriminate between schizophrenics who describe themselves as actively psychotic (especially delusional) and those who describe themselves as discouraged, but without florid symptomatology.

Helmes and Barilko (1988) gleaned symptom descriptions from the files of 109 psychiatric inpatients who had completed the MCMI. Of relevance to the present review, the symptom "delusions" occurred in 25% of the cases. Discriminant analyses (evidently using all MCMI scales) correctly classified 79% of the cases as delusional or nondelusional, but this accuracy rate was not statistically significant. Also, neither the BPI nor MMPI classified delusional cases at a level of statistical significance.

Hogg, Jackson, Rudd, and Edwards (1988) investigated personality disorders among schizophrenics diagnosed with a semistructured interview. The investigators measured personality dysfunction according to the MCMI and a semistructured interview for personality disorders; patients were tested when stable and close to discharge. Agreement between the two personality instruments was poor. The MCMI results suggested that dependent, narcissistic, and avoidant personality disorders were most common among schizophrenics.

In an attempt to explain the insensitivity of the MCMI to the diagnosis of schizophrenia, Jackson, Greenblatt, Davis, Murphy, and Trimakas (1991) used a brief checklist to establish whether psychiatric inpatients were symptom "reporters" or "nonreporters." The sample included 258 psychiatric inpatients with a discharge diagnosis of schizophrenia. The authors hypothesized that symptom reporters would attain higher scores on the MCMI scales used to assess schizophrenia. A multivariate analysis of variance and follow-up univariate tests revealed that symptom reporters scored higher than non-reporters on the Asocial, Avoidant, Schizotypal, and Psychotic Thinking scales; no significant differences were found for the Paranoid or Psychotic Delusions scales. Willingness to report distress or deviant behavior thus influences patients' MCMI profiles. No effects were found for the Paranoid or Psychotic Delusions scales based on reporter/nonreporter status.

In another study using a brief symptom checklist, Greenblatt and Davis (1992) used the MCMI personality scales to predict self-reports of psychotic symptoms in 1,050 Black and White psychiatric inpatients. The MCMI predicted self-reports of psychotic symptoms accurately in nearly 70% of both Black and White patients; the accuracy rate was statistically significant for both races. The Avoidant scale was the only important predictor.

These studies provide some support to the notion that the MCMI can accurately describe patients who are willing to report their symptoms. Not surprisingly, schizophrenics appear as a diverse group, and no single pattern of findings emerges from these data. The MCMI distinguished between schizophrenics with psychotic thinking, delusional thinking, substance abuse, mild personality dysfunction, or severe personality dysfunction; yet, these findings were inconsistent across studies. The MCMI demonstrated some ability to predict psychosis, yet the predictors were inconsistent—either delusional thinking or a mildly dysfunctional personality style, avoidant.

Case Examples

We present these cases in the spirit of assessment as a way of evaluating one's hypotheses about patients, and of generating otherwise unconsidered hypotheses. These cases are of psychiatric inpatients well known to one author of this chapter. As such, they tend to be chronically and seriously disturbed patients. These were not especially difficult diagnostic cases, but instead, represented our psychiatric inpatients. The benefit of selecting well known patients is that they present a wealth of clinical information on which to evaluate the "fit" between the MCMI and clinical status. Still, the measure of fit is informal, and the adequacy of the MCMI in describing and suggesting new ideas is linked inextricably to our own clinical conjectures about these patients.

Case 1

CS is a single White, male, Viet Nam veteran with 11 years education and a GED. He first took the MCMI in 1986 when he was 37-years-old, was retested in 1987, and took the MCMI-II in 1989. The discharge diagnoses that most often concluded his multiple psychiatric hospitalizations were schizophrenia, paranoid type, or schizophrenia, undifferentiated type. He has had a history of substance abuse, but these episodes have become unusual.

CS's presenting complaints usually included dysphoria, often accompanied by an unusual belief such as thinking that people are staring at him because they think he is homosexual. He bases his belief on his observation of the way people sit and talk among themselves. At times he has believed that he had a family residing in his body. He maintained regular communication with the family when they were "in residence."

His social relations can be best characterized as self-deprecating. He gives away money and has even given away a house, saying he does not deserve it and does not need it. As an inpatient, when CS is not withdrawn, his social interactions are, at best, superficial. He has frequently expressed fears of being "cornered" and of hurting someone else.

MCMI-I Code (1986)
2 *1* 3 8 ** − * − + − " 7 6 5 4 // S ** − * //
D A ** B * // ** − SS * //

MCMI-I Code (1987)
2 1 *3* 8 ** − * 6 5 + 7 " 4 // − ** P S * //
B A ** D * // PP SS ** − * //

MCMI-II Code (1989)
2 8B 3 8A ** 1 6A * 4 + 5 *6B* " 7 // C ** S * //
T ** D * // − ** − * //

The three administrations represent both consistency and change. The testings consistently reflected his avoidant personality style, and MCMI-II scale 8B best captures his self-deprecation and feelings of unworthiness. The elevations on SS are also a clear "hit" for the MCMI, as are the elevations on the symptom scales D and A.

Still, the absence of elevations on any of the MCMI-II severe clinical syndrome scales is a clear "miss." Although CS's clinical status can change, we do not believe that his thinking was ever clear or that he was free of delusions. Perhaps CS wanted to emphasize his dysphoria, but then an elevation on CC seems warranted.

We must be more equivocal in evaluating how accurately the remaining elevations describe CS. For example, the elevation on 6A might suggest his fears of acting out, instead of any recent episodes of overt, physical, aggression. The elevation on the pathological personality scale S captures CS's fantasy laden cognitive style and social isolation, but the inconsistent elevations of scales P and C probably reflect more acute conditions, although the scales are not intended to describe acute states. The elevations on the Alcohol and Substance Abuse scales reflect history rather than a current problem, and the inconsistent elevations on PP seem to reflect CS's changing clinical state or preoccupation.

Case 2

KM, a Black, divorced, male, was 43-years-old in 1985 when he first completed the MCMI. The patient has had over 100 psychiatric admissions, with diagnoses primarily of paranoid schizophrenia. He has not worked for many years. He reports his years of education as 17 or 23.

KM's presenting complaints to the hospital are often of a dramatic nature, either homicidal or suicidal ideation, although no evidence exists that the patient aggressed against others or hurt himself. The patient feels rejected and angered by his family's misuse of money and refusal to house him, though he has given them financial and emotional support. KM has often introduced himself as a doctor, preacher, and educator. He has also stated repeatedly that he is God. He can discuss abstract ideas at length and over many occasions. The patient has abused alcohol and drugs (mainly cocaine, recently) for many years. The patient has believed that the FBI is out to get him. Auditory hallucinations usually tell him to harm himself or others. He also has diabetes mellitus that is often out of control because of poor medication and dietary compliance.

The patient completed the MCMI three times.

> MCMI-I (1985)
> 5 6 ** − * 4 2 8 + 7 " 1 3 // P ** − * //
> T N ** − * // − ** PP * //
>
> MCMI-I (1985)
> 6 ** 5 * 4 + 7 2 8 3 " 1 // P ** − * //
> ** − T * // ** − PP * //
>
> MCMI-I (1986)
> 6 ** 5 * 4 7 + 1 3 " 8 2 // P ** − * //
> T ** − * // − ** − * //

The profiles are remarkably consistent across the three administrations. The patient's paranoid style came through consistently, capturing his resistance to external influences, belligerence, suspiciousness, and continuously delusional thinking. The elevation on 5 suggests how the patient's expansive and grandiose nature flavor the delusional contents of his thinking. Scale 5 suggests also his inflated self-image and lack of understanding of reciprocity in relationships. His hostility and projective approach coincide with the elevations on 6. Still, I am aware of no recent evidence for outright aggressiveness toward others. Perhaps the coolness of affect and presentation suggested by scale 5 moderate the impulsivity suggested by scale 6. The MCMI well reflects the patient's drug abuse. The one nonelevated PP scale is likely a test miss, as I have not known the patient to be without frankly delusional symptoms. It is also interesting that unlike most patients, KM does not does not show elevations on A or D. Possibly his well sustained delusional structure is sufficient to leave him free from clinically significant depression or anxiety.

Case 3

PP, a 29-year-old single, White, male, completed the MCMI in 1987. He has had 25 admissions between 1985 and 1990, primarily for schizophrenia, paranoid type. The patient is a high school graduate. Though usually unemployed, he had pumped gas prior to his last admission.

While on the unit, PP has attended no activities and stayed in the quiet room. He reported a gamut of auditory and visual hallucinations and bizarre delusions, involving visitors from other planets and special messages. PP has gone for weeks with a minimum of nourishment because of fears that people were poisoning his food. He once barricaded himself in his apartment because of his fear of being harmed, and the police had to remove him forcibly. He often tries to elope from the unit, although he usually "manages" to get caught. He uses marijuana as often as he can, and lacks desire to stop. When less withdrawn, PP discusses these events with a bit of laughter. The admission during which the patient completed the MCMI was during one of his less withdrawn and paranoid conditions.

MCMI-I (1987)
− ∗∗ 3 ∗ 4 7 1 + 5 8 2 ″ 6 // − ∗∗ − ∗ //
− ∗∗ − ∗ // − ∗∗ − ∗ //

This profile of a mildly dependent individual with no clinically significant pathology bears no resemblance to this patient, and is the single clear-cut "miss" in the cases presented. Clinicians can use assessment instruments to modify prior clinical hypotheses, and one indeed could be enlightened to see this patient as a compliant and conciliatory individual. Yet, even if this patient does see himself as counting on others for support, his dependency is more likely of the histrionic type rather than passive-dependent type; he repeatedly takes action (such as eloping from the unit) to engage others. More significantly, the MCMI profile addresses nothing about the strong schizotypal or paranoid components of PP's personality. Moreover, despite PP's relatively stable condition at testing, he affirmed "Thoughts that I might be harmed or plotted against" on a brief checklist. The MCMI gave no indication that this patient harbored these suspicions. Finally, the MCMI gave no indication of this patient's rampant marijuana abuse.

Case 4

TT is a 34-year-old single, Black male who completed the MCMI in 1987. He is a high school graduate and is usually unemployed. This patient has had 40 hospitalizations between 1985 and 1990, usually with a diagnosis of schizophrenia, paranoid type. His behavior on the unit has included standing in defensive positions in his room or the hallway. He is isolative and rarely engages others socially. The occasions when he does converse with others are brief, and the patient can walk away from the conversation in midsentence. He repeatedly steals shirts (and perhaps other items) from other patients. He usually denies that his mother is truly his mother. He rarely complies with treatment after discharge. TT is a regular abuser of marijuana.

TT had taken the MCMI twice in 1986, both times responding affirmatively to the validity item about flying over the Atlantic, thus generating reports of questionable validity. In 1987, his profile was valid.

MCMI Code (1987)
$6\,5\,** - *\,4\,7 + 8\,3\,''\,1\,2 // - ** - *//$
$- **\ T\ * // - ** - *//$

The MCMI accurately captured TT's impulsiveness, arrogance, and substance abuse. The profile failed to represent the remainder of his symptomatology, including persecutory delusions, thought disorder, and his paranoid stance. TT presents a challenge to objective assessment, as he stays with tasks for only a short period. Perhaps his concentration and cooperativeness were sufficient to allow him to express his current concern with the salient problem of substance abuse, but not the more integral problem of psychosis. Still, as scales 5 and 6 are positively correlated with T, we might be seeing more an expression of personality than a recognition of substance abuse.

Case 5

EQ was a 40-year-old Hispanic, single male when he completed the MCMI-II in December, 1989. He is an honorably discharged Viet Nam veteran. He is a GED recipient who has not worked regularly in over 5 years. The patient had 12 psychiatric admissions between 1984 and 1990. He describes his primary problem as post traumatic stress disorder (PTSD), and indeed, that has been a consistent discharge diagnosis. He has also heavily abused cocaine and heroin. EQ talks about wanting to change his values and gain acceptance from others; he refers vaguely to guilt feelings.

MCMI-II Code (1989)
$6A\ 6B\ 8A\ 5\ ** * 4 * 2 + 8B\ 1\ 7\ ''\ 3\ //\ P\ C\ ** - * //$
$T\ A\ N\ D\ B\ **\ H\ * //\ CC\ SS\ PP\ ** - * //$

This is a valid, but remarkably elevated profile. Elevations occur on every symptom scale and two of the three pathological personality scales. The patient does report psychotic-like symptoms related to his PTSD, and does report depressive-like symptoms. Still, no evidence exists that this patient is either schizophrenic or has a delusional disorder. He had led an antisocial-like lifestyle, resists external controls and societal rules, yet reports painful emotional anguish. One cannot interpret every symptom scale as significant in its own right; certainly, an accurate diagnosis for this patient is not simultaneously schizophrenia, psychotic depression, and delusional disorder. Instead, one might interpret this completely elevated profile as suggesting a marked state of despair and confusion. One also must consider a "fake bad" profile, although the profile did pass the MCMI-II validity checks.

SUMMARY

The MCMI contains items that describe the experiences of patients suffering from various thought disorders. The scales comprising these items were derived from an explicit theoretical position and attained acceptable internal consistency. The research supports the contention that some patients who are in distress because they are aware of their unusual experiences and behaviors, and who want others to know about their distress, will affirm the relevant items.

We ordinarily want tests such as the MCMI to identify not only those patients who readily admit their symptomatology, but those who do not. The research reviewed here suggests that the MCMI is not better than other tests in ferreting out patients who are not distressed or conceal their symptomatology.

Clinicians must ask another question about a test of psychopathology. "Does the test incorrectly classify people as schizophrenic when they are not?" The consequences of incorrectly classifying people as schizophrenic can be at least as grave as not identifying them correctly. The few studies with racially mixed samples suggest that the MCMI, even with "Black" norms, incorrectly classifies nonpsychotic Black patients as suffering from a thought disorder.

The MCMI is a relatively new instrument and lacks the rich, 4-decade, research base of the other popular objective test of psychopathology, the MMPI. Accordingly, we cannot conclusively evaluate the MCMI's diagnostic efficacy based on the few studies completed to date. Investigators should conduct more studies, including studies of a different kind, with the MCMI. The following are directions that we recommend for future research.

An immediate need is for data reporting the accuracy of classification for the Thought Disorder and Delusional Disorder scales under optimal conditions. As the data reported in the MCMI-II manual contain criterion contamination, we remain unaware of classification accuracy rates derived from clinicians who are thoroughly familiar and experienced with the MCMI and their patients.

As a test designed for assessment in general clinical populations, the low prevalence of schizophrenia in the MCMI construction sample presents a difficult and perhaps impossible hurdle in the MCMI's attempts to achieve satisfactory classification rates. For example, with a prevalence of .04 for Thought Disorder, one's accuracy will be 96% by calling all patients "non-thought disordered." Possibly, the calculation of local base rates and optimal cutting scores, especially for inpatient samples, might boost the clinical usefulness of the MCMI. Rorer and Dawes (1982) describe methods for establishing local cutting scores.

Another uncharted area of investigation is the incremental validity (e.g., Sines, 1959) of the MCMI in a clinical context. That is, one can assess the validity of the MCMI not only in terms of superiority to chance or prevalence, but in comparison to information that is more readily available, or that clinicians collect by necessity. As no test should be used *blindly* in a clinical setting, diagnoses derived from biographical data and a brief clinical interview define the baseline upon which the MCMI must improve diagnostic accuracy.

Studies of expert decision making suggest a different research approach that might benefit MCMI interpretation. These studies (e.g., Goldberg, 1965; Kleinmuntz, 1990) used statistical or computer models to capture and implement the decision strategies of the most valid clinicians. Capturing the decision rules of expert MCMI users also might serve to increase the diagnostic accuracy at the expert-test junction.

Despite these suggestions for future research, unusual symptoms define schizophrenia, and the underdeveloped theory of symptomatology embodied in the MCMI might hinder the assessment of schizophrenia. Millon (1983, 1987) clearly articulates the personality theory underlying the test, in proposing that the symptoms arising in schizophrenia and other Axis-I diagnoses occur in the context of maladaptive patterns of behavior. Although an intriguing assertion, this is an open empirical issue. Asking a brief psychometric inventory such as the MCMI to measure accurately the full range of personality and symptomatology found in clinical settings might be over ambitious. Personality variables are the central focus of the underlying theory, and perhaps should remain the focus of the test.

In summary, the MCMI is a good identifier of schizophrenics who are willing to admit their symptoms. Yet, the evidence shows that non-thought disordered patients will be identified as schizophrenic, as well. The MCMI is not a good diagnostic tool for the identification of schizophrenics and other, similar, disorders if the patients want to conceal their symptoms. Further, the MCMI will misclassify nonpsychotic Black and, probably, other underprivileged minorities, as suffering from schizophrenia or some related disorder, an uncomfortably large proportion of the time.

ACKNOWLEDGMENTS

This study was supported by Department of Veterans Affairs basic institutional research funds.

REFERENCES

American Psychiatric Association (1987). Diagnostic and statistical manual of mental disorders (3rd ed.—rev). Washington, DC: American Psychiatric Association.

Bonato, D. P., Cyr, J. J., Kalpin, R. A., Prendergast, P., & Sanhueza, P. (1988). The utility of the MCMI as a DSM-III Axis I diagnostic tool. Journal of Clinical Psychology, 44, 867–875.

Choca, J. P., Peterson, C. A., & Shanley, L. A. (1986). Factor analysis of the Millon Clinical Multiaxial Inventory. Journal of Consulting and Clinical Psychology, 54, 253–255.

Davis, W. E., Greenblatt, R. L., & Pochyly, J. M. (1990). Test of MCMI black norms for five scales. Journal of Clinical Psychology, 46, 175–178.

Goldberg, L. R. (1965). Diagnosticians vs. diagnostic signs: The diagnosis of psychosis vs. neurosis from the MMPI. Psychological Monographs, 79, (9; Whole No. 602), 1–28.

Greenblatt, R. L., & Davis, W. E. (in press). Accuracy of MCMI classification of angry and psychotic black and white patients. Journal of Clinical Psychology.

Helmes, E., & Barilko, O. (1988). Comparison of three multiscale inventories in identifying the presence of psychopathological symptoms. *Journal of Personality Assessment, 52,* 74–80.

Hogg, B., Jackson, H. J., Rudd, R. P., & Edwards, J. (1988). Diagnosing personality disorders in recent-onset schizophrenia. *Journal of Nervous and Mental Disease, 178,* 194–199.

Jackson, J. L., Greenblatt, R. L., Davis, W. E., Murphy, T. J., & Trimakas, K. (1991). Assessment of schizophrenic inpatients with the MCMI. *Journal of Clinical Psychology, 47,* 505–510.

Josiassen, R. C., Shagass, C., & Roemer, R. (1988). Somatosensory evoked potential correlates of schizophrenic subtypes identified by the Millon Clinical Multiaxial Inventory. *Psychiatry Research, 23,* 209–219.

Kleinmuntz, B. (1990). Why we still use our head instead of formulas: Toward an integrative approach. *Psychological Bulletin, 107,* 296–310.

McMahon, R. C., & Davidson, R. S. (1986). Concurrent validity of the clinical symptoms syndrome scales of the Millon Clinical Multiaxial Inventory. *Journal of Clinical Psychology, 42,* 908–912.

Millon, T. (1981). *Disorders of personality: DSM-III, Axis II.* New York: Wiley.

Millon, T. (1983). *Millon Clinical Multiaxial Inventory Manual* (3rd ed.). Minneapolis, MN: National Computer Systems.

Millon, T. (1984). *Millon Clinical Multiaxial Inventory Manual Supplement.* Minneapolis, MN: National Computer Systems.

Millon, T. (1987). *Manual for the MCMI-II* (2nd ed.). Minneapolis, MN: National Computer Systems.

Patrick, J. (1988). Concordance of the MCMI and the MMPI in the diagnosis of three DSM-III Axis I disorders. *Journal of Clinical Psychology, 44,* 186–190.

Rorer, L. G., & Dawes, R. M. (1982). A base-rate bootstrap. *Journal of Consulting and Clinical Psychology, 50,* 419–425.

Sexton, D. L., McIlwraith, R., Barnes, G., & Dunn, R. (1987). Comparison of the MCMI and MMPI-168 as psychiatric inpatient screening inventories. *Journal of Personality Assessment, 51,* 388–398.

Silverstein, M. L., & McDonald, C. (1988). Personality trait characteristics in relation to neuropsychological dysfunction in schizophrenia and depression. *Journal of Personality Assessment, 52,* 288–296.

Sines, L. K. (1959). The relative contribution of four kinds of data to accuracy in personality assessment. *Journal of Consulting Psychology, 23,* 483–492.

6 Affective Disorders and the MCMI

James Choca, Ph.D.
Linda Bresolin, Ph.D.

The unique advantage of the MCMI over other self-report psychological inventories is that it provides an effective measure of personality structure. This chapter focuses on using the MCMI to assess affective disorders. However, the value of personality style assessment in diagnosing affective disorders will also be emphasized, since to do otherwise would be to overlook the greatest strength of the MCMI.

Perhaps no other group of diagnoses has been more vehemently debated than the affective disorders. Associated with the development of effective biological treatments for depression has been a search for biological markers and chemical imbalances. Nevertheless, affective disorders have well recognized psychosocial corollaries, as reflected in the DSM-III-R by the diagnoses of uncomplicated bereavement and adjustment disorder with depressed mood. The issue of predisposing factors, including genetic and familial influences and personality traits, has also been repeatedly raised. It is interesting to explore the ways in which MCMI research has supported one side or the other in these controversies. We first review, however, the MCMI scales that are designed to measure mood, the validity and reliability of these scales, and the scale profile patterns typical of affective disorder patients.

MOOD SCALES OF THE MCMI

Moods can fluctuate along a bipolar continuum, from severe depression to mania. The MCMI has two primary scales designed to measure mood states. The Hypomania, or Bipolar Manic Scale (N), was constructed to assess elevated mood. The psychomotor aspects of mania are tapped by statements dealing with restlessness, overactivity, irritability, pressured speech, and impulsivity. To assess the affective elements of mania, the MCMI also asks subjects to describe their tendency to experience intense emotions or to demonstrate erratic behavior and moods. Cognitive items deal with the subjects' perception of themselves as superior to others or as psychologically insensitive. Items dealing with gregariousness and attention-seeking tendencies evaluate social behavior. A few items inquiring about heightened sensitivity to sounds and tendency toward alcohol abuse are also included.

An apathetic, irritable, or dejected mood is the cardinal feature assessed by items of the Dysthymic Disorder Scale (D), together with feelings of discouragement, guilt, or hopelessness. Low self-confidence, suicidal thoughts, and tearfulness also contribute to the scale score. Vegetative signs measured include physical and emotional exhaustion, sleep difficulties, and lack of personal initiative. To a lesser degree, distrust of others and a perfectionistic attitude are also assessed.

The MCMI has two additional scales that relate to affective symptomatology. The Psychotic Depression, or Major Depression, Scale (CC) was designed to measure depressive symptoms at the severe, psychotic level. The scale items include assessment of a dysphoric mood of such magnitude that it prevents the individual from functioning. This depressed mood may be accompanied by tension or confusion, difficulty sleeping, feelings of hopelessness, fear of the future, agitation, and psychomotor retardation. Other features measured include feeling physically drained, becoming angry or tearful with little provocation, feeling unworthy or undeserving, self-destructive behaviors, and being socially withdrawn or sexually inhibited. Goldberg and his associates factor analyzed the items of this scale and identified three factors: Mood Disturbance, Suicidal Ideation, and Dependency Conflicts. They criticize this scale for neglecting the vegetative symptoms of depression (Goldberg, Shaw, & Segal, 1987).

Originally, the MCMI also had a Cycloid, or Cyclothymia, Scale that was designed to measure a pervasive pattern of bipolar mood instability. This scale was eventually renamed the Borderline Scale (C) and was substantially altered in the MCMI-II revisions to better reflect the characteristics of that personality disorder. This included adding items addressing identity confusion, resentment of control, anger, and destructive or self-defeating tendencies. Items in the MCMI-II that still deal with mood disturbance assess impulsive, over-emotional behaviors, labile affective responses, apathy and numbness, low self-esteem, self-doubt, sadness, guilt, hopelessness, and aimlessness.

Reliability and Validity

Reliability coefficients for the Bipolar Manic Scale range from .62 to .79, depending on the study, the population measured, and the length of time between test and retest. Reliability coefficients for the Dysthymia, Major Depression, and Borderline scales range from .32 to 78, .52 to .79, and .27 to .84 respectively (McMahon, Flynn, & Davidson, 1985; Millon, 1987; Piersma, 1986). The lower figures were consistently obtained with inpatient populations and may reflect improvement of the subjects over time, rather than test-retest instability.

Operating characteristics that have been reported for each of these scales are displayed in Table 6.1. Millon's (1987) data suggests that the Dysthymia Scale has the best predictive power of the four—the ability to identify the presence of a disorder when the disorder is present. The Manic Scale was found to have the poorest positive predictive power. Each of the scales performed well on tests of negative predictive power—not identifying the disorder when the disorder is absent.

We used the MCMI-I to evaluate 270 psychiatric patients with major affective disorders. We found the Dysthymia and Mania scales to be diagnostically useful, identifying 65% and 56% of patients in depressed and manic states, respectively (Choca, Bresolin, Okonek, & Ostrow, 1988). Other studies have also reported good validity scales for the Dysthymia Scale (Goldberg, et al., 1987; Wetzler, Kahn, Strauman, & Dubro, 1989) using the MCMI-I. Flynn and McMahon (1983), however, found only modest correlations between the scale and three items dealing with depression and suicidality on an unstandardized survey.

The Psychotic Depression Scale of the MCMI-I is seldom elevated in any of the available samples. Many authors have felt it to be of little clinical utility (Choca et al., 1988; Goldberg, et al., 1987; Wetzler et al., 1989). Flynn and McMahon (1983) reported a modest correlation between the Psychotic Depression Scale and their three items dealing with depression and suicidality.

In a recent study, Piersma (1991) examined the effectiveness with which the Dysthymia and Major Depression Scales of the MCMI-II distinguish between major depression and other forms of depression. Using a cutoff BR score of 75, he reported that the Major Depression Scale missed 39% of individuals with major depression in his sample. With this exception, however, his data generally supported the validity of the scales (see Table 6.1).

In a sample of patients with affective disorders, the Cycloid Scale of the MCMI-I (Borderline Scale) seemed to respond properly to the presence of depressed mood. It appeared to be fairly insensitive to mood elevation. This scale, then, is felt to be somewhat redundant to the Dysthymia Scale as a measure of affective stability (Choca et al., 1988).

Other studies have indirectly addressed the validity of the MCMI for assessing mood disorder. McMahon and coworkers, for example, have demonstrated that the MCMI-I can be used to discriminate between alcoholics experiencing transient depressive episodes from those for whom depression may be more enduring and problematic (McMahon & Davidson, 1985a, 1986; McMahon & Tyson, 1989, 1990). MCMI scores have also been found to be related to patients'

TABLE 6.1
Operating Characteristics, in Percentiles, of the Affective Scales of the MCMI

	Mania			Dysthymia					Major Depression						Borderline		
Scale ――>	Gibertini	Choca	Millon	Gibertini	Choca	Wetzler	Millon	Piersma	Gibertini	Choca	Goldberg	Wetzler	Millon	Piersma	Gibertini	Choca	Millon
MCMI Version ――>	I	I	II	I	I	I	II	II	I	I	I	I	II	II	I	—	II
Prevalence	8		4	41		41	46	77	6		35	41	14	77	20		11
Sensitivity	56		42	91		71	81	86	41			4	68	61	77		67
Specificity	96		99	88		70	83	32	97			97	96	52	92		95
Positive Predictive Power	55	56	55	84	87	77	80	81	46	20	18	59	73	81	71	24/65*	60
Negative Predictive Power	96		98	93		63	84	40	96			50	97	28	94		96
Overall Diagnostic Power	93		82	89		69	82	73	94			58	92	59	89		92

*The first rate is for manic bipolar patients, the second rate is for depressed unipolar patients.

response to tricyclic antidepressants (Joffe & Regan, 1989a) and to the possible assessment of suicidal behavior (Joffe & Regan, 1989b).

PROFILE INTERPRETATION

Millon (1987) has stated that patients experiencing an adjustment disorder with depressed mood are distinguishable by their fairly low overall profile. He further predicts that these individuals will obtain low scores on the Dysthymic Disorder and Major Depression scales. However, Malec and his associates found significant elevations on the Dysthymia Scale of the MCMI-I, even when these symptoms were not pronounced enough to meet the DSM-III criteria for a major depressive episode (Malec, Wolberg, Romsaas, Trump, & Tanner, 1988). The following case history illustrates a patient with an adjustment disorder with depressed mood:

> A.D. was a 72-year-old male who was psychiatrically hospitalized when he became withdrawn, lost interest in life activities, had a poor appetite, and sustained weight loss over a few months. A sleep disturbance was also reported, and A.D. reported that he would often remain in pajamas all day. The symptoms appeared gradually, 6 months after he lost his wife of 44 years. This was the first time that A.D. had ever experienced any emotional or psychiatric problems.
>
> Although he had been a below average student, he had managed to graduate from high school and to attend one year of college. After serving in the Air Force, A.D. worked at a railroad business office for 34 years, retiring 11 years before his admission. Mental status exam was remarkable only for dysphoric mood. Some range of affect was seen, with A.D. being able to smile faintly from time to time.
>
> The projective protocol was short and contained some death themes. However, he was also able to provide more neutral responses. A.D.'s MCMI-II scores are listed in Table 6.2. Scale elevations suggest depression, anxiety, and some somatic preoccupation. In view of these findings, the dependent-compulsive personality style can be linked to the difficulty A.D. was having in coping with his wife's death. Dependent traits may have caused him to feel the loss of his wife more deeply than otherwise. Compulsive traits may have been threatened by his inability to control or prevent her death. It should be noted, however, that depressed mood may have contributed directly to A.D.'s dependent tendencies.

Millon (1987) indicates that patients suffering from dysthymia will obtain their highest elevation on the Dysthymic Disorder Scale of the MCMI-II, with the Avoidant and Passive-Aggressive Scales also being elevated. The following case history illustrates this pattern:

> Mr. D., a 40-year-old male, reported having felt depressed for the last 15 years, although the problem had worsened just before his evaluation. The depression involved a chronic unhappiness with his marriage, with his job, and with life in

TABLE 6.2
MCMI-II Scores for the Illustrative Cases

	A.D.	D.	M.D.	M.
Personality Style Scales				
1 - Schizoid	73	70	<u>115</u>	16
2 - Avoidant	57	<u>94</u>	<u>110</u>	15
3 - Dependent	<u>93</u>	61	<u>85</u>	55
4 - Histrionic	44	27	5	94
5 - Narcissistic	5	36	68	98
6A - Antisocial	0	61	52	64
6B - Aggressive/Sadistic	25	53	66	70
7 - Compulsive	<u>83</u>	40	<u>85</u>	71
8A - Negativistic	22	<u>99</u>	73	24
8B - Self-Defeating	41	45	<u>79</u>	60
Severe Personality Scales				
S - Schizotypal	66	65	<u>112</u>	35
C - Borderline	46	<u>82</u>	44	50
P - Paranoid	21	45	71	64
Clinical Symptom Scales				
A - Anxiety	<u>75</u>	<u>97</u>	92	44
H - Somatoform	73	61	56	60
N - Bipolar Manic	10	49	41	83
D - Dysthymia	<u>89</u>	<u>102</u>	<u>78</u>	44
B - Alcohol dependence	51	71	53	68
T - Drug dependence	25	63	49	66
SS - Thought disorder	0	65	<u>80</u>	38
CC - Major depression	60	<u>78</u>	64	43
PP - Delusional	0	39	64	68
Modifier Indices				
X - Disclosure	35	70	<u>84</u>	72
Y - Desirability	46	56	50	78
Z - Debasement	52	71	<u>90</u>	43
V - Validity	OK	OK	OK	OK

general. The depression "came and went," in that there were days when he felt less unhappy, but the dissatisfaction invariably returned. Mr. D. complained of low self-esteem, indecisiveness, crying spells, and feelings of hopelessness. A sleep disorder was present at one time but had responded to a trial of the antidepressant Pamelor.

Mr. D. reported that he had been a shy and nervous individual all of his life. He recalled that he would avoid eating before any big event in his life, because he tended to feel nauseated otherwise. This temperament developed to the considerable disappointment of his gregarious, outgoing father, who had difficulty understanding his son's timidity. Mr. D.'s distaste for any kind of confrontation led him to very secretive, especially toward his father. There were many occasions when Mr. D. arranged for his mother to discuss a problem with his father before approaching his father personally. Mr. D. now feared that he had become the type of individual who avoids discussing many issues and who tends to seethe over unre-solved conflicts. The patient had not received any mental health treatment until very recently.

Mr. D.'s medical history was remarkable for a long history of asthma and allergies. He was adopted as an infant and was raised as an only child. He claimed to have had a trauma-free, happy childhood. He had been married for 16 years. Although his 38-year-old wife was said to be a good and competent person, Mr. D. criticized her for being "unemotional." He felt the marriage had gradually lapsed into a convenient living arrangement, with little sexual contact and mutual disin-terest in the other person's activities. The couple had a 10-year-old who had presented no problems, by Mr. D.'s report.

Mr. D. was a college graduate. He recalled that he was not a self-motivated student, had had difficulty concentrating, and did not excel in school. He had always felt insecure about his writing, a problem that had persisted into adulthood. For the past 15 years Mr. D. had worked as a salesman in a men's store. He stated that he "abhorred" this job, but admitted that he had never made a serious effort to secure a different position.

The results of the MCMI-II supported Mr. D.'s report of dysphoria. All the scales measuring depression were elevated. This depression was accompanied by moderate anxiety, judging from the elevation on the Anxiety Scale. Mr. D.'s character structure may have been partly responsible for the problems he presented. Low self-esteem often led him to make unsatisfying compromises in his life. Moreover, his negativism meant that he was usually dissatisfied with and resentful toward more facets of his life. This negativistic element, as well as the avoidant tendencies of his personality, placed him in constant internal conflict. In Mr. D.'s case, the characterologic discomfort and the dissatisfaction with his life situation may have brought about the chronic state of dysphoria that is inherent to Dysthymic Disorder.

The MCMI profiles of patients with major depression have their highest elevations on the Dysthymic and Major Depression Scales, according to Millon (1987). These elevations are followed by lesser ones on the Anxiety, Self-Defeat-ing, Avoidant, and Dependent Scales. Work by Wetzler and colleagues tended to support this contention. They reported that the 23 depressed patients they studied scored higher than 24 nondepressed subjects on the Schizotypal, Borderline, Anxiety, Somatic Preoccupation, Dysthymic, Psychotic Thinking, and Psychotic Depression Scales of the MCMI-I (Wetzler, Kahn, Cahn, van Praag, & Asnis, 1990). An example of patient with major depression is the following:

M.D., a 62-year-old female, was evaluated while hospitalized on a psychiatric unit. On admission she was dysphoric and felt that "everything" in her life "was worthless." She feared she was doomed and that she would spend the rest of her life "in a state hospital." She complained of being tired all the time, having a poor appetite, and having trouble sleeping. Suicidal ideas often bothered her, though she felt that she would never harm herself. M.D. stated that she was not "glad to see anybody anymore." This social withdrawal was very different from her premorbid pattern. She was described as an active individual who was very involved with other family members and was always doing things for others.

Together with the symptoms of depression, M.D. was experiencing a great deal of anxiety and apprehension. She had become very irritable and nervous, and she complained of difficulty walking and thinking clearly. She also claimed to have panic attacks, in which she became dizzy and experienced shortness of breath, palpitations, and trembling. During these episodes she feared she was losing her mind.

M.D. had become depressed for the first time 3 years previously. She denied any emotional problems before that time. She was treated as an outpatient by her family physician, using Ludiomil and Xanax. After one month of treatment the symptoms resolved, and the medications were discontinued. M.D. continued to take Xanax on occasion when she felt anxious.

Coincident to the onset of the present episode, M.D. sustained a fall that resulted in a fractured vertebra and pain. She was wearing a brace to immobilize her back at the time of evaluation. M.D. also suffered from degenerative joint disease in her spine, diverticulosis, and rectocele.

She was the second of four sisters. Her father was a heavy drinker, although M.D. claimed that his drinking was controlled. Her mother was reportedly devoted to caring for her children, and M.D. described her childhood years as good. She completed 2 years of high school and recalled being a poor student. Her husband of 41 years, age 65, had a history of alcoholism and compulsive gambling. He had reportedly been abstinent from both these behaviors in the 10 years before M.D.'s evaluation. The couple had no children. M.D. retired from her 30 year's work as a government clerk 5 years previously.

On mental status exam, M.D.'s thought process was disorganized. She was very preoccupied and accused the examiner several times of laughing at her. Mood was serious and worried, with frequent complaints of being sick. She was mildly agitated, repeatedly standing up, pacing, and sitting at the far end of the room.

Elevations on the Dysthymia and Major Depression Scales of M.D.'s MCMI-II are consistent with the presence of major depression. The elevations on the Disclosure and Debasement Modifier Indices suggest that M.D. tended to emphasize her psychopathology and support a diagnosis of depression. The anxiety she evidenced was reflected in an elevated score on the Anxiety Scale. The elevation on the Psychotic Thinking Scale provides further evidence for the presence of psychotic features.

The personality scores obtained were probably elevated by acute symptoms emanating from depression and the psychotic features. Nevertheless, it is likely that the schizoid, schizotypal, avoidant, dependent, and compulsive self-defeating traits were present premorbidly. These traits may explain the type of decompensation the patient was experiencing. Although M.D. had apparently not experienced significant psychiatric problems until recently, the MCMI results suggest that she had probably had a marginal adjustment in her social activities and general level of functioning throughout her life.

Finally, Millon (1987) expects manic patients to demonstrate elevations in both the Bipolar Manic and Dysthymic Scales. This pattern has been corroborated in our own work (Choca et al., 1988). Millon also states that bipolar patients will obtain high scores on the Histrionic and Negativistic personality scales. A case illustration of a manic patient follows:

Mr. M. is a 34-year-old male who was evaluated while hospitalized on a psychiatric unit. He had become grandiose, stating that he was the "instigator of great schemes" and had "amazing powers." He was not eating consistently and had consequently lost weight. He was very talkative, rambling from topic to topic. Eventually he had become paranoid, wearing disguises. Mr. M. had been hospitalized seven years previously, while serving in the military. At that time he became psychotically suspicious of the men with whom he was serving. After three weeks hospitalization, Mr. M. was transferred to another squadron, resulting in a resolution of his symptoms.

Mr. M. was born in the Midwest, the youngest of four children. Both parents were immigrants to the United States, with little formal education. Mr. M.'s father supported the family by working as a coal miner. Mr. M. reports a "wonderful childhood" and denied any family psychiatric history. He had been married and divorced.

He was a high school graduate and had completed a few college courses. After working for several years he was drafted into the Army and completed his military tour. On return to civilian life, he worked as a salesman and was eventually promoted to regional sales manager. Shortly before his hospitalization, new management in his company had resulted in decreased benefits at work and in Mr. M. feeling less appreciated in his job.

The mental status exam was remarkable for hyperverbality. Attention and concentration were impaired. Thought process was very disorganized, with much circumstantial thinking. However, Mr. M. was able to keep track of questions and generally managed to provide an acceptable response if given enough time to do so. Affect was inappropriately elated. Mr. M. evidenced little anxiety and was disinhibited in his behavior. Psychomotor activity was also elevated.

As predicted, Mr. M.'s MCMI-II shows an elevation on the Bipolar Manic Scale. Slight elevation on the Desirability Scale of the MCMI may also be related to Mr. M.'s mania. As appears to be typical of many individuals with bipolar disorder (Alexander, Choca, Bresolin, DeWolfe, Johnson, & Ostrow, 1987), Mr. M.'s personality style had prominent narcissistic and histrionic elements.

ETIOLOGY OF DEPRESSIVE DISORDERS
AND THE MCMI

Much recent research on affective disorder has concentrated on identifying organic markers for and biological contributors to mood disturbance. Although most hypotheses attempt to link organic markers to affective symptomatology, it is possible that biological factors affect personality traits, which in turn may be precursors to mood fluctuations.

Shaughnessy and her coworkers, for example, compared women with high vs.

low lithium ratios. She used the Clinical Analysis Questionnaire and a non-psychiatric sample. The authors report that the high lithium ratio group was significantly more dominant, assertive, stern, and stubborn. They were more likely to withdraw from people and were more immune to criticism by others. These women enjoyed conflict, needed less sleep, and were less disturbed by being considered deviant (Shaughnessy, Dorus, Pandey, & Davis, 1980). In our own work, we have been able to demonstrate that the Narcissistic and Histrionic Scales of the MCMI can be used as significant predictors of sodium-dependent lithium efflux in patients with affective disorder (Choca, Okonek, Ferm, & Ostrow, 1982).

Another long-standing argument in the area of affective disorder has been whether there are personality traits that predispose individuals to mood fluctuations. Chodoff's (1972) review of this literature traces the idea that mood disorders are associated with underlying personality patterns back to the pioneers of our field. Research has indicated that unipolar depression may occur in individuals with predominant obsessive traits, such as orderliness, rigidity, and guilt (Bech, Shapiro, Sihm, Nielson, Sorenson, & Rafaelsen, 1980; Charney, Nelson, & Quinlan, 1981; Hirschfeld & Klerman, 1979; Julian, Metcalfe, & Coppen, 1969; Kendell & DiScipio, 1968; Nystrom & Lindegard, 1975; Palmer & Sherman, 1938; Rosenthal & Gudeman, 1967). Other investigators have demonstrated a connection between depression and dependence (Strandman, 1978) or social introversion (Donnelly, 1976; Hirschfeld & Klerman, 1979; Murray & Blackburn, 1974; Nystrom & Lindegard, 1975; Perris, 1966).

Bipolar affective disorders have been linked to hysterical character traits, such as the need for attention expressed in a dramatic, impulsive, and emotional manner (Charney et al., 1981; Cohen, Baker, Cohen, Fromm-Reichmann, & Weigert, 1954; Lazare & Klerman, 1968). The presence of premorbid personality characteristics seen in individuals with bipolar disorder, however, is more controversial than in the case of unipolar disorders. Several studies have shown relatively normal personality profiles when bipolar patients were evaluated during an asymptomatic period (Bech et al., 1980; Donnelly, 1976; Murray & Blackburn, 1974; Nystrom & Lindegard, 1975; Perris, 1966, 1971; Strandman, 1978; von Zerssen, 1982).

Using DSM-III and DSM-III-R personality categories, depressed individuals without anxiety have been associated with schizoid and avoidant personality structures (Alnaes & Torgerson, 1990). Personality disorders have also been frequently found in depressed individuals (Charney, Nelson, & Quinlan, 1981; Koenigsberg, Kaplan, Gilmore, & Cooper, 1985). McMahon and Davison (1985b) found a significant relationship between depression and the Avoidant and Negativistic Scales of the MCMI-I.

The reverse relationship, however, may also be true—mood state may influence personality traits. Hirschfeld, Klerman, Clayton, Keller, McDonald-Scott, and Larkin (1983) examined the personality patterns of affective disorder patients at intake and at 1 year follow-up. Patients were grouped according to whether or not they had recovered from their affective disturbance. Personality traits were measured on 19 scales that assessed emotional strength, interpersonal dependency, and extroversion. The findings indicated that depression strongly influences scores on those three personality constellations. The authors point to the need to measure personality patterns when patients are in a symptom-free, euthymic state.

Alexander et al. (1987) found that bipolars in remission were more narcissistic and histrionic than normal controls, as measured by the MCMI-I. Euthymic unipolar patients, in contrast, scored significantly higher than psychiatric normals on the Avoidant, Dependent, and Negativistic Scales. The authors concluded that affective disorder patients tend to develop personality traits associated with their mood disorder, which remain even after the acute episode has resolved.

This conclusion conflicts with the findings of Reich and Troughton (1988), who reported no MCMI differences between normal controls and those of individuals with depressive disorders who were currently asymptomatic. The conclusions of Wetzler et al. (1990) corroborated those of Alexander et al. (1987) in finding that depressed mood led to elevations in the Schizoid, Avoidant, and Negativistic Scales. Mania, on the other hand, did not seem to be associated with elevations in any of the basic personality scales of the MCMI-I.

In other words, people who suffer from depression tend to be more avoidant, dependent, and negativistic, even when they are asymptomatic. Depressed mood itself further increases the Schizoid, Avoidant, and Negativistic scales in both unipolar and bipolar patients.

Bipolar patients tend to be more narcissistic and histrionic after symptoms have abated, but mania alone does not seem to have much effect on MCMI personality scores. Caution should be used in interpreting elevations on the Schizoid, Avoidant, and Negativistic scales of depressed individuals. These scores can be expected to moderate as the acute affective episode resolves. Less concern is needed in interpreting elevated scores in individuals experiencing mania.

A different way of examining the relationship between mood disorder and personality style is to conceptualize personality traits as defining different depressive styles. Goldberg and his associates, for example, found two such styles (Goldberg, Segal, Vella, & Shaw, 1989). The first of these styles is characterized by an elevated Negativistic Scale score on the MCMI and is similar to Beck's "autonomous" depressive (Beck, 1983). These individuals feel misunderstood and unappreciated. They tend to anticipate disappointment and precipitate failures through their own obstructional behavior. The other depressive style conceptualized by Goldberg et al. is marked by elevations on the Dependant and Avoidant scales of the MCMI. These individuals are seen as similar to Beck's "sociotropic" subtype. They are thought to be self-effacing, noncompetitive people who constantly seek relationships in which they can depend on others for guidance and security.

Overholser, Kabakoff, and Norman (1989) examined the difference between dependent and nondependent depressed individuals. Their data indicate that dependent depressed subjects were more likely to be older and female than were the nondependent psychiatric controls. Dependent depressed subjects were also more likely to have reduced activity and energy levels than the nondependent depressed controls.

CONCLUSION

By far the greatest advantage of the MCMI as an inventory is its measure of personality structure. Personality disorder and some specific personality traits have been associated with important differences in both affective symptomatology and patients' response to treatment (Faravelli, Ambonetti, Pallanti, & Pazzagli, 1986; Frank, Kupfer, Jacob, & Jarrett, 1987; Joffe & Regan, 1989a, 1989b; Pfohl, Stangl, & Zimmerman, 1984; Weissman, Prusoff, & Klerman, 1978). Additionally, taking into account a patient's personality configuration can contribute to insight about the way that person functions. Understanding the role of personality in defining behavior may ultimately contribute to a general understanding of mood disorders.

REFERENCES

Alexander, G. E., Choca, J. P., Bresolin, L. B., DeWolfe, A. S., Johnson, J. E., & Ostrow, D. G. (1987, May). *Personality styles in affective disorders: Trait components of a state disorder.* Paper presented at the convention of the Midwestern Psychological Association, Chicago.

Alexander, G. E., Choca, J. P., DeWolfe, A. S., Bresolin, L. B., Johnson, J. E., & Ostrow, D. G. (1987, August). *Interaction between personality and mood in unipolar and bipolar patients.* Paper presented at the convention of the American Psychological Association, New York.

Alnaes, R., & Torgerson, S. (1990). MCMI personality disorders among patients with major depression with and without anxiety disorders. *Journal of Personality Disorders, 4,* 141–149.

Bech, P., Shapiro, R. W., Sihm, F., Nielsen, B. M., Sorenson, B., & Rafaelsen, O. J. (1980). Personality in unipolar and bipolar manic-melancholic patients. *Acta Psychiatrica Scandinavica, 62,* 245–257.

Beck, A. T. (1983). Cognitive therapy of depression: New perspectives. In P. Clayton & J. E. Barrett (Eds.), *Treatment of depression: Old controversies and new approaches* (pp. 265–290). New York: Ravens Press.

Charney, D., Nelson, J. C., & Quinlan, D. M. (1981). Personality traits and disorder in depression. *American Journal of Psychiatry, 138,* 1601–1604.

Choca, J., Bresolin, L., Okonek, A., & Ostrow, D. (1988). Validity of the Millon Clinical Multiaxial Inventory in the assessment of affective disorders. *Journal of Personality Assessment, 53*(1), 96–105.

Choca, J., Okonek, A., Ferm, R., & Ostrow, D. (1982, May). *The relationship of personality style and lithium efflux in affective disorders.* Paper presented at the convention of the American Psychiatric Association, Toronto, Canada.

Chodoff, P. (1972). The depressive personality. *Archives of General Psychiatry, 27,* 666–673.

Cohen, M. B., Baker, G., Cohen, R. A., Fromm-Reichmann, F., & Weigert, E. V. (1954). An intensive study of twelve cases of manic depressive psychosis. *Psychiatry, 17,* 103–137.

Donnelly, E. F. (1976). Cross-sectional and longitudinal comparisons of bipolar and unipolar depressed groups on the MMPI. *Journal of Consulting and Clinical Psychology, 44,* 233–237.

Faravelli, C., Ambonetti, A., Pallanti, S., & Pazzagli, A. (1986). Depressive relapses and incomplete recovery from index episode. *American Journal of Psychiatry, 143,* 888–891.

Flynn, P. M., & McMahon, R. C. (1983). Indicators of depression and suicidal ideation among drug abusers. *Psychological Reports, 52,* 784–786.

Frank, E., Kupfer, D., Jacob, M., & Jarrett, D. (1987). Personality features and response to acute treatment in recurrent depression. *Journal of Personality Disorders, 1,* 14–26.

Goldberg, J. O., Shaw, B. F., & Segal, Z. V. (1987). Concurrent validity of the Millon Clinical Multiaxial Inventory depression scales. *Journal of Consulting and Clinical Psychology, 55,* 785–787.

Goldberg, J. O., Segal, Z. V., Vella, D. D., & Shaw, B. F. (1989). Depressive personality: Millon Clinical Multiaxial Inventory profiles of sociotropic and autonomous subtypes. *Journal of Personality Disorders, 3,* 193–198.

Hirschfeld, R. M. A., & Klerman, G. L. (1979). Personality attributes and affective disorders. *American Journal of Psychiatry, 136,* 67–70.

Hirschfeld, R. M. A., Klerman, G. L., Clayton, P. J., Keller, M. P., McDonald-Scott, P., & Larkin, B. H. (1983). Assessing personality: Effects of the depressive state on trait measurement. *American Journal of Psychiatry, 140,* 195–199.

Julian, T., Metcalfe, M., & Coppen, A. (1969). Aspects of personality of depressive patients. *American Journal of Psychiatry, 115,* 587–589.

Joffe, R., & Regan, J. (1989a). Personality and response to tricyclic antidepressants in depressed patients. *Journal of Nervous and Mental Disease, 177,* 745–749.

Joffe, R., & Regan, J. (1989b). Personality and suicidal behavior in depressed patients. *Comprehensive Psychiatry, 30,* 157–160.

Kendell, R. E., & DiScipio, W. J. (1968). Eysenck Personality Inventory scores of patients with depressive illness. *British Journal of Psychiatry, 114,* 767–770.

Koenigsberg, H., Kaplan, R., Gilmore, M., & Cooper, A. (1985). The relationship between syndrome and personality disorder in the DSM-III: Experience with 2,462 patients. *American Journal of Psychiatry, 142,* 207–212.

Lazare, A., & Klerman, G. L. (1968). Hysteria and depression: The frequency and significance of hysterical personality features in hospitalized depressed women. *American Journal of Psychiatry, 124,* 48–56.

Malec, J., Wolberg, W., Romsaas, E., Trump, D., & Tanner, M. (1988). Millon Clinical Multiaxial Inventory (MCMI) findings among breast clinic patients after initial evaluation and at four or eight month follow-up. *Journal of Clinical Psychology, 44,* 175–180.

McMahon, R., & Davidson, R. (1985a). Transient versus enduring depression among alcoholics in inpatient treatment. *Journal of Psychopathology and Behavioral Assessment, 7,* 317–328.

McMahon, R., & Davidson, R. (1985b). An examination of the relationship between personality patterns and symptom/mood patterns. *Journal of Personality Assessment, 49,* 552–556.

McMahon, R., & Davidson, R. (1986). An examination of depressed vs. nondepressed alcoholics in inpatient treatment. *Journal of Clinical Psychology, 42,* 177–184.

McMahon, R., Flynn, P.M., & Davidson, R. S. (1985). Stability of the personality and symptom scales of the Millon Clinical Multiaxial Inventory. *Journal of Personality Assessment, 49,* 231–234.

McMahon, R., & Tyson, D. (1989, August). *Transient versus enduring depression among alcoholic women.* Paper presented at the convention of the American Psychological Association, New Orleans, LA.

McMahon, R., & Tyson, D. (1990). Personality factors in transient versus enduring depression among inpatient alcoholic women: A preliminary analysis. *Journal of Personality Disorders, 4,* 150–160.

Millon, T. (1987). *Manual for the MCMI-II* (2nd ed.). Minneapolis, MN: National Computer Systems.

Murray, L. G., & Blackburn, I. M. (1974). Personality differences in patients with depressive illness and anxiety neurosis. *Acta Psychiatrica Scandinavica, 50,* 183–191.

Nystrom, S., & Lindegard, B. (1975). Predisposition for mental syndromes: A study comparing predisposition for depression, neurasthenia, and anxiety state. *Acta Psychiatrica Scandinavica, 51,* 69–76.

Overholser, J. C., Kabakoff, R., & Norman, W. H. (1989). The assessment of personality characteristics in depressed and dependent psychiatric inpatients. *Journal of Personality Assessment, 53,* 40–50.

Palmer, H. D., & Sherman, S. H. (1938). Involutional melancholia process. *Archives of Neurology and Psychiatry, 40,* 762.

Perris, C. (1966). A study of bipolar (manic depressive) and unipolar recurrent depressive psychosis: A multidimensional study of personality traits. *Acta Psychiatrica Scandinavica Supplement, 194,* 68–82.

Perris, C. (1971). Personality patterns in patients with affective disorders. *Acta Psychiatrica Scandinavica Supplement, 221,* 43–51.

Pfohl, B., Stangl, D., & Zimmerman, M. (1984). The implications of the DSM-III personality disorders for patients with major depression. *Journal of Affective Disorders, 7,* 309–318.

Piersma, H. L. (1986). The stability of the Millon Clinical Multiaxial Inventory for psychiatric inpatients. *Journal of Personality Assessment, 50,* 193–197.

Piersma, H. L. (1991). The MCMI-II depression scales: Do they assist in differential prediction of depressive disorders? *Journal of Personality Assessment, 56,* 478–486.

Reich, J., & Troughton, E. (1988). Comparison of DSM-III personality disorders in recovered depressed and panic disorder patients. *Journal of Nervous and Mental Disease, 176,* 300–304.

Rosenthal, S. H., & Gudeman, J. E. (1967). The endogenous depressive pattern: An empirical investigation. *Archives of General Psychiatry, 16,* 241.

Shaughnessy, R., Dorus, E., Pandey, G. N., & Davis, J. M. (1980). Personality correlates of platelet monoamine oxidase activity and red blood cell lithium transport. *Psychiatric Research, 2,* 63.

Strandman, E. (1978). "Psychogenic needs" in patients with affective disorders. *Acta Psychiatrica Scandinavica, 58,* 16–29.

von Zerssen, D. (1982). Personality and affective disorders. In E. S. Paykel (Ed.), *Handbook of affective disorders* (pp. 212–228). New York: Guilford Press.

Weissman, M., Prusoff, B., & Klerman, G. (1978). Personality and the prediction of long term outcome of depression. *American Journal of Psychiatry, 135,* 797–800.

Wetzler, S., Kahn, R. S., Cahn, W., van Praag, H. M., & Asnis, G. M. (1990). Psychological test characteristics of depressed and panic patients. *Psychiatry Research, 31,* 179–192.

Wetzler, S., Kahn, R., Strauman, T., & Dubro, A. (1989). Diagnosis of major depression by self-report. *Journal of Personality Assessment, 53,* 22–30.

7 The MCMI/MCMI-II with Substance Abusers

Robert J. Craig, Ph.D.

Although the clinical interview remains the most frequently used procedure to assess substance abuse (Craig, 1988a), there are a number of structured instruments that are also available for this purpose. Two types of assessment inventories have appeared in the literature: (a) Instruments have been developed that were explicitly designed to assess substance abuse and its consequences. Examples of these include the *Addiction Severity Index*, the *Michigan Alcoholism Screening Test*, the *Comprehensive Drinkers Profile*, and the *Substance Abuse Problem Checklist*, and (b) Objective Personality tests that include scales that also assess substance abusing tendencies or problems. The more popular of these include the *Minnesota Multiphasic Personality Inventory-2 (MMPI-2)*, and the *MacAndrew Alcoholism Scale-R*, derived from the MMPI.

The MCMI-II may be used with substance abusers to (a) identify a patient who has a drug abuse problem, (b) assess the personality of a known abuser, and (c) predict meaningful dimensions related to outcome, such as response to treatment, program attrition, or correlates or predictors of abstinence or relapse. The Drug and Alcohol Dependence Scales of the test, independently or in combination with test patterns or configurations, are potentially useful for these purposes.

This chapter reviews the research published to date with the MCMI-II with both alcohol and drug abusing patients, and then provides clinical presentations to demonstrate the utility of this instrument with substance abusers.

Use with Alcoholics

Table 7.1 presents a summary of studies published that has used the MCMI with alcoholics. Rather than present the details of these studies, it is assumed that the

TABLE 7.1
MCMI Studies With Alcoholics

Authors	Population	Sample Size	Type of Study	Results
Bartsch and Hoffman (1985)	male inpatients	125	cluster analysis	5 distinct clusters based on personality style differences
McMahon and Davidson (1985)	predominantly white males; inpatient	96	comparative	alcoholics with enduring depression were more seriously distressed than alcoholics with transient depression
Craig, Verinis, and Wexler (1985)	inpt. black alcoh. inpt. black opiate addicts	106 100	comparative	clusters aligned by personality style and not by drug of choice
McMahon, Flynn, and Davidson (1985a)	inpatient	96	outcome	MCMI scale scores decreased after treatment
McMahon, Flynn, and Davidson (1985b)	inpatient	96	reliability/stability	Scales relatively stable after 30–45 days
McMahon and Davidson (1986a)	predominantly white male inpatients	144	comparative	Depressed alcoholics had different personality styles than nondepressed alcoholics
McMahon and Davidson (1989b)	inpatients	243	correlational	Symptom scales correlated moderately with 5 POMS scales
McMahon, Davidson, and Flynn (1986)	mostly white male inpatients	256	comparative	Low social functioning alcoholics had more severe MCMI profiles than high functioning alcoholics
Hyer et al. (1987)	inpatient	80	descriptive	Alcoholic depression rated as mild
Warner (1987)	alcoholics in treatment	13	descriptive	Dependent and Narcissistic styles most prevalent
Millon (1987)	alcoholics	20; 43	descriptive	presented MCMI-II modal profile
Jaffe and Archer (1987)	undergraduates	190	predictive validity	Scale B significantly correlated with a variety of drug use patterns and categories

Study	Sample	N	Type	Findings
Gualitieri et al. (1987)	inpatient males and females	175	rating narrative reports	Computer generated reports rated as accurate by alcoholism counselors
Retzlaff and Gibertini (1987)	mostly males	250	factor analysis	Found a 3-factor solution: aloof/asocial aggressive/submissive labile/restrained
Tamkin et al. (1987)	male inpatients	67	concurrent validity	MCMI adequately assessed depression in alcoholics
Gibertini and Retzlaff (1988)	Air Force cadets in alcohol rehab	250	factor analysis	4-factor solution: general distress social acting out submissive/aggressive psychotic detached
Lundholm (1989)	undergraduate females	135	predictive validity	Scale B significantly predicted eating disorder
Lorr, Retzlaff, and Tarr (1989)	inpatients	185	factor analysis	Found 6 dimensions for personality scales and 5 for symptom scales when factored separately at item level
McMahon, Gersh, and Davidson (1989)	male inpatients	256	comparative	Continuous drinkers showed different MCMI personality style than episodic drinkers
Miller and Streiner (1990)	psychiatric inpts. with and without alcohol abuse	175	concurrent validity	Scale B identified only 43% of patients with alcohol abuse
McMahon and Tyson (1990)	females	53	comparative	Passive-aggressive style seen among continuous drinkers; compulsive styles seen among episodic drinkers; results similar to males
Bryer et al. (1990)	adult psychiatric (about 20% alcoholic)	561	concurrent validity	Scale B identified 43% of alcoholics
McMahon et al. (1991)	inpatient white males	125	comparative	Continuous drinkers showed different personality styles from episodic drinkers

reader is primarily a clinician, and therefore we present just a summary of this evidence.

MCMI-II Modal Profile with Alcoholics

Assessing alcoholism with any instrument or method is very complex because alcoholism is not a unitary syndrome. There are heterogeneous subpopulations each with distinguishing features. Also, the syndrome covaries with demographic, personality, familial, sociocultural, medical, and other factors that affect its course and development. These facts are to be considered in evaluating the information presented here.

Millon (1987) reported median MCMI-II base-rate (BR) scores for a total of 63 alcoholics. This profile peaked on Passive-Aggressive (8A) and Borderline (C) and had symptom scale elevations on Alcohol Dependence (B) and Drug Dependence (T).

Subsequent studies generally have confirmed Millon's initial modal profile. However, median scores are consistently lower by an average of 20 BR scores on the personality scales, and are consistently lower on the symptom scales as well. Scales P (Paranoid) and 6A (Antisocial) have also been clinically elevated, as have scales A (Anxiety) and D (Dysthymia), although these latter two scales have been ranging higher than Millon's initial data (Bartsch & Hoffman, 1985; Craig, Verinis, & Wexler, 1985; McMahon & Davidson, 1985, 1986a; McMahon, Davidson, & Flynn, 1986; McMahon, Davidson, Gersh, & Flynn, 1991; and McMahon, Gersh, & Davidson, 1989). The reasons for these differences are not immediately obvious, but probably are due to population differences. For example, female alcoholics (N = 53) had elevated scores on scales 3, 8A, C, A, B, and T (McMahon & Tyson, 1990), and ideographic analysis of MCMI profiles reveals individual variations and different personality styles compared to the modal profile (Warner, 1987).

Alcoholic Subtypes

Bartsch and Hoffman (1985), using cluster analysis, found five distinct subtypes, including an antisocial/aggressive type (6A6BT), a narcissistic/histrionic/ antisocial-aggressive type (546ABT), a negativistic/unstable/borderline/passive-aggressive style with neurotic anxiety and depression (8CPBAD), a narcissistic/ antisocial and gregarious type (6A54BT) similar to cluster three, except they showed more discomfort and psychic distress, and a schizoid/avoidant/ dependent group with anxiety and depression (32SDB). Craig et al. (1985) compared alcoholics with opiate addicts and found that the alcoholics scored higher on scales 2, 8A, S, C, SS, and PP. Cluster analysis among 106 alcoholics and 100 opiate addicts aligned by personality style and not by drug of choice, and partially replicated the clusters found by Bartsch and Hoffman (1985).

Depressed alcoholics score differently than nondepressed alcoholics. They have a "detached" personality style (avoidant/asocial) with disorganized thinking and disturbed cognition, that may be a residual effect of chronic drinking, with mild anxiety and depression (Hyer, Harrison, & Jacobsen, 1987; McMahon & Davidson, 1986a; McMahon & Tyson, 1990). Episodic drinkers score higher on Scale 7 (Compulsive) than continuous drinkers, who score higher on Scales 8A, 2, SS, and CC (McMahon et al., 1991; McMahon, Gersh, & Davidson, 1989; and McMahon & Tyson, 1990). Alcoholics whose depression remained clinically elevated after 6 weeks of inpatient treatment scored higher on scales 2, SS, and PP (McMahon & Davidson, 1985). Higher functioning alcoholics score higher on Scale 7, whereas lower functioning alcoholics scored higher on scales 2, S, 8A, SS, CC, B, and C (McMahon, Davidson, & Flynn, 1986).

Scale B (Alcohol Dependence)

Although a modal alcohol MCMI profile may exist, there are too many variables that interact with alcoholism and too many subpopulations of alcoholics to suggest that only one MCMI profile code would reflect all of these variations. However, Scale B would hopefully be more sensitive to these nuances.

Scale B is a 46-item scale whose content deals with excessive drinking, loss of control, impulsivity, guilt, feelings of failure, and family and work problems. The scale is reasonably stable over short intervals, with a median test-retest correlation of .70 across all studies (Craig & Weinberg, 1991).

Scale B shows low to moderate correlations with MMPI Pd (.31), Ma (.39), and MAC (.44) (Millon, 1987), no associations with any of the scales from the Profile of Mood States, but correlated .35 with the Anxiety scale of the Symptom Checklist-Revised (McMahon & Davidson, 1986b).

Millon (1987) reported that Scale B was 89% accurate in identifying the presence of alcoholism, and median BR scores across all studies for Scale B is 92 (Craig & Weinberg, 1991). However, two studies have found that Scale B was not effective in identifying alcoholism in psychiatric patients, though it was quite accurate in identifying patients who do not have an alcohol problem (Bryer, Martines, & Dignan, 1990; Miller & Streiner, 1990). It is important to state that all of this research has been conducted with alcoholics in treatment. No study has used the MCMI in a population motivated to deny alcohol problems. This is a more common problem for clinicians, especially among patients in the early stages of alcoholism.

In summary, the MCMI has been given to over 1,800 alcoholics in the published literature. Preliminary findings indicate that Scale B has good positive predictive power in identifying primary alcoholics and good negative predictive power in identifying patients who do not have alcoholism. It may be less successful in identifying alcohol abuse in psychiatric patients. Stability of Scale B is good over short intervals.

Median MCMI-II profile codes for alcoholics reflect a Passive-Aggressive (8A) and Antisocial (6A) personality style with paranoid (P), and borderline (C) features, with subjective distress characterized by anxiety (A), depression (D) and secondary drug abuse (T). Cluster analysis, however, reveals several distinct MCMI codes suggesting that alcoholism is not a unitary syndrome and one cannot expect to find a code that would be applicable to all alcoholics.

Most of these findings pertain to adult male alcoholics in treatment and it remains to be seen whether these findings generalize to other subpopulations of alcoholics.

We now present examples of how the MCMI-II may be useful in the assessment of individual alcoholics.

Case # 1.   This is a 40-year-old, divorced White male who initially sought outpatient therapy for marital problems associated with his drinking. Due to the insistence of his therapist, he attended an AA meeting but did not return. After several years of sporadically attended therapy, the patient finally agreed to a 28-day inpatient, private, alcohol rehabilitation hospital and remained abstinent for 5 months following discharge. He relapsed and has been drinking daily ever since. He continued to attend marital therapy, drinking before and after each session, and his wife eventually divorced him. He remains depressed, tearful, and guilty at causing the dissolution of his marriage, but continues to drink about five beers at lunch and about ten vodkas after supper. He is steadily employed in the skilled trades and has a supervisor, who is a recovering alcoholic and "supportive" but enabling of this employee's behavior at work. He has also a girlfriend who enables by "not minding" that he drinks. The patient continues to be replete with rationalizations, denial, nervous tension, and depressive-like affect, clouded by a pleasant demeanor and sense of humor, all designed to

TABLE 7.1A
40-Year-Old Male MCMI-II Scores

MCMI-II Scale Scores

Scales	BR Scores	Scales	BR Scores
X	77	S	64
Y	25	C	93
Z	80	P	75
1	74	A	78
2	78	H	55
3	21	N	58
4	61	D	88
5	71	B	93
6A	83	T	87
6B	112	SS	60
7	34	CC	66
8A	111	PP	50
8B	73		

maintain his current behavior and drinking. His MCMI-II scores appear in Table 7.1A:

The MCMI-II modifier indices suggest a slight tendency to exaggerate the severity of his problem, but yet a feeling of vulnerability in being unable to manage his present condition. It suggests he is likely to be self-pitying.

His clinical behavior, suggested by test results, reflects unpredictable moods, a pessimistic outlook, feelings of being cheated and unappreciated, and an irritability stemming from feelings of resentment. He is likely to be hostile and unpredictably angry, negativistic and stubborn, along with periodic outbursts followed by expressions of contrition. Passive-aggressive behaviors and an irascible demeanor can be expected. He is likely to be seen by others as a malcontent who makes those around him miserable with his constant complaining. Alcoholism for this patient may serve the psychological function of containing his frustrations and disappointments, yet it may also produce a disinhibited state where these traits are actually exacerbated. He is inclined to be abusive towards others, perhaps emotionally through his drinking, and maybe even physically, particularly when drunk, since he seems to lack empathy and struggles with issues of self-assertion. While he has a significant amount of anxiety and depression, it cannot be determined if these are alcohol-induced via chronic drinking or if they are related to poor psychological adjustment stemming from his divorce.

Case # 2.   This is a 32-year-old unmarried Mexican American male in an alcohol rehab program. He had been living with his mother but stole her TV and VCR to get money for cocaine. Although she will not allow him back in the house, he has been sleeping on her front porch.

He has a 7-year history of alcohol abuse, but recently switched to cocaine freebasing for the past 2 years. He becomes belligerent under the influence of alcohol, walking into bars wielding a gun or knife and threatening various people he does not know, though he had never harmed anyone. He has a history of physical abuse from his father of rather long duration. He witnessed his father hang his stepbrother upside down as a punishment, and father was also physically abusive towards patient's mother, who later separated and divorced her husband due to his alcoholism. In high school the patient was sexually abused and retains much guilt over this matter. He cried when revealing this information, but otherwise did not show any signs of depression.

He has held a series of odd jobs and was treated for alcohol abuse on three other occasions, but relapses immediately after discharge. He was also treated for alcoholism while in the Army. He has never dated and seems to lack sexual interest.

In the treatment program he was a loner, rarely relating to any patient or staff, expressed a degree of uncomfortableness in group therapy, and did not generally participate or become involved in this modality. He seemed to do better in individual sessions. His MCMI-II scores appear in Table 7.1B.

TABLE 7.1B
32-Year-Old Mexican American

MCMI-II Scale Scores

Scales	BR Scores	Scales	BR Scores
X	83	S	71
Y	50	C	67
Z	70	P	67
1	117	A	77
2	112	H	55
3	90	N	35
4	22	D	79
5	37	B	94
6A	53	T	65
6B	62	SS	61
7	74	CC	58
8A	67	PP	58
8B	116		

The MCMI-II profile suggests a person who is basically an introversive, dependent, compliant, and placating person who blends into the background. Though he tries not to be a burden and is reluctant to ask for help, he has a strong need to be dependent on others, viewing himself as weak and ineffectual. He has a mildly anxious but chronic dysphoria, and is particularly vulnerable to threats of separation and loss of security. There is a compulsive and self-defeating aspect to his behavior. He is not inherently antisocial in personality but has begun to engage in antisocial behavior in order to acquire money for cocaine. This resulted in his loss of security and threatened permanent separation. Hence he sought a supportive institution to restore his needs for security, probably more so than for treatment of his alcohol and drug problem.

Case # 3.   This patient is a 26-year-old, never-married, White male seen in an outpatient mental health setting. His psychological state, upon initial contact, was characterized by extreme evasiveness, anxiety, headaches, mood-congruent obsessions with religious and occasional delusional thoughts (frightened by the Apocalypse, concerns about sorcery), withdrawn behavior, and excessive bible reading. His personality was described as reserved, sensitive to criticism, shy, (never dated), and emotionally detached. He acts like a door mat, but seems to have become depressed, and then delusional. He has 3 DUIs and recently lost his job in an auto repair garage. His MCMI-II scores appear in Table 7.1C.

The MCMI-II reflects a Schizoid personality pattern with pervasive Dysthymia and recurring periods of anxiety, dependent behaviors, and difficulties in coping with societal and familial demands and responsibilities. This patient seeks people who will take care of him, avoids autonomous behaviors, suppresses his anger and resentment over his caretakers, and assumes a passive, submissive role

TABLE 7.1C
26-Year-Old White Male

MCMI-II Scale Scores

Scales	BR Scores	Scales	BR Scores
X	66	S	69
Y	43	C	51
Z	73	P	48
1	121	A	80
2	85	H	56
3	77	N	12
4	06	D	85
5	38	B	75
6A	52	T	54
6B	41	SS	69
7	71	CC	67
8A	47	PP	57
8B	70		

in relationships in order to fulfill his dependency needs. He is conciliatory, overly concerned with social rebuff, and prefers to maintain an emotional distance in interpersonal relationships. He tends to become absorbed in daydreams and appears sluggish and aloof. His needs for closeness and affection are denied and he shows a depressive blandness that masks a mix of inhibited anger, anxiety and resentment. The pattern suggests severe maladjustment, blunted affect and eccentric behavior. He seems caught between feelings of loneliness and social apprehension. We can speculate that alcohol serves to produce self-assurance and increased confidence, and reduces social anxiety while in social contact, thereby allowing him to relate more comfortably to others. It may also temporarily reduce his psychic pain and feelings of loneliness. It was somewhat surprising that the Schizotypal Scale (S) and Thought Disorder Scale (SS) were not in the clinically significant range, given his psychotic-like thinking.

Use with Drug Abusers

Table 7.2 presents a listing of all studies that have used the MCMI with a drug abusing population. Once again, we present the essential conclusions from this evidence.

MCMI Modal Profile with Drug Abusers

Millon (1987) presented the median MCMI-II profile for drug dependent patients, based on a total of 78 cases. This profile showed peak elevations on Antisocial (6A), and secondary elevations on Aggressive/Sadistic (6B), Passive-Aggressive (8A), Narcissistic (5), Histrionic (4), and Borderline (C). Clinically

TABLE 7.2
MCMI Studies With Drug Abusers

Authors	Population	Sample Size	Type of Study	Results
Flynn and McMahon (1983a)	Drug abusers (unspecified)	161	Reliability study of the Drug Dependence Scale	Stability coefficients ranged from .45 to .74, depending on temporal interval studied
Flynn and McMahon (1983b)	Addicts on methadone; drug free outpatient; or in residential treatment	88	Criterion validity study for the two depression scales	Dysthymia and major depression scales had low correlations with survey intake data dealing with depression and suicidal ideation
Craig (1984a)	Opiate addicts	100	Compared program dropouts with completers	No significant differences between groups on any scale
Flynn and McMahon (1984a)	Addicts on methadone; drug free outpatient; or in residential treatment	139	Stability of Drug Dependence Scale	Mean BR score was 83; Drug Dependence Scale was stable after 1 and 3 months of treatment
Flynn and McMahon (1984b)	Same as above sample	139	Factor analysis	Three factor-structure was found that were similar to the factors found with other populations
McMahon, Flynn, and Davidson (1985)	Same as above sample	86	Stability estimates in scale scores with 1 to 3 months of treatment	Addicts showed few changes in personality scores and no changes in symptom scale scores
Craig, Verinis, and Wexler (1985)	Opiate addicts Alcoholics	100 106	Comparative study	Cluster analysis showed four basic personality styles grouped by personality pattern and not by drug of choice
McMahon and Davidson (1986b)	Mixed addicts and alcoholics in inpatient treatment	243	Concurrent/ convergent validity	Moderate associations between the symptom scales and the POMS
Siddall (1986)	MCMI profiles from 100 substance abusers	100	Descriptive utility of computer reports	Clinicians rated MCMI reports as accurate and useful

Study	Sample	N	Approach	Findings
Jaffe and Archer (1987)	College students	186	Predictive validity	Alcohol Dependence Scale had associations in predicting college drug use than Drug Dependence Scale
Calsyn and Saxon (1988)	Opiate addicts and polydrug abusers	45 31	Cluster analysis	Opiate addicts scored higher on Scale 6A; polydrug abusers scored higher on Scales 1, 2, and 8A
Marsh et al. (1988)	Addicts on methadone	159	Convergent validity	Drug Dependence Scale did not identify 51% of addicts in treatment; MCMI scales had low correlations with MMPI
Craig (1988b)	Opiate addicts	121	Study of prevalence rates of personality disorders	Rates were comparable to those determined from structured psychiatric interviews
Stark and Campbell (1988)	Polydrug abusers in outpatient clinic	100	Predictive validity	Program completers scored higher on 7 scales, showing more psychopathology
Dougherty and Lesswing (1989)	Inpatient cocaine addicts	100	Descriptive	Mixed, Borderline, and Narcissistic disorders accounted for 50% of the cases
Craig and Olson (1990)	Cocaine abusers	107	Comparative	4 different personality styles revealed by cluster analysis; prevalence rates of personality disorders similar between groups
Calsyn, Saxon, and Daisy (1990)	Opiate addicts Cocaine addicts	49 22	Concurrent validity	Drug Dependence Scale classified correctly 39% of addicts
Calsyn and Saxon (1990)	Opiate and cocaine inpatient addicts	243	Descriptive	Both groups had high rates of Narcissistic and Antisocial, Dependent and Withdrawn/Negative disorders
Bryer et al. (1990)	Adult psychiatric with drug abuse problems	561	Concurrent validity	43% of alcoholics and 49% of drug abusers successfully identified by Scales B and T

elevated scores appeared on the Drug Dependence Scale (T) and a secondary elevation on Alcohol Dependence (B). An inspection of studies that reported BR scores for drug abusing populations have tended to corroborate this modal profile (Craig, 1984b; Craig & Olson, 1990; Craig, Verinis, & Wexler, 1985; Marsh, Stile, Stoughton, & Trout-Lamden, 1988; and Stark & Campbell, 1988). Both the Narcissistic and Antisocial Scales are among the two most often elevated personality disorder scales, along with Paranoid (P), which may be an artifact, and Drug Dependence (T) as the most elevated clinical syndrome scale with Alcohol Dependence (B) showing secondary elevations. This pattern appears for both opiate and cocaine addicts and reflects a character disorder with little subjective distress. This finding is interesting because it provides a level of consensual validation for the MCMI-II in this area, since the finding is similar to that observed with median MMPI profiles for the same kinds of patients (Craig, 1982, 1984b).

Although MCMI studies have found few differences between opiate and co-caine addicts in terms of personality style (Craig & Olson, 1990; Calsyn & Saxon, 1988; Calsyn, Saxon, & Daisy, 1990), and although both groups show significant narcissistic and antisocial traits that are similarly reflected on other major personality instruments, it would be a mistake to believe that such findings represent *the* addict personality. Cluster analysis of addict profiles reveal mean-ingful subgroups or "types" that align, not by drug of choice, but rather by underlying personality style. Although the narcissistic/antisocial style represents a large subgroup, research also found a passive-aggressive/withdrawn style, a basically dependent type, and addicts with significant underlying psycho-pathology who would be considered psychiatric patients (Calsyn & Saxon, 1988, 1990; Craig & Olson, 1990; and Craig, Verinis, & Wexler, 1985). Similar find-ings also appear in the MMPI literature (Craig & Olson, 1992), suggesting that these findings are veridical.

Drug Dependence Scale (T)

Scale T is a 58-item scale that assesses recent or recurrent drug abuse. Item content deals directly with drug abuse behaviors and indirectly, by assessing problems with impulse control, difficulties adhering to societal standards, and the traits of extroversion, mania, and paranoia. Median stability coefficients for Scale T range from .41 to .83, with a median of .73, and an internal consistency estimate of .87. The scale correlates .37 with MMPI Pd, .59 with Ma, .51 with MAC, .43 with Wiggins HOS, and .42 with AUT (Craig & Weinberg, 1991). McMahon and Davidson (1986b) found that it correlated .27 with Profile of Mood States (POMS) Anger-Hostility, and .20 with Vigor-Activity. The scale is relatively stable, suggesting it is measuring enduring personality traits in addition to substance abuse.

Validity Studies

The evidence is mixed with respect to Scale T's concurrent validity. Drug addicts, both opiate and cocaine, have mean BR scores in the 70s and 80s in all studies that reported the data (Craig, 1984b; Craig & Olson, 1990; Craig et al., 1985; Flynn & McMahon, 1984a; Marsh et al., 1988; and Stark & Campbell, 1988). Yet studies have found some difficulty in the ability of this scale to detect drug abuse. Only 39%–49% of patients in treatment for drug abuse have been successfully identified by the scale (Bryer et al., 1990; Calsyn et al., 1990; and Marsh et al., 1988). Millon (1987) reported the sensitivity of Scale T was 72% with a specificity of 98% when the BR score was >74, and 62% when the BR score was >84.

Prevalence Rates of Personality Disorder

When one compares the prevalence rates of personality disorders among drug addicts, determined by the MCMI, with those determined by structured personality instruments, these rates are quite concordant (Craig, 1988b; Craig & Olson, 1990; and Dougherty & Lesswing, 1989). However, there is some evidence that the MCMI overdiagnoses paranoia among substance abusers (Craig & Olson, 1990; Craig et al., 1985; and Siddall, 1986). This may be due to the 17 redundant items that appear on both Scales T and P. This may not be as serious as it appears. Drug addicts have many false positives on initial screening for venereal disease. Physicians, knowing this, then order a more refined test for diagnostic accuracy. Similarly, clinicians, knowing that the MCMI may provide "false positive" elevations on Paranoid among drug abusers can simply ignore it, or, more probably, conduct a closer clinical evaluation with the patient to determine its accuracy.

Predictive Validity

There is a dearth of research with the MCMI in the area of predictive validity. One study found no differences between program completers and dropouts on MCMI scales (Craig, 1984a), while another study found that program completers had more psychopathology across seven different MCMI scales (Stark & Campbell, 1988). Jaffe and Archer (1987) reported that the Drug Dependence Scale was significantly associated with a number of drug use categories among college students, but the Alcohol Dependence accurately predicted more categories of use.

In summary, the MCMI has been given to over 2,000 drug abusers in the published literature. The Drug Dependence Scale generally is elevated in the clinical ranges among addicts in treatment, yet ideographic analysis indicates that the scale has had some problems in reliably detecting drug abuse, with "hit rates" hovering around 50%. No study has reported on the Scale's ability to detect drug abuse in a person who is motivated to deny it. There seems to be a reliable modal MCMI profile that reflects an Antisocial/Narcissistic character type, but cluster analysis also reveals at least four common personality types appear with this population. Prevalence rates of personality disorders among addicts determined by the MCMI are quite similar to those established by structured psychiatric interviews. So far there has been little predictive validity research with this population.

The following cases illustrate how the MCMI-II can be helpful in assessing drug abusers.

Case # 1. The patient is a 37-year-old, Black, male in a drug abuse treatment program. He is married and has two children. Although he is employed full time as a laborer, he has a law degree but has been unable to pass the bar exam.

Drug use began in Viet Nam, where he was in combat. He has a history of PTSD symptoms but none currently. He has been taking heroin for the past 11 years, using a $10.00 bag every week. This is his first time in treatment but alleges depression since age 19, when he joined the military. He sought outpatient treatment prior to service for "shyness," but never followed through after the initial appointment. He says he has an inferiority complex and has been withdrawing from people since childhood. He was the 9th of 11 children and described his parents as "beautiful people." He came for drug rehab due to pressure from wife, who also complained that he spends an inordinate time in the basement watching TV and not conversing with her. On a Patient Goals checklist, he listed the following items for treatment: Increase my self-respect, feel more self-confident, feel more cheerful and optimistic, avoid the use of drugs, and avoid depression. His MCMI-II scores appear in Table 7.2A.

TABLE 7.2A
37-Year-Old Black Male

MCMI-II Scale Scores

Scales	BR Scores	Scales	BR Scores
X	66	S	64
Y	43	C	53
Z	65	P	47
1	116	A	61
2	105	H	54
3	102	N	00
4	26	D	81
5	19	B	55
6A	13	T	48
6B	00	SS	65
7	61	CC	67
8A	44	PP	40
8B	73		

The patient's MCMI-II profile seems quite isomorphic with his case history. He has an emotionally detached personality style with chronic dysphoria. Interestingly, his drug abuse seems quite mild and this is correlated with frequency and amount of use. His wife was more upset with his interpersonal behavior than with his drug abuse. This behavior can be characterized by a general sluggishness, aloofness, and social awkwardness in social interaction. He seems to be a person who wants affection, closeness, and intimacy but is so concerned with social rebuff that he anticipates rejection and thereby does not initiate any autonomous behaviors, in order to protect himself from this perceived threat. We can expect him to be conciliatory and submissive, seeking out dependent relationships so that he can maintain a passive role in order to be nurtured by others. We can speculate that this interpersonal style was learned in childhood, perhaps because he did not receive close attention to basic needs due to the large number of children in his family and to other parental factors, thereby experiencing parental deprivation of affectional needs. His heroin use keeps him in a dependent and self-defeating pattern, though momentarily it provides him with a drug-induced ego state that provides him with a good feeling about himself that he does not normally experience.

The next two cases integrate MCMI-II findings with the MMPI-2, and illustrates how these two tests may be used as an objective test battery to refine the overall assessment (see Antoni's chapter, in this book for additional details.)

Case #2.   Patient is a 49-year-old, married, Black female, evaluated while in a 21-day residential treatment program for drug abuse. She has an MA in Education and has worked as an elementary school teacher for over 20 years. Though presently married, her husband is in jail awaiting his release.

Her pattern of drug abuse reflects sporadic alcohol and marijuana use as a teen ager, amphetamine use in college for weight control and to "improve study habits," and IV cocaine abuse, (onset 10 years ago) introduced to her by her current husband, who supplied her drugs and gave her the injections. Her use was initially confined to weekends, increased during the summers, after which she would reduce the frequency of use prior to returning to her job as a school teacher, but she eventually became dependent on heroin and cocaine. About 5 years ago her husband was imprisoned and she found other addicts to inject her. She had a 2-year period of methadone maintenance. Recently her attempts to control illicit drug use were unsuccessful and her employer insisted she complete a drug rehabilitation program. She is currently on an unpaid leave of absence.

She reports a family history where she was catered to and spoiled by her parents. She married in her early 20s, but her husband was a womanizer. She insisted on fidelity, leading to a separation and divorce after 3 years. Some years later, she remarried a man 10 years her junior, describing him as attractive, exciting, charismatic, and attentive. However, as their relationship developed, he became domineering, exploiting and physically abusive. He was also a drug

TABLE 7.2B
49-Year-Old Black Female

MMPI-II
Scores

Scales	T Score	Scales	T Score	Scales	T Score
L(R2)	43	ANX	64	WRK	63
F(R#)	48	FRS	59	TRT	59
K(R9)	37	OBS	53	MAC-R	R21
Hs	63	DEP	62	A	62
Dep	64	HEA	72	R	44
Hy	43	BIZ	47	Es	41
Pd	58	ANG	64	Hy2	34
Mf	40	CYN	69	Pd5	72
Pa	39	ASP	66	Ma1	70
Pt	51	TPA	73	Si3	69
Sc	53	LSE	52		
Ma	53	SOD	52		
Si	32	FAM	57		

MCMI-II Scores

Scales	BR Score	Scales	BR Score
X	65	S	58
Y	45	C	64
Z	78	P	67
1	66	A	87
2	73	H	63
3	98	N	49
4	77	D	88
5	37	B	62
6A	60	T	71
6B	66	SS	60
7	49	CC	64
8A	78	PP	60
8B	96		

addict. His physical abuse was often brutal. She reports that he held a shotgun to her head on the bed, beat her and threatened to kill her if she ever left him. When he was jailed, her life improved somewhat, though all of her friends are drug abusers. Her husband will soon be released from prison and she is faced with what to do about the relationship.

Her operative diagnosis is Opioid Dependence, severe and Cocaine Dependence, moderate. Precipitating stresses were threatened job suspension and marital conflict pending release of husband from jail. Her test scores appear in Table 7.2B.

Her MMPI-2 profile reflects a person with low self-esteem, who is overly self-critical with feelings of inadequacy, some somatic concerns that are probably related to drug withdrawal states, low self-esteem, and mild anxiety and depression. Interpersonally, she appears to be passive-dependent in relationships, requires much reassurance due to her feelings of alienation, and cynical and negative in her attitudes towards life. She admits to engaging in antisocial practices, but this appears to be socially determined rather than an intrinsic personality trait. This pattern seems quite stable and not situationally based. She does not appear to be under much manifest immediate stress at the present time and level of symptom expression at this time appears to be low.

Her MCMI-II profile reflects a woman whose behavior is characterized by excessive dependency and martyr-like behaviors. She shows dependency, an anxious seeking of reassurance from others coupled with behaviors that undo the support she seeks. She tends to allow others to exploit and mistreat her, though this has resulted in periodic occasions where she becomes erratically moody and withdrawn. She seems to seek relationships where she can conclude that she "deserves" to suffer. She vacillates between being pleasant and agreeable and passive-aggressive, trying to induce guilt in people for their disinterest or for their abuse. Although she appears self-sacrificing and obliging, she may actually provoke people by questioning the sincerity of their support for her. Anxiety and depression seem paramount clinical symptoms, while her drug abuse is of moderate intensity.

Both tests reflect her dependency, low self-esteem, need for reassurance, anxiety and depression, and sense of personal alienation. The MCMI-II adds the self-defeating aspect not tapped by the MMPI-2.

Case # 3.   The patient is a 39-year-old divorced, White male in drug rehab. He has a 21-year history of episodic heroin abuse and a current 3-year history of cocaine freebasing. He has been treated twice before for drug abuse problems and maintained substantial periods of remission (9 years and 7 years, respectively) after each treatment episode.

Each drug use episode has been associated with significant stressful events. Initially he began drug use in Viet Nam where he was bored, scared, and seeking acceptance from fellow soldiers, who offered him the drug. Some time later, he relapsed after losing his job, his marriage, and his mother, who died from natural causes, all within a few months of each other. At this time he also made an unsuccessful suicide attempt by tying a basketball net around his neck and tried to hang himself from the basketball rim. The precipitant for his most recent treatment episode was that his girlfriend, with whom he had been living for 3 years, left him for another man. He has been on a 3-year cocaine run ever since.

The patient does not appear depressed, but he does become pensive with apparent remaining grief when discussing his mother's death. There were no other clinical signs of importance upon mental status exam. His test scores appear in Table 7.2C.

The MMPI-2 reflects a person who was quite defensive in responding to the test items, and who tried to place himself in a favorable light. The one area of exception is his complaints about physical malfunctioning, vague physical com-

TABLE 7.2C
39-Year-Old White Male

MMPI-II
Scores

L R(8)	T 70	ANX	T 57
F R(3)	T 45	FRS	T 51
K R(26)	T 72	OBS	T 37
Hs	T 77	DEP	T 58
D	T 74	HEA	T 60
Hy	T 89	BIZ	T 39
Pd	T 84	ANG	T 36
Mf	T 50	CYN	T 32
Pa	T 75	ASP	T 37
Pt	T 70	TPA	T 36
Sc	T 58	LSE	T 35
Ma	T 47	SOD	T 45
Si	T 48	FAM	T 41
A	T 43	WRK	T 48
R	T 63	TRT	T 47
MAC-R	R 23	OH	T 62

MCMI-II Scores

Scales	BR Score	Scales	BR Score
X	40	S	46
Y	75	C	53
Z	42	P	55
1	48	A	65
2	41	H	63
3	71	N	44
4	69	D	35
5	69	B	63
6A	59	T	65
6B	54	SS	45
7	64	CC	67
8A	22	PP	59
8B	33		

plaints without a coherent symptom picture, and general fatigue. Also, he feels that others are not sympathetic to his perceived health problems. He is an exploiting, self-centered, and dependent person who may be controlling others by his complaints of physical symptoms. He is quite passive-aggressive, sullenly angry, and projects much of the blame for his problems onto others. The MMPI-2 suggests a somatoform disorder in a dependent, passive-aggressive personality, though the possibility exists of malingering associated with insurance claims.

The MCMI-II reflects his dependent personality, fears of abandonment, his submissive stance in interpersonal relationships, and his desire to avoid conflict. He seems alert to rejection and tries to be conciliatory. However, he has a self-centeredness and oppositional stance that is likely to protrude in moments of stress and the histrionic component to his complaints, plus the manner in which he tries to elicit support via dramatic demands, are more likely to elicit an antagonistic response from those whose support he is trying to maintain.

The combined use of the MMPI-2 and the MCMI-II gives us a clearer picture of this patient. Both tests detected his oppositional and exploiting nature, his underlying dependency, and the histrionic quality to much of his behavior. Though the MMPI-2 presented a more severe pattern of somatoform disorder than that portrayed by the MCMI-II, we can surmise that his physical complaints are more of the histrionic variety, designed to draw attention to himself and to elicit sympathy and support, thereby recapturing his security and providing him with a haven that will continue to cater to his dependency. This interpersonal style correlates with the stressful events that preceded the onset of his drug use and with the periods of remission when those dependency needs had been fulfilled once again.

REFERENCES

Bartsch, T. W., & Hoffman, J. J. (1985). A cluster analysis of Millon Clinical Multiaxial Inventory (MCMI) profiles: More about a taxonomy of alcoholic subtypes. *Journal of Clinical Psychology, 41*, 707–713.

Bryer, J. B., Martines, K. A., & Dignan, M. A. (1990). Millon Clinical Multiaxial Inventory Alcohol Abuse and Drug Abuse scales and the identification of substance-abuse patients. *Psychological Assessment: A Journal of Consulting Psychology, 4*, 438–441.

Calsyn, D., & Saxon, A. J. (1988). Identification of personality disorder subtypes among drug abusers using the Millon Clinical Multiaxial Inventory. 49th Annual Scientific Meeting of the Committee on Problems of Drug Dependence, 1987. *National Institute on Drug Abuse: Research Monograph Series*. Rockville, MD, p. 299.

Calsyn, D. A., & Saxon, A. J. (1990). Personality disorder subtypes among cocaine and opioid addicts using the Millon Clinical Multiaxial Inventory. *International Journal of the Addictions, 25*, 1037–1049.

Calsyn, D. A., Saxon, A. J., & Daisy, F. (1990). Validity of the MCMI Drug Abuse Scale with drug abusing and psychiatric samples. *Journal of Clinical Psychology, 46*, 244–246.

Craig, R. J. (1982). Personality characteristics of heroin addicts: Review of empirical research. *International Journal of the Addictions, 17*, 227–248.

Craig, R. J. (1984a). Can personality tests predict treatment dropouts? *International Journal of the Addictions, 19*, 665–674.

Craig, R. J. (1984b). A comparison of MMPI profiles of heroin addicts based on multiple methods of classification. *Journal of Personality Assessment, 48*, 115–120.

Craig, R. J. (1988a). Diagnostic interviewing with drug abusers. *Professional Psychology: Research and Practice, 19*, 14–20.

Craig, R. J. (1988b). A psychometric study of the prevalence of DSM-III personality disorders among treated opiate addicts. *International Journal of the Addictions, 23*, 115–124.

Craig, R. J., & Olson, R. E. (1992). MMPI subtypes of cocaine abusers. *American Journal of Drug and Alcohol Abuse*, 197–205.

Craig, R. J., & Olson, R. E. (1990). MCMI comparisons of cocaine abusers and heroin addicts. *Journal of Clinical Psychology, 46*, 231–237.

Craig, R. J., Verinis, J. S., & Wexler, S. (1985). Personality characteristics of drug addicts and alcoholics: Admission, discharge, and outcome comparisons. *Journal of Personality Assessment, 49,* 156–160.

Craig, R. J., & Weinberg, D. (1991). *The Millon Clinical Multiaxial Inventory: A clinical information synthesis.* Unpublished manuscript. Chicago, Illinois.

Dougherty, R. J., & Lesswing, N. J. (1989). Inpatient cocaine abusers: An analysis of psychological and demographic variables. *Journal of Substance Abuse Treatment, 6,* 45–47.

Flynn, P., & McMahon, R. C. (1983a). Stability of the Drug Misuse Scale of the Millon Clinical Multiaxial Inventory. *Psychological Reports, 52,* 536–538.

Flynn, P., & McMahon, R. C. (1983b). Indicators of depression and suicidal ideation among drug abusers. *Psychological Reports, 52,* 784–786.

Flynn, P., & McMahon, R. C. (1984a). An examination of the Drug Abuse Scale of the Millon Clinical Multiaxial Inventory. *International Journal of the Addictions, 19,* 459–468.

Flynn, P., & McMahon, R. C. (1984b). An examination of the factor structure of the Millon Clinical Multiaxial Inventory. *Journal of Personality Assessment, 48,* 308–311.

Gibertini, M., & Retzlaff, P. D. (1988). Factor invariance of the Millon Clinical Multiaxial Inventory. *Journal of Psychopathology and Behavioral Assessment, 10,* 65–74.

Gualtieri, J., Gonzales, E., & Baldwin, N. (1987). The accuracy of MCMI computerized narratives for alcoholics. In C. Green (Ed.), *Conference on the Millon inventories (MCMI, MBHI, MAPI)* (pp. 263–268). Minneapolis: National Computer Systems.

Hyer, L., Harrison, W. R., & Jacobsen, R. H. (1987). Later-life depression: Influences of irrational thinking and cognitive impairment. *Journal of Rational-Emotive Therapy, 5,* 43–48.

Jaffe, L. T., & Archer, R. P. (1987). The prediction of drug use among college students from MMPI, MCMI and Sensation Seeking Scales. *Journal of Personality Assessment, 51,* 243–253.

Lorr, M., Retzlaff, P. D., & Tarr, H. C. (1989). An analysis of the MCMI-I at the item level. *Journal of Clinical Psychology, 45,* 884–890.

Lundholm, J. K. (1989). Alcohol use among university females: Relationship to eating disordered behavior. *Addictive Behaviors, 14,* 181–185.

Marsh, D. T., Stile, S. A., Stoughton, N. L., & Trout-Landen, B. L. (1988). Psychopathology of opiate addiction: Comparative data from the MMPI and MCMI. *American Journal of Drug and Alcohol Abuse, 14,* 17–27.

McMahon, R. C., & Davidson, R. S. (1985). Transient versus enduring depression among alcoholics in inpatient treatment. *Journal of Psychopathology and Behavioral Assessment, 7,* 317–328.

McMahon, R. C., & Davidson, R. S. (1986a). An examination of depressed vs. nondepressed alcoholics in inpatient treatment. *Journal of Clinical Psychology, 42,* 177–184.

McMahon, R. C., & Davidson, R. S. (1986b). Concurrent validity of the clinical symptom syndrome scales of the Millon Clinical Multiaxial Inventory. *Journal of Clinical Psychology, 42,* 908–912.

McMahon, R. C., Davidson, R. S., & Flynn, P. M. (1986). Psychological correlates and treatment outcomes for high and low social functioning alcoholics. *International Journal of the Addictions, 21,* 819–835.

McMahon, R. C., Davidson, R. S., Gersh, D., & Flynn, P. M. (1991). A comparison of continuous and episodic drinkers using the MCMI, MMPI, and ALCEVAL-R. *Journal of Clinical Psychology, 47,* 21–31.

McMahon, R. C., Flynn, P. M., & Davidson, R. S. (1985). The personality and symptom scales of the Millon Clinical Multiaxial Inventory: Sensitivity to posttreatment outcomes. *Journal of Clinical Psychology, 41,* 862–866.

McMahon, R. C., Gersh, D., & Davidson, R. S. (1989). Personality and symptom characteristics of continuous vs. episodic drinkers. *Journal of Clinical Psychology, 45,* 161–168.

McMahon, R. C., & Tyson, D. (1990). Personality factors in transient versus enduring depression among inpatient alcoholic women: A preliminary analysis. *Journal of Personality Disorders, 4,* 150–160.

Miller, H. R., & Streiner, D. L. (1990). Using the Millon Clinical Multiaxial Inventory's Scale B and the MacAndrew Alcoholism Scale to identify alcoholics with concurrent psychiatric diagnosis. *Journal of Personality Assessment, 54,* 736–746.

Millon, T. (1987). *Millon Clinical Multiaxial Inventory-II: Manual for the MCMI-II.* Minneapolis: National Computer Systems.

Retzlaff, P. D., & Gibertini, M. (1987). Factor structure of the MCMI basic personality scales and common-item artifact. *Journal of Personality Assessment, 51,* 588–594.

Siddall, J. W. (1986). Use of the MCMI with substance abusers. *Noteworthy Responses, 2,* 1–3.

Stark, M. J., & Campbell, B. K. (1988). Personality, drug use, and early attrition from substance abuse treatment. *American Journal of Drug and Alcohol Abuse, 14,* 475–485.

Tamkin, A. S., Carson, M. F., Nixon, D. H., & Hyer, L. A. (1987). A comparison among some measures of depression in male alcoholics. *Journal of Studies on Alcohol, 48,* 176–178.

Warner, J. S. (1987). Use of the Millon Clinical Multiaxial Inventory (MCMI) in an alcoholism halfway house program. In C. Green (Ed.), *Conference on the Millon clinical inventories (MCMI, MBHI, MAPI)* (pp. 269–272). Minneapolis: National Computer Systems.

8 The Use of the MCMI with Eating Disorders

Martha Tisdale, Ph.D.
Linda Pendleton, Ph.D.

There have been relatively few studies utilizing the MCMI with an eating disordered population. Chandarana, Holliday, Conlon, and DeSlippe (1988), looking at pre- and post-gastric stapling surgery patients, found that the postsurgery group had lower mean scores on the Schizoid and Schizotypal scales. Both groups were above the normal range on the Anxiety scale. Identifying an eating disordered group within the university population, Lundholm (1989) utilized the MCMI to determine alcohol abuse within this group. Alcohol abusers were noted to be dissatisfied with themselves whereas infrequent users of alcohol were generally dissatisfied with others; these conclusions were based on Eating Disorder Inventory (EDI; Garner & Olmsted, 1984) scores. The MCMI scores were only employed in identifying level of alcohol use, not for purposes of personality description.

In one study utilizing the MCMI with an eating disordered population, Tracy, Norman, and Weisberg (1987) compared MCMI scores of anorexics with bulimics. Anorexics were found to score significantly higher on the Schizoid and Avoidant scales whereas the bulimic group scored higher on the Histrionic and Narcissistic scales. Both groups showed elevation on the Passive Aggressive scale and relatively high numbers of bulimics and anorexics fell above the cutoff for the Borderline or Schizotypal scales. Both anorexic and bulimic patients demonstrated high levels of anxiety, depression, and a tendency towards somatization. However, conclusions to be drawn from this are limited by the small sample size (21 bulimics, 10 anorexics). Even more problematic is the fact that, as noted by the authors, "very few" of the anorexic sample were purely restricting. Previous literature suggests anorexics with bulimic symptoms are more similar in personality structure to bulimics than they are to restricting anorexics (Johnson & Connors, 1987). An additional difficulty with this study is the absence of report of actual scale elevations.

Lepkowsky (1987) compared MCMI profile elevations of anorexics, bulimics, and depressed neurotic controls. In comparing anorexics with bulimics, bulimics were found to score significantly lower on the Compulsive scale but higher on the Histrionic scale. Although this difference was not significant, the bulimics scored higher than anorexics on the Borderline scale. No significant differences were found between bulimics and anorexics on the Clinical Symptom Syndrome and Psychotic Features scales. Relative to depressed neurotics, bulimics scored significantly higher on the Avoidant, Borderline, and Schizotypal Scales as well as on the Somatoform scale.

In a second study comparing anorexics, bulimics, and compulsive overeaters, bulimics scored significantly higher than compulsive overeaters on the Avoidant, Dependent, Antisocial, and Borderline scales. The bulimics also scored higher on the Anxiety, Somatoform, Dysthymic, and Psychotic Depression scales. In comparing bulimics and anorexics, bulimics again scored higher on the Histrionic scale. Other differences between anorexics and bulimics that did not appear in the first study include higher elevation for the bulimics on the Antisocial and Passive-Aggressive scales as well as a greater elevation reaching statistical significance on the Borderline Scale. There were no differences between anorexics and bulimics on the Clinical Symptom Syndrome scales.

In one of three studies comparing eating disordered women with normal controls, Lundholm, Pellegreno, Wolins, and Graham (1989) examined individual item content on the MCMI and found that women receiving treatment for bulimia were characterized by social withdrawal and depression. Tisdale, Pendleton, and Marler (1990) reported profile elevations on the Basic Personality Patterns and Pathological Personality Disorders of the MCMI for bulimics, general psychiatric outpatients, and normal controls. Bulimic women were found to score higher than the other groups on the Schizoid, Avoidant, and Dependent Scales. They also scored lower than the other two groups on the Antisocial Scale. Both the bulimic and the outpatient groups scored significantly higher than the normal control group on the Borderline Scale. Pendleton, Tisdale, and Marler (1990) also examined bulimics, general psychiatric outpatients, and normal controls on these same scales but looked at percentage of subjects exceeding a cutoff of 84. A significantly greater percentage of bulimics scored above the cutoff on the Avoidant and Dependent Scales than did the outpatients and normals. In addition, the percentage of bulimics scoring above the cutoff was greater than that of normals on the following scales: Schizoid, Passive-Aggressive, Schizotypal, and Borderline.

Studies comparing performance of bulimics and anorexics on the MCMI have consistently reported greater elevations for bulimics on the Histrionic Scale. The Narcissistic, Antisocial, Passive-Aggressive, and Borderline Scales have also been reported to be more elevated for bulimics than anorexics. Personality characteristics of bulimics contrasted with anorexics appear to reflect a greater impulsivity, hostility, affective dysregulation, and interpersonal intensity.

Comparison of bulimics with both outpatients and normals produces a much different picture of bulimics than when compared with anorexics. Bulimics have more schizoid, avoidant, and dependent character pathology. They display more passive-aggressive, schizotypal, and borderline characteristics than normals but they are similar to general psychiatric outpatients on these same dimensions. These profile elevations seem to suggest bulimics experience a strong conflict between an intense interpersonal neediness and a wish to disavow such needs entirely and retreat into isolation. Affectively, they appear tense, dysphoric, and in turmoil. Although there have not been efforts to systematically compare bulimics and normals on the Clinical Symptom Syndrome scales, in our experience bulimics typically demonstrate elevations on these scales that are consistent with or which might be predicted from the affective dimension of Basic Personality Pattern elevations. Typically, bulimics' MCMI profiles show elevations on Anxiety and Dysthymia.

The foregoing literature can be applied in developing an approach to interpreting the MCMI profiles of bulimics. We have selected three profiles of patients in treatment for their bulimia in a hospital based eating disorders program. The first case presented reflects the most common clinical presentation of bulimia seen in treatment settings. Because bulimia accompanied by borderline personality disorder is also commonly encountered in clinical practice, we have included one such case. Perhaps less commonly encountered but clinically problematic is a case of psychotherapy-resistant bulimia nervosa, the third case we describe.

A CASE OF TYPICAL BULIMIA NERVOSA

A. W. was an 18-year-old single White female who was self-referred for treatment of her bulimia nervosa. She first began binge eating at age 15, 4 months after she began to diet. At the onset of her binge eating she weighed 132 pounds at her height of 5 ft. 8 inches. She perceived herself as "fat." Her weight at the start of treatment was 135 pounds and she perceived herself to be overweight. Although the patient had a history of self-induced vomiting and laxative abuse, at the time of presentation she was occasionally inducing vomiting but primarily starving herself the day after a binge and engaging in excessive exercise. Binging was occurring on average two times a week at the onset of treatment and invariably occurred if the patient was spending any amount of time alone. Patient had never received any form of psychiatric treatment before and was free of serious medical problems. She denied drug or alcohol use. Affect and mood were noted to be within the normal range and she denied suicidal ideation.

Patient was raised in a strictly observant Jewish family. There was no family history of eating disorder, substance abuse, or any other psychiatric disorder. At

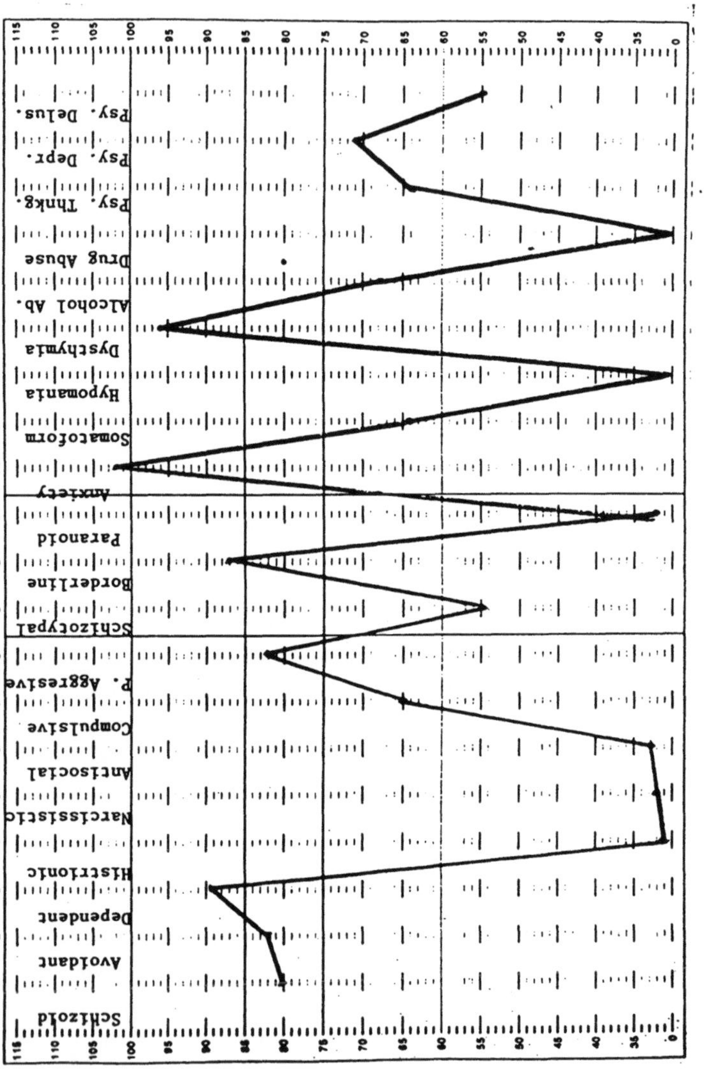

FIG. 8.1. A case of typical bulimia nervosa.

the time of treatment, patient was enrolled in college. Although she indicated that she had some friends, she also noted that she had no close relationships.

The patient's MCMI profile (Fig. 8.1) reflects typical elevations within the group of personality pathology scales. As is typically the case with bulimic profiles, the Dependent scale shows the greatest elevation of personality pathology scales. Elevation on this scale reflects passivity, conflict avoidance, eagerness to please, a self-sacrificing quality, a poor self-image, and a Pollyanna cognitive style. There is also elevation on the Avoidant scale characterized by dysphoric and tense affective undercurrent, self-alienation, social anxiety and avoidance, and hypersensitivity to criticism and rejection. The elevation on the Schizoid scale is associated with interpersonal detachment, lack of emotional responsiveness, diminished energy and spontaneity, minimal self-awareness and mild cognitive slippage. Irritability, low frustration tolerance, peevish and oppositional behavior characterize the elevation on the Passive-Aggressive scale. Other descriptors include a gloomy, victimized outlook on self and life, emotional capriciousness and reactivity, ambivalence in object relations including vacillation from being dependent to being counterdependent.

On the Pathological Personality Disorders scales, the sole elevation was on the Borderline scale. Because these patients commonly display an underlying borderline conflict in object relations, even those who do not meet DSM-III-R criteria for borderline personality disorder frequently show some elevation on this scale. This conflict is manifest in ambivalence about dependency and attachment.

Among the Clinical Symptom Syndrome scales, elevations are seen on the Anxiety and Dysthymia scales. The elevation on Anxiety describes this patient's globally anxious mood along with restlessness, indecisiveness, and physical complaints. The elevation on the Dysthymia scale indicates a disheartened, guilt-ridden, apathetic, and self-critical individual.

The constellation of personality characteristics seems to represent bulimic traits that have been described elsewhere. Striegel-Moore, Silberstein, and Rodin (1986) describe bulimic women as "dependent, unassertive, eager to please, and concerned with social approval" (p. 249). Others have noted the same need for social approval in addition to external locus of control, lack of assertiveness, and hypersensitivity to others' expectations and criticisms of them (Connors, Johnson, & Stuckey, 1984; Katzman & Wolchik, 1984; Love, Ollendick, Johnson, & Schlesinger, 1985; Nagleberg, Hale, & Ware, 1984).

This is typical of the MCMI elevations among the bulimic group, illuminating a complex interplay of personality variables reflecting a strong conflict over autonomy. Avoidant characteristics would appear to conflict with strong needs for nurturance reflected in the bulimic's dependent stance. The tension between fear of engulfment and fear of abandonment reflected in the MCMI scores may lead to resentment and anger, which is expressed passive-aggressively (as reflected in scores on this scale) rather than through hostility towards others (low scores on the Antisocial scale). The elevations on the Anxiety and Dysthymia scales in conjunction with the elevation on the Avoidant scale and the Passive-Aggressive scale indicate a quality of affective instability that is consistent with that identified by Johnson and Connors (1987).

A CASE OF BORDERLINE PERSONALITY DISORDER AND BULIMIA NERVOSA

L. M. was a 24-year-old divorced White female who was referred by her family physician for treatment of her bulimia nervosa. The onset of her bulimic symptoms occurred at age 19, at which time the patient weighed 137 pounds with a height of 5 feet 2 inches. Weight at the onset of treatment was 107 pounds. Her binge frequency at the beginning of treatment was 4 to 7 times per day, with binges invariably followed by self-induced vomiting. She reported that binge episodes typically occurred when she was feeling depressed and were more frequent in the evenings. She denied any history of laxative abuse but did admit to periods of several days where she would completely restrict her food intake. The patient expressed a terror of gaining weight. She had a history of alcohol dependence and was completing a substance abuse treatment program at the time of her presentation for treatment of her bulimia. The patient also had a history of suicidal ideation with two attempts at age 17 and age 19.

Patient was adopted at infancy and had no knowledge of her biological parents. Adoptive parents were described by the patient as "overcontrolling." The patient married at age 18 and divorced at 21 but only lived with her husband for 8 months. At the time of treatment, she was living with her boyfriend and operating a dog-grooming business. Although she had received previous treatment for her psychiatric problems, neither her bulimia nervosa nor her borderline personality disorder improved significantly. The patient had a high school education and had attended some business school and a half-year of college.

This profile (Fig. 8.2) is characteristic of borderline bulimic profiles in that there are greater elevations overall. The configuration of the Basic Personality Pattern scales does not differ from that of the typical bulimic profile except in magnitude of the specific elevations. An amplification of the conflict around dependency needs in this patient is seen in the concurrent elevations of the Schizotypal and Borderline scales. This patient is in intense turmoil over her yearning for interpersonal contact juxtaposed with her extreme sense of interpersonal alienation. She would appear to vacillate between dealing with this through interpersonal withdrawal or, alternately, through self-destructive acting out. Intense emotional states including rage, despondency, and panic are characteristic of such individuals. The elevation on Alcohol Abuse also suggests she may attempt to medicate these affective states in order to achieve some degree of emotional equilibrium. Likewise, engaging in bulimic behavior may be an attempt to regulate intense negative affect.

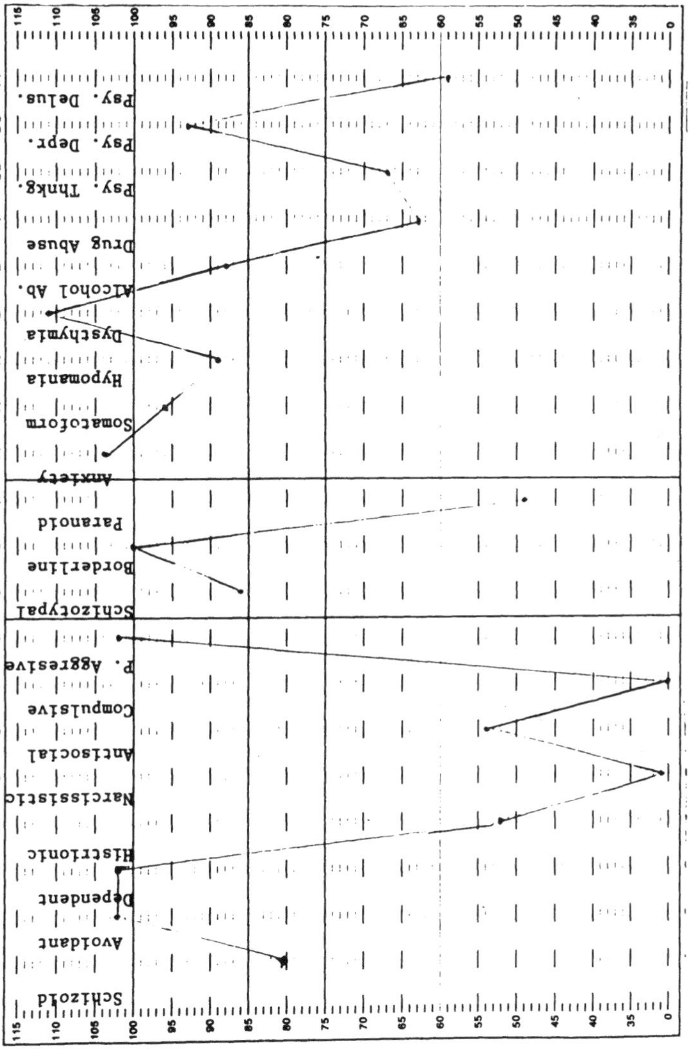

FIG. 8.2. A case of borderline personality disorder and bulimia nervosa.

153

The score on the Somatoform scale indicates an attempt to somatize her psychological conflicts although, given the overall level of distress reported, this defense is not likely to be effective. Somatic complaints may also represent commonly observed physiological epiphenomena of bulimic behavior.

A CASE OF PSYCHOTHERAPY-RESISTANT
BULIMIA NERVOSA

J. K. was a 22-year-old single White female who was self-referred at the suggestion of her family for treatment of bulimia nervosa. She reported an onset of bulimia at the age of 19 following a diet. Prior to the diet, the patient weighed 181 pounds at her height of 5 feet 11½ inches. She achieved a weight of 156 on the diet but had regained back to 181 at the time she presented for treatment. The patient had a history of laxative abuse and abuse of diet pills as well as self-induced vomiting, but only the vomiting was current at the time of treatment. At the onset of treatment, bulimic episodes were reported to occur 3 times per day on average and were triggered by "nervousness" or occasions on which the patient had to interact with men. The patient had been hospitalized twice for her bulimia but had never had any previous outpatient psychotherapy. She was treated briefly with antidepressants during one of her hospitalizations but indicated that this was not helpful. No depressive symptoms were noted at the time of treatment and she was not suicidal. She denied substance abuse.

The patient was raised within a lower middle-class urban family which was quite enmeshed. Family history was negative for eating disorder or psychiatric disorder, but one uncle died from complications of alcoholism. The patient had entered a nursing program upon high school graduation and had made the Dean's list prior to the onset of her bulimia. However, when the bulimia developed, it interfered significantly with her studying and she dropped out of school following her first hospitalization. At the time of treatment she was working 25–30 hours a week at a hotel and 30 hours or more a week at a hospital. The patient indicated that she liked working so many hours as she tended to isolate herself when working fewer hours. J. K. indicated that she had virtually no friends and that this had pretty much always been the case for her.

This profile (Fig. 8.3) presents the characteristic avoidant-dependent conflict as reflected on the Avoidant and Dependent scales but is notable for the complete absence of any other scale elevations. The absence of elevations commonly seen in the typical bulimic profile (Anxiety and Dysthymia) suggests a level of comfort with the bulimic symptoms that presents an obstacle to psychotherapeutic treatment. Although the avoidant-dependent conflict exists and is expressed through bulimic symptoms, such patients seem to lack the psychological structures to examine this in psychotherapy. Relative to the typical bulimic patient, the score on the Borderline scale is quite low, suggesting that the absence of affective

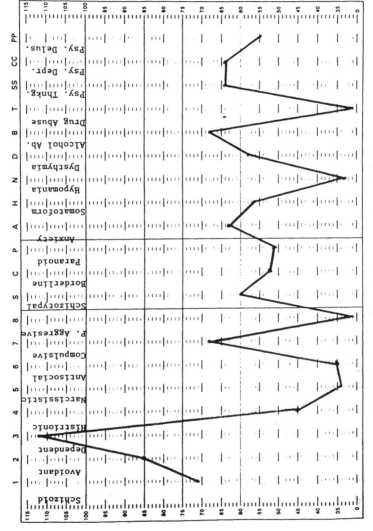

FIG. 8.3. A case of psychotherapy-resistant bulimia nervosa.

155

distress is more than situational, and may be seen as a characterlogical deficit. In psychotherapy sessions, they are alexithymic and markedly nonpsychologically minded. Such individuals are frequently urged by others to seek treatment and have little motivation to follow through, usually terminating treatment prematurely.

SUMMARY

The MCMI can be useful in identifying subtypes of bulimic psychopathology and assisting the clinician not only in better understanding the personality dynamics of individual bulimic patients, but also in formulating appropriate treatment strategies. Patients with the more common type of profile may be approached with the more standard therapy methods for bulimia nervosa, whereas other subtypes may require alternative approaches to treatment. For the borderline bulimic, the focus of treatment may need to be on the borderline pathology rather than the bulimic symptoms and the clinician should anticipate a relatively lengthy treatment before appreciable change in bulimic symptomatology occurs. For these patients, bulimic symptoms may be viewed as yet another example of self-destructive behavior aimed at regulating intense affective states. The psychotherapy-resistant bulimic patient may have a better response to psychopharmacological treatment than to talking therapy. In our experience, these patients may be responsive to fluoxetine even with a history of failed treatment with other pharmacological agents.

REFERENCES

Chandarana, P., Holliday, R., Conlon, P., & DeSlippe, T. (1988). Psychosocial considerations in gastric stapling. *Journal of Psychosomatic Research, 32*, 85–92.

Connors, M. E., Johnson, C. L., & Stuckey, M. K. (1984). Treatment of bulimia with brief psychoeducational group therapy. *American Journal of Psychiatry, 141*, 1512–1516.

Garner, D. M., & Olmsted, M. P. (1984). Manual for eating disorders inventory (EDI). Odessa, FL: Psychological Assessment Resources.

Johnson, C., & Connors, M. E. (1987). *The etiology and treatment of bulimia nervosa.* New York: Basic Books.

Katzman, M., & Wolchik, S. (1984). Bulimia and binge eating in college women: A comparison of personality and behavioral characteristics. *Journal of Consulting and Clinical Psychology, 52*, 423–428.

Lepkowsky, C. M. (1987). Personality pathology in eating disorders. In C. Green (Ed.), *Conference on the Millon clinical inventories (MCMI, MBHI, MAPI)* (pp. 215–220). Minneapolis, National Computer systems.

Love, S. Q., Ollendick, T., Johnson, C. L., & Schlesinger, S. (1985). A preliminary report of the prediction of bulimic behaviors: A social learning analysis. *Bulletin of the Society of Psychologists in Addictive Behaviors, 4*, 93–101.

Lundholm, J. K. (1989). Alcohol use among university females: Relationship to eating disordered behavior. *Addictive Behaviors, 14*, 181–185.

Lundholm, J. K., Pellegreno, D. D., Wolins, L., & Graham, S. L. (1989). Predicting eating disorders in women: A preliminary measurement study. *Measurement and Evaluation in Counseling and Development, 22,* 23–30.

Nagelberg, D., Hale, S., & Ware, S. (1984). The assessment of bulimic symptoms and personality correlates in female students. *Journal of Clinical Psychology, 40,* 440–445.

Pendleton, L., Tisdale, M. J., & Marler, M. (1991). Personality pathology in bulimics versus controls. *Comprehensive Psychiatry, 32,* 516–520.

Striegel-Moore, R. H., Silberstein, L. R., & Rodin, J. (1986). Toward an understanding of risk factors for bulimia. *American Psychologist, 41,* 246–263.

Tisdale, M. J., Pendleton, L., & Marler, M. (1990). MCMI characteristics of DSM-III-R bulimics. *Journal of Personality Assessment, 55,* 477–483.

Tracy, H., Norman, D., & Weisberg, L. (1987). Anorexia and bulimia: A comparison of MCMI results. In C. Green (Ed.), *Conference on the Millon clinical inventories (MCMI, MBHI, MAPI)* (pp. 195–197). Minneapolis, National Computer Systems.

9 Post-Traumatic Stress Disorders and MCMI-Based Assessment

Leon Hyer, Ed.D.
Mary Melton, Ph.D.
Cheryl Gratton, Ph.D.

This chapter addresses issues of the trauma response, especially that of chronic combat-related victims with Post-Traumatic Stress Disorder (PTSD). We consider four areas. First, the complexity of this form of trauma is considered. In an effort to simplify, our second section considers assessment and treatment. Third, we argue for personologic primacy in the transcoding of trauma within the victim and provide a rough typology based on the MCMI. Fourth, we outline three therapeutic considerations: (a) the importance of the relationship; (b) the need to understand the person of the trauma victim, personality styles, and symptoms; and (c) the work of therapy on core personality processes and evolving symptoms. Finally, examples are given.

There is one truth that emerges: the prepotency of the person in the organization of the trauma response. This is basically a constructionist conceptualization of the processing of trauma. Even in the decompensation process due to combat trauma, singularly devastating and unforgiving, the dynamics of the person are logical and understandable.

POST-TRAUMATIC STRESS DISORDER

Diagnostic Criteria. The current form of PTSD as given in the DSM-III-R (American Psychiatric Association, 1980) includes three categories encompassing 17 symptoms, in addition to the trauma. With varying degrees of dissent, researchers have endorsed and validated these symptoms in its current composition. Sufferers of PTSD fail to habituate despite persistent imagined reexposure in the form of reexperiencing, intrusion, and/or flashbacks. Category B (reex-

159

perience of symptoms), therefore, receives the most interest, as these symptoms are extremely painful and disturbing to normal living. These symptoms are considered more pronounced than "avoidance-numbing" (Category C) according to many studies (Pitman, Orr, Forgue, DeJong, & Claiborn, 1987) and are considered most important to clinicians who work with combat trauma. Category D (increased arousal) are highly related to category B (Peterson et al., 1987).

It is Category C, however, that perpetuates PTSD problems. In fact, avoidance and constriction seem to represent an uneasy adaptation and a continuance of the trauma response. The avoidance response perpetuates resistant and noxious elements of this disorder; the trauma is never fully reexperienced and is periodically reconditioned, thus reinforcing the process. Peterson, Prout, and Schwartz (1991) note that the end state of avoidance is psychic numbing. Initially, the client tries to avoid thoughts, images, and feelings directly related to the disorder (first order association). Different internal stimuli, however, remind the person of this first order association. This is also avoided. Eventually, via this process, anxiety becomes controlled. The sufferer never fully reexperiences the stressor and therefore accommodates poorly.

Prevalence.   The prevalence rates of PTSD among combat related Vietnam veterans is of concern. As a function of the kind of trauma, definition of adjustment, the sample used, and the overall evaluation method, there has evolved a range of morbidity among combat Vietnam veterans from 3% to 23% (Boyle, Decoufle, & O'Brien, 1989). The study of most note is the National Vietnam Veteran Re-adjustment Study (NVVRS) (Kulka et al., 1988). The focus was prevalence and incidence of psychiatric problems among this population. Face-to-face interviews with a nationally representative sample (>3000) of Vietnam theater veterans, Vietnam era veterans, and nonveterans or civilian counterparts were conducted. The non-veterans or civilian counterparts were matched to the theater veterans with regard to age, sex, race (ethnicity) for men, and by occupation only for women. This study also conducted preliminary validation on all measures of PTSD. It used multiple measures on carefully derived samples in the assessment of PTSD.

Highlights of these findings are given in Table 9.1. Roughly one in two combat veterans will experience some form of psychiatric syndrome or PTSD symptoms over his or her life time. This study also revealed that combat intensity is the most important determinant of the trauma response in this group. Prevalence increases with longer tours of duty, being wounded, more heroism (decorations in combat), being younger in Vietnam, having less education, having a low SES, living in a large city, and having no religious preference (Kulka et al., 1990).

As a result of this study, we can draw some simple truths regarding this disorder's complexity and considerable needs for care. First, the problem of trauma at both clinical and subclinical levels is massive. This means that there

TABLE 9.1
NVVRS Results

30% of male Vietnam veterans have had PTSD *at some time* since the end of the war.

50% have had at least one other diagnosable psychatric disorder.

15.2% of male theater veterans (479,000) currently suffer from PTSD.

11.1% have significant symptoms of the disorder but not not meet DSM-III-R criteria (Partial PTSD).

27.9% of Hispanic Vietnam theater veterans currently have PTSD.

20.6% of Black male theater veterans have the disorder.

8.5 of female theater veterans corrently have PTSD.

7.8% o female theater veterans have Partial PTSD.

are many victims with various levels of trauma problems. Second, the variable that consistently *wins* in the battle for variance explanation is level of combat experience. And, although this factor is not sufficient by itself, it is prepotent. There appears to be an etiological link between combat exposure and the emergence of subsequent problems that is driven by the trauma and formed by the person. Third, there appear to be many subtypes of trauma problems, not just separated by clinical/subclinical or combat/noncombat dimensions, but by other person dimensions. This means that the phenomenology of trauma comes from the person, an idiographic response at adaptation. And, fourth, it is reasonable to postulate that effects of this trauma are stubborn and resistant to change. This means that as therapists, we must know the "right" person factors *and* trauma factors and intervene according to some plan.

ASSESSMENT

Excellent reviews on the assessment of chronic PTSD (Litz, Penk, Gerardi, & Keane, in press; Lyons, Gerardi, Wolfe, & Keane, 1988) are available. They emphasize the need for a multimodal approach, including structured interviews, clinical ratings, psychometric scales, collateral reports, psychophysiological indices, and even biological markers, along with a complete record review. Due to the chronicity of this disorder, a continuous assessment over time is also recommended. In addition, Eldridge (1991) has pointed out the many pragmatic issues confounding assessment. As with few other disorders, the purposes of assessment, treatment, sequelae of assessment results, attitude of the assessor, and typical clients evaluated by the assessor, assert a powerful influence on results. In addition, Eldridge recommends that the evaluator respect the experiences of

TABLE 9.2
Assessment of PTSD

---

1. Structured Interview
   SCID-NP-V - (PTSD)
   CAPS
   PTSD - Interview (PTSD-1)
       DSM-III-R

2. Psychometric Measures
   Mississippi Scale for Combat Related PTSD
   MMPI-PTSD (Keane)
   MMPI-PTSD (Schlenger)
   Impact of Events

3. Combat Exposure
   Combat Exposure Scale (Keane et al., 1989)
   Perceived Stress Scale (Linn, 1986)

4. Psychophysiological Measures
   Measures of heart rate to neutral and combat scripts

5. Psychohistory (objective factors)
   Pre trauma
   Trauma description (objective)
   Social support after trauma

6. Personality Measures
   MCMI or MCMI-II

---

the victim, be prepared for intense experiences, be sensitive to his or her own values and vulnerabilities, and be aware of the unique idiom of this disorder, especially cultural or social ones.

The recommended protocol for trauma evaluation is given in Table 9.2. Currently, the "gold standard" of the assessment of PTSD is the clinical interview. The structured or clinical interview should be viewed as one that provides optimal flexibility with various decision trees branching off from central interview questions. These should be rigorously followed, but should never be so rigid or limited as to provide just a diagnosis or classification (except for research purposes). The trained clinician should be able to assess trauma related issues (including the DSM-III-R criteria), associated symptoms and disorders, treatment issues, and make treatment judgments. Three structured interviews are recommended: Structured Clinical Interview for the DSM-III-R (SCID) (Spitzer, & Williams, 1985), Clinician Administered PTSD Scale (CAPS) (Blake, Keane, Wine, Mora, Taylor, & Lyons, 1990), and the PTSD Interview (Watson, Juba, Manifold, Kucala, & Anderson, 1991). All three are clinician rated and anchored firmly to the DSM-III-R criteria for PTSD.

All other measures in this table (except history) are psychometric ones and should be viewed as tools that assist in the clinical validation of the diagnosis. The Mississippi Scale for Combat Related PTSD is especially noteworthy, followed by the special MMPI scales (MMPI and MMPI-2) (Litz et al., in press).

Measures of combat exposure are also important as these provide the clinician with basic information on the nature of the combat experience. In addition, the scale provided by Lynn (1968) evaluates perceived stress, unexpectedness of the event, perceived responsibility, and degree of support. This information, along with the history, nicely mixes with other data for a total picture of the response to trauma.

Where possible, psychophysiological measures should be taken, particularly heart rate. In studies of trauma victims, a basic paradigm involves the presentation of trauma related and neutral stimuli, measurement of multimodal response channels, self-reports of arousal, and possibly behavioral responses. In the absence, however, of any psychological stimuli capabilities, the clinician may monitor blood pressure and heart rate, as there is some evidence that, even in the absence of trauma events, victims are hyperaroused (Litz et al., in press). Personality measures are addressed next.

Person-Event Model.   Over the past decade extensive research has examined variables related to personal characteristics and combat experience in attempting to understand the development of PTSD among Vietnam combat veterans. Foy, Resnick, Sipprelle, and Carroll, (1987) reviewed 13 retrospective studies that examined premilitary, military, and postmilitary etiologic factors in combat-related PTSD among Vietnam veterans. Their review concludes that a diagnosis of PTSD and/or PTSD symptom severity is most strongly associated with indices of the extent and intensity of exposure to combat in Vietnam. In contrast, research in different samples of Vietnam veterans examining associations between various premilitary vulnerability characteristics (e.g., adolescent psychosocial adjustment, alcohol and drug problems, family stability) and PTSD has produced contradictory and inconclusive results (Foy et al., 1987). These findings have led some investigators to favor the extreme event argument as a model for explaining the origins of PTSD among Vietnam combat veterans, and to minimize the etiologic role of premilitary social and personality characteristics (Watson, Kucala, Manifold, Juba, & Vassar, 1988).

As emphasized by a number of authors, however, to view the two explanations as mutually exclusive or diametrically opposed is too simplistic and impedes development of more comprehensive etiologic models (Escobar, 1987). One promising research paradigm that attempts to integrate both explanations is the person/event interaction model, in which individual variability in response to extreme life events is viewed as a function of the dynamic interaction of both internal and external factors (Keane, 1989). Acknowledging that extreme events can elicit significant distress in anyone exposed, advocates of this model postulate that the severity and persistence of adverse psychological reactions will vary depending on the magnitude of the event relative to the individual's coping resources. Up to a certain threshold, premorbid factors variably assert a considerable influence on the response to trauma.

Traumatic Personality and MCMI Test Results.   Much of the research on PTSD during the 70s and 80s has been directed at symptoms (Lyons et al., 1988). Increasingly, however, there has developed an awareness of the importance of personality in the diagnosis and treatment of victims. Most notable among these studies is the work of Horowitz (Horowitz, Marmar, Krupnick, Wilmer, Kaltreider, & Wallestein, 1984), who developed a method of treatment of PTSD based on information processing of stressors and the character structure of the individual. In the extant literature there also exists a small group of studies on the character adaptation of the Vietnam veteran using the MCMI. Several studies have reported the existence of the passive aggressive and avoidant profile (8/2 or 2/8) in this population (e.g., Choca, Peterson, & Shanley, 1986; Sherwood, Funari, & Piekorski, 1990). In the Sherwood study 189 male Vietnam veterans who were categorized as having PTSD according to the MMPI-PTSD scale were evaluated on the MCMI. The character styles passive aggressive, schizoid, avoidant, and borderline were significantly related to PTSD patients, but not to non-PTSD patients. Once again, the most common 2-point profile was the 8/2 or 2/8. In this sample a hit rate of 80% would be obtained if the sample was classified as having PTSD on the basis of scales 8 and 2 on the MCMI (BR $\geq$ 85). The authors concluded that the surprising homogeneous character styles among this group represented adaptive patterns to cope with the traumas of Vietnam. These styles were viewed, therefore, as *defenses* which better enable the veteran to manage high levels of anxiety.

The Hyer group at the Augusta War Trauma Project used the MCMI and MCMI-2 on PTSD veterans and emphasized the role of personality in a different way (Hyer, Woods, & Boudewyns, 1991). In one study, "A Three Tier Evaluation of PTSD Among Vietnam Combat Veterans," Hyer et al. (1991) attempted a careful disaggregation of the clinical components of this chronic population. Tier 1 consisted of life style analysis according to the methods of Adler. Basically, this was an attempt to understand the person of the victim. Tier 2 involved the use of the MCMI. Resultant personality styles of the trauma victim were conceived as a direct outgrowth of the life style. Tiers 1 and 2, therefore, reflect the idiographic character of the person. (Table 9.3 presents the MCMI and MCMI-II profiles for 100 Vietnam veterans with PTSD.)

The highlight of Tier 2 was a typology of the MCMI based on a sorting procedure outlined by Millon (1983). Only the eight basic personality codes were used. Initially, a code was arrived at by prominence of a style; that is, any of the eight mild personality styles beyond BR-84 was included in that code. Next, each veteran was sorted into additional codes based on presence (BR $>$ 74). As a result of these two procedures, a parent code, the 8–2 (Traumatic Personality), was identified, as well as three additional codes (Table 9.4).

This is a clinical taxonomy and represents anything but perfect classification. All codes possess the Traumatic Personality plus others. The importance, therefore, is in the incremental information provided by the other codes (3, 6, 1, 8B).

TABLE 9.3
Means and MCMI and MCMI II

	MCMI Mean	MCMI-II Mean
Schizoid	81.65	89.547
Avoidant	89.80	92.267
Dependent	44.15	34.942
Histrionic	30.07	40.640
Narcissistic	38.01	61.593
Antisocial	64.80	86.291
Sadistic		50.61
Compulsive	33.15	50.605
Passive Aggressive	94.62	101.767
Self-Defeating		82.28
Schizotypal	64.98	86.465
Borderline	76.84	85.186
Paranoid	60.00	68.570
Anxiety	97.88	88.733
Somatoform	67.50	60.000
Hypomanic	37.29	44.709
Dysthymic	93.70	91.535
Alcohol abuse	76.27	82.651
Drug abuse	64.23	79.477
Psychotic thinking	68.75	80.523
Psychotic depression	73.94	89.465
Psychotic delusions	60.20	58.733
Disclosure		35.12
Desirability		91.99
Debasement		89.54

n = 100

These additional codes then provide distinctive clinical information. It is further noteworthy that severe personality styles were also present and measurably influence these milder styles.

Tier 3 addressed symptoms, both psychosocial and trauma related. These symptoms were explained according to Millon's model (1969; 1981); that is, they

TABLE 9.4
Traumatic Personality
(8/2 or 2/8)

The "8" style, passive aggressive, is characterized by labile affectivity, behavioral contrariness, discontented self-image, deficient regulatory controls, and interpersonal ambivalence. In fact, this style is conceptually close to, but less severe than the borderline personality as represented in Millon's theory. The "2" style, avoidant, is represented by alienated self-image, affective dysphoria, mild cognitive slippage, aversive interpersonal behavior, and perceptual hypersensitivity. Adjectives used to describe this 8-2 profile are: oversensitive, fearful, self-preoccupied, disgruntled, uneasy, irritable. neat traditional, moody, unsettled, negativistic, anxious, complaining, and powerless. It is noteworthy, too that the 8-2 code is a symptom exaggeration or overreporting code.

Schizoid influence:	8A-2-1
Dependent influence:	8A-2-1-3
Antisocial influence:	8A-2-1-6A
Self-Defeating influence:	8A-2-1-8B

are logical extensions of embedded and long-term personality styles of the individual. They are "ego dystonic," but logical from inner stimuli of the person. Psychosocial symptoms included the DSM-III-R criteria and correlated symptoms characteristic of this disorder. The psychosocial symptoms are the "squeaky" wheels in treatment. The therapeutic goal is to reframe these in the context of the personality style of the person (Tiers 1 and 2).

Trauma symptoms were similarly considered. They are separate because they represent the essence of PTSD and because this symptom involves distinctive treatment (e.g., direct therapeutic exposure). Results of this study (Hyer et al., 1991) showed further that four trauma questions were important: (a) whether intrusive symptoms were present; (b) what controls were present; (c) how avoidance was manifested; and (d) whether access to the memory was allowed. Based on this information, a decision on whether and how to treat the trauma could be made.

The advantages of the three tier approach are many. First, this is an evaluation process, an analysis that provides a blueprint for action. It is a new beginning regardless of past treatment. Second, the thrust is for a case formulation from the person-event model. Emphasis is placed on the person of the trauma victim and psychological ways that PTSD and its symptoms are processed. The character of the person influences and is influenced by trauma. Finally, the processing of information is disaggregated according to meaningful person components. Treatment, then, can occur on the *ready* parts of the person, while others *prepare* for their time.

PTSD TREATMENT

Treatment Model.   Components in the treatment of PTSD include the relationship, an understanding by the client of his/her personality and role, and the tasks and goals of treatment.

There is no other component of therapy more accepted than the first treatment factor, the working alliance between patient and therapist. In fact, it is a virtual impossibility to find a description of psychotherapy with the trauma victim without the heavy endorsement of a positive relationship. Basically, this therapy component creates an atmosphere for dialogue. It allows for the collaborative process to occur and for the work of therapy to proceed within safe bounds. Relationship and technique have long been the two touchstones for organizing the phenomenon of successful therapy. Neither is complete without the other. Necessarily, this relationship involves attendant nonspecific features: hope, care, unconditional acceptance, listening, genuineness and the like; as well as a commitment to "interiority," the inward and interpersonal press involving the tasks of therapy (Component 3) (Bugental, 1987). These are the elements that keep the client open, cooperative, and nondefensive.

The understanding of self and role is perhaps the simplest but most difficult to apply consistently. There are two features, the client road map (self-understanding) and the tasks or role in therapy. Client understanding of his/her personality dynamics, based on the MCMI (MCMI-II) and the PTSD topology, is a condition for the change process. In working with personality disorder patients, it is helpful to be *sure* that there is a clear understanding of components, both core cognitions and affective/behavioral/interpersonal styles, and of the role one plays in the effort to unearth these. This is labor intensive since a main goal is for the client to be a collaborator. Accordingly, this type of care must include strong supportive components. Trauma victims universally show various degrees of lack of self-observation, poor motivation, lack of skill, secondary gain considerations, fear of vulnerability or views of hopelessness, fears that others will not accept change, and characterological rigidity. The ultimate goal in collaboration is for both client and therapist to participate in the ongoing experience of the client occurring in therapy and currently in life.

Component 3 involves both personality and symptom issues. The more important focus is personality, which includes two elements of therapy. The first is the judicious pursuit of the core cognitions of the client. These beliefs are based on enduring and embedded learnings that are often tacit and must be unearthed, repeatedly tagged, challenged, and hopefully altered. Based on the Millon model (1969), the core beliefs for the milder personality disorders follow developmental learnings and self-reinforced patterns (of each personality style). These are reasonably anchored to DSM-III-R, Axis II. For the more severe personality styles, schizotypal, borderline and paranoid, the content and experience of the core beliefs follow from the milder personality styles.

In addition to the core cognitions, interpersonal patterns and modal styles of the personality need to be addressed. These are the behavioral/affective/interpersonal styles that foster and maintain the personality styles. Young (1990) labels these as "maintenance behaviors." We have chosen not to specify these since they are addressed by Millon (1969). They too need to be exhumed, tagged repeatedly, challenged, and hopefully altered.

Finally, there are symptoms. Again, the distinction between personality and symptoms is important for both conceptualization and treatment purposes. The former involves the person; the latter (symptoms), the perturbations of the person that often are all consuming. The former necessitates the careful monitoring of the collaboration and understanding (of self and role); the latter is technique directed, with remission as its immediate goal. Cognitive behavioral therapy (CBT) divides these into schema therapy and symptom therapy (Freeman & Leaf, 1990). Schemas are conceptually close to personality patterns and are considered more central to the person. Should symptoms override the person ("cognitive shift"), then symptom therapy is required. Symptoms *demand* attention from the therapist. In trauma work, typical symptom theories include direct therapeutic exposure, eye movement desensitization/reintegration, stress reduction, or grief/trauma therapy. Although it is appropriate to conceive of schema therapy as more long term, symptom therapy is just as important with trauma victims. The differences are ones of focus (symptoms) and technology.

Symptoms of the trauma victim require both assessment and intervention. They include psychosocial symptoms, the litany of DSM-III-R symptoms specific to each person, and trauma symptoms. Remember that both forms of symptoms are ego dystonic. Each type of symptoms should be addressed separately. The clinician should outline and treat these depending on the degree of intensity or frequency. The therapeutic goal, however, is to return to "schema therapy." Because both psychosocial symptoms and trauma memories represent protypical exemplars of the personality, these should flow naturally. Finally, it should be noted that trauma memories are not absolutely accurate accounts of the patient's history; rather, they are reasonable outgrowths of the person's unique way of processing trauma. What is important is the meaning of the memory to the patient and not the details of the memory.

CASE EXAMPLE

A case example is presented, representing one of our codes. As we use CBT routinely to challenge core cognitions and modal styles, these are addressed briefly but not emphasized. Remember, our focus is understanding, relationship, and techniques (trauma vs. psychosocial). Treatment always begins with the first two, deferring to techniques only if the symptoms are prepotent. When the symptom is less in evidence, the more important work of treatment ensues.

Self-Defeating Influence.   JM was the only child of a mother who had a number of conflicted relationships with men. At an early age, he learned to meet his mother's needs. JM was distraught when his mother divorced the man that he thought was his father. As a young adolescent he had to cope with the divorce and the discovery of a different biological father.

JM left high school at age 15 because he had conflicts with peers and believed he needed a job to help out with his mother's financial problems. At 17 he convinced his mother to allow him to join the army. There he was trained as a medic and had one tour in Vietnam. He identified several trauma memories in which he was unable to perform due to excessive turmoil, lack of training, inability to overcome the inevitable, or procrastination. JM retains guilt about events in Vietnam, believing he could have done more. He is exquisitely sensitive to the anti-Vietnam sentiment into which he returned.

JM has not been able to keep jobs and moved his family frequently throughout the past 20 years. There appears to be a consistent pattern of failure to accomplish tasks and the elicitation of negative responses from others without clear reason. He could perform adequately for only a short time, until confusion or failure resulted. His long marriage recently ended in divorce due to flashbacks that resulted in dangerous behavior.

MCMI II: 8B28A**1*36A6B+754//SC* //ADB** //CCSS*

Core Cognitions

I am a failure; self sacrifice is my only way.
I both need others and hate others.
When I feel stuck, I act against myself.
I am misunderstood, an innocent victim.

Modal Styles:

Interpersonally doleful and inconsistent.
Behaviorally slow and ineffectual.
Affectively irritable and depressive.

PTSD Symptoms:

Psychosocial	*Trauma*
Negative therapeutic attitude	
	Frequent intrusions
Anxiety/hyperarousal	
Self-anger	He will only minimally allow access and memories are frequent and he has few controls.

JM is self defeating, avoidant, and passive aggressive in ways. A common belief in the Trauma Personality is a feeling of being a misunderstood victim. This clearly applies to JM. In addition, there is also a drive to compensate overtly for the *bad* self by sacrificing himself for others. He is never good enough and always angry about this condition. He realizes too that he must interact with others for assistance. But his need for others is only met through caretaking, thus reinforcing distance. He possesses an undeserving self-image with cognitions that endorse his fear of failure, ineptitude, neediness, and lack of ability to control himself. His role as caretaker and the need to subvert himself seriously interfere with his ability to benefit as a patient in therapy.

Because he experiences high levels of trauma symptomology, Eye Movement Desensitization/Reintegration was employed to reduce his pain levels and alter self-statements. When his hyperactivity was lessened somewhat, his core cognitions and modal styles were confronted. CBT was utilized to heighten his awareness of his self-defeating patterns and to assist him in altering such behavior. Use of the "downward arrow" technique was especially helpful, as he could view his self defeating styles in particular situations. Anger, feelings of ineffectiveness, and misplaced ideas of self-control (by defeat) were gradually altered.

CONCLUSION

The problem of trauma is universal. Increasingly, it appears that even *smaller* trauma powerfully impacts on the person. We have emphasized that the person must be understood and that the way to approach this is through an "unpacking" of the personality. The information currently available on the person, personality (cognition and model styles), as well as trauma, allows us to muddle through with skill and efficacy. This information gives way to an integrated model of care providing the clinician with appropriate vision and tools.

REFERENCES

American Psychiatric Association. (1980). *Diagnostic and Statistical Manual of Mental Disorders* (3rd ed.), Washington, DC, Author.

Blake, D. D., Keane, T. M., Wine, P. R., Mora, C., Taylor, K. L., & Lyons, J. A. (1990). Prevalence of PTSD symptoms in combat veterans seeking medical treatment. *Journal of Traumatic Stress, 3,* 15–27.

Boyle, C. A., Decoufle, P., & O'Brien, T. R. (1989). Long-term health consequences of military service in Vietnam. *Epidemiologic Reviews, 11,* 1–27.

Choca, J., Peterson, S., & Shanley, L. (1986). Factor analysis of the MCMI. *Journal of Consulting and Clinical Psychology, 44*(5), 760–763.

Eldridge, G. (1991). Contextual issues in the assessment of posttraumatic stress disorder. *Journal of Traumatic Stress, 4*(1), 7–24.

Escobar, J. I. (1987). Posttraumatic stress disorder and the perennial stress-diathaesis controversy. *Journal of personality, 57,* 311–341.

Foy, D. W., Resnick, H. S., Sipprelle, R. C., & Carroll, E. M. (1987). Premilitary, military, and postmilitary factors in the development of combat-related posttraumatic stress disorder. *Behavior Therapist, 10,* 3–9.

Freeman, A., & Leaf, R. (1990). Cognitive therapy applied to personality disorders. In C. Gurman (Ed.), *Handbook of cognitive therapy.*

Horowitz, M., Marmar, C., Krupnick, J., Wilmer, N., Kaltreider, M., & Wallestein, R. (1984). *Personality styles and brief psychotherapy.* New York: Blair Books.

Hyer, L., Woods, G., & Boudewyns, P. (1991). A three tier evaluation of posttraumatic stress disorder. *Journal of Traumatic Stress, 4*(2), 165–194.

Keane, T. M. (1989). Posttraumatic stress disorder: Current status and future directions. *Behavior Therapy, 20,* 149–153.

Kulka, R. A., Schlenger, W. E., Fairbank, J. A., Hough, R. L., Jordan, B. K., Marmar, C. R., & Weiss, D. S. (1988). *Contractual report of findings from the National Vietnam Veterans Readjustment Study.* Research Triangle Institute, NC: Research Triangle Institute.

Linn, M. W. (1968). Modifiers and perceived stress scale. *Journal of Consulting Clinical Psychology, 54,* 507–513.

Litz, B., Penk, W., Gerardi, R., & Keane, T. (in press). The assessment of posttraumatic stress disorder. In P. Saigh (Ed.), *Posttraumatic stress disorder: A behavioral approach to assessment and treatment.* New York: Pergamon Press.

Lyons, J. A., Gerardi, R. J., Wolfe, J., & Keane, T. (1988). Multidimensional assessment of combat-related PTSD: Phenomenological, psychometric, and psychophysiological considerations. *Journal of Traumatic Stress, 1,* 373–394.

Millon, T. (1969). *Modern psychopathology.* Philadelphia: Saunders.

Millon, T. (1981). *Disorders of personality: DSM-III Axis II.* New York: Wiley.

Millon, T. (1983). *Millon clinical multiaxial inventory manual* (3rd ed.). Minneapolis: National Computer Systems.

Millon, T. (1987). *Millon Clinical Multiaxial Inventory-II: Manual for the MCMI-II.* Minneapolis, MN: National Computer Systems.

Peterson, K., Prout, M., & Schwartz, R. (1991). *Post-traumatic Stress Disorder: A clinician's guide.* New York: Plenum Press.

Pitman, R. K., Orr, S. P., Forgue, D. F., DeJong, J. B., & Claiborn, J. M. (1987). Psychophysiologic assessment of posttraumatic stress disorder imagery in Vietnam combat veterans. *Archives of General Psychiatry, 44,* 970–975.

Sherwood, R., Funari, D., & Piekorski, A. (1990). Adapted character styles of Vietnam veterans with posttraumatic stress disorder. *Psychological Reports, 66,* 623–31.

Spitzer, R. L., & Williams, J. B. (1985). *Structured clinical interview for DSM-III-Revised,* SCID. Version prepared for the National Vietnam Veterans Readjustment Study. New York: State Psychiatric Institute, Biometrics Research Department.

Young, J. (1990). *Cognitive therapy for personality disorders: A schema focused approach.* Saratoga, FL: Professional Resource Exchange.

Watson, C. G., Kucala, T., Manifold, V., Juba, M., & Vassar, P. (1988). The relationship of posttraumatic stress disorder to adolescent illegal activities, drinking, and employment. *Journal of Clinical Psychology, 44,* 592–598.

Watson, C. G., Juba, M. P., Manifold, V., Kucala, T., & Anderson, P. E. (1991). The PTSD interview: Rationale, description, reliability, and concurrent validity of a DSM-III-based technique. *Journal of Clinical Psychology, 47,* 179–188.

10 The MCMI and DSM-III Anxiety Disorders

James Reich, M.D., M.Ph.

The MCMI has now gained wide use and acceptance as a clinically useful tool for clinicians and has also been used in numerous research studies. So far there has not been a useful summary of reports of its use in the anxiety disorders. Millon himself does not report in this area (Millon, 1987). This chapter tries to rectify this lack. The chapter is divided into several areas: first, demographics, or how the MCMI personality scales covary with DSM-III anxiety disorder populations and whether they predict outcome of treatment. The second section describes a report of a personality disorder occurring secondary to chronic panic disorder. The third section examines the relationship of anxiety, personality, and family history; the last section offers a clinical vignette. The MCMI scaled score of >85 was used in the cited studies to define a personality disorder. All axis I disorders in these studies were measured by standardized interviews administered by a masters level research assistant. Although many of the subject areas covered have literature available on other personality disorder instruments, they are not the focus of this chapter. It should be kept in mind that different DSM-III personality measurement instruments do not always agree with each other (Reich, Noyes, & Troughton, 1987b). The literature is a bit sparse and only reports using the original MCMI version are available.

THE RELATIONSHIP OF MCMI PERSONALITY SCALES TO DSM-III ANXIETY DISORDERS

There is one large study that compares the frequency of personality disorders in an outpatient, panic disorder, and nonpsychiatric population (Reich & Troughton, 1988b). In this study the MCMI was given to 88 panic disorder, 82 new outpatient psychiatric clinic intakes (excluding panic disorder, schizophrenic and organic brain syndrome disorders), and 40 normals who were recruited by advertising and screened to exclude depressive and psychotic disorders. Personality measurements on patients were taken upon entry and before treatment had commenced. In this study 62.7% of the panic population qualified for at least one personality disorder. In terms of the DSM-III clusters, there were 12.1% who qualified for a Schizoid cluster diagnosis, 27.7% who qualified for a Dramatic cluster diagnosis, and 59.8% qualified for an Anxious cluster diagnosis.[1] The following individual personality disorders had a prevalence of greater than 10%: Schizoid (10.8%), Histrionic (12.1%), Borderline (10.8%), Dependent (31.3%), Avoidant (15.7%), Passive-Aggressive (24.1%), and Compulsive (10.8%). (The percentages add up to greater than 100 since diagnoses were not mutually exclusive.) There were no significant differences between the nonpsychotic outpatient group and the panic disorder group in terms of prevalence of personality disorders. The panic group had significantly more disorders than controls in the following disorders Anxious cluster (54.2% vs. 20.0%, $p < .0006$), dependent (31.3% vs. 12.5%, $p < .04$), avoidant (15.7% vs. 2.5%, $p < .04$), and passive-aggressive (24.1% vs. 0%, $p < .002$).[2] As a part of this study a logistic regression was performed to determine which variables predicted the presence of personality disorder diagnoses in subjects. To qualify as a personality disorder for this analysis subjects had to have the personality disorder on the MCMI and also have the same personality disorder on another self report instrument. In this analysis the presence of panic disorder predicted the presence of an Anxious cluster personality disorder diagnosis ($p = .04$).

There is one study with the MCMI examining the degree of phobic avoidance in panic disorder and its relationship to the Anxious cluster personality disorder (Reich, Noyes, & Troughton, 1987a). This study examined 88 panic disorder patients recruited for a panic disorder treatment trial and who were free of psychotic disorder and organic brain syndrome. Measurements for this study were taken at intake before treatment. The MCMI measure of dependent personality disorder was significantly higher for those patients with uncomplicated panic versus limited phobic avoidance (11% vs. 42.9%, Chi square = 4.8, df = 1, $p < .03$) with similar finding for extensive phobic avoidance (agorophobia) (11.1% vs. 40.0%, Chi square = 5.0, df = 1, $p < .03$). A similar finding was found for the Anxious cluster personality disorder. Other personality measures

---

[1]The DSM-III divides the personality disorders into three clusters. The Schizoid cluster consists of the Schizoid, Schizotypal, and Paranoid personality disorders: the Dramatic cluster consists of the borderline, narcissistic, antisocial and histrionic personality disorders; while the Anxious cluster consists of the avoidant, dependent, passive-aggressive and compulsive personality disorders. For the purposes of this report any subject who qualifies for one of the diagnoses in the cluster qualifies for the cluster diagnosis.

[2]Comparisons between two groups of categorical data in this document use Fisher's exact test unless otherwise specified.

were also used and the results were generally consistent. Basically, panic patients with some phobic avoidance appear to have a much higher level of dependent personality disorder than patients with no phobic avoidance.[3]

There is one report of the frequency of MCMI personality disorders in social phobia (Reich, Noyes, & Yates, 1989). In this study, 14 DSM-III social phobics were diagnosed with the MCMI. In this population 50% had a Schizoid cluster personality disorder diagnosis, 50% a Dramatic cluster personality disorder diagnosis, and 64.3% an Anxious cluster personality disorder diagnosis. Individual personality disorders exceeding 10% prevalence were: schizoid 21.4%, schizotypal 28.5%, narcissistic 14.3%, borderline 21.4%, dependent 28.5%, avoidant 35.7%, passive-aggressive 35.7%, and compulsive 21.4%. When the prevalence in personality disorders is compared with the panic population previously cited the social phobic group had significantly more schizoid cluster (50% vs. 11.4%, $p = .002$) and schizotypal personality disorder diagnoses (28.5 vs. 1.1, $p = .001$). When compared to the control group of non patients cited earlier the social phobic group had significantly more Schizoid cluster diagnoses (50.0% vs. 2.5%, $p = .0001$), schizotypal personality disorder (28.5 vs. 0%), $p = .003$), borderline personality disorder (21.4% vs. 0%), Anxious cluster personality disorder (64.3% vs. 20.0%, $p = .004$), avoidant personality disorder (35.7% vs. 2.5%, $p = .003$) and passive-aggressive personality disorder (35.7% vs. 0%, $p = .001$). In general these findings appear consistent with clinically expected findings, with the possible exception of the high prevalence of passive aggressive personality disorder.

One problem that has caused concern for personality test developers is the problem caused by distortions in measurement due the acute illness state. There is clearly evidence that, in some circumstances, the effects of acute illness can make personality pathology appear more pervasive (Reich, Noyes, Hirschfeld, Coryell, & O'Gorman, 1987). Another question of interest is whether a personality instrument can differentiate the anxiety and depressive disorders. There are two reports that focus on this question. The first examines patients with panic disorder and major depression with patients in the acutely ill state (Reich & Noyes, 1987). The second examines a population of panic and depressed patients after recovery (Reich & Troughton, 1988a). The first study shows that in the acutely ill state there are significant personality differences between depressed and panic patients. Results indicate that the depressed patients are more personality disordered. Depressed patients have higher levels of any personality disorder (87.5% vs. 62.7%, $P < .05$), schizoid personality disorder (29.2% vs. 10.8%, $p < .05$), avoidant personality disorder (37.5% vs. 15.7%, $p < .05$), and dependent personality disorder (54.2% vs. 31.3%, $p < .05$). Interestingly, when

---

[3]This distinction is important as when agorophobic patients are compared with patients without agorophobia the results may be nonsignificant if there are a large number of limited avoidance patients in the nonagorophobic group.

panic disorder and major depression are examined in the recovered state the total number of personality disorders decreases by about a third and there are no longer any significant differences between the personalities of panic and depressed patients. This appears to indicate that the MCMI one is in some circumstances susceptible to state bias and that possibly that this bias is differential, depending on the disorder.

One of the interesting aspects of personality research is the relationship of personality to treatment outcome. There is only one study using the MCMI to determine the effect of outcome of treatment in panic disorder (Reich, 1988c). This study examined how MCMI personality traits measured at baseline predicted outcome of 52 panic disorder patients treated with benzodiazepines in a double blind treatment trial. In this case the scaled score of histrionic personality disorder correlated negatively with positive outcome ($r = -.28, p < .04$). There was no predictive effect on spontaneous panic attacks. This finding is in agreement with the general finding that personality disorders tend to create worse outcomes for treatment of Axis I disorders (Reich & Green, 1991).

PERSONALITY DISORDERS OCCURRING SECONDARY TO AN ANXIETY DISORDER

Although there are many theoretical etiologies to personality disorders and I do not argue the merits of them in this chapter, clinicians have often wondered whether, upon occasion, a severe chronic stressor could cause a personality disorder in patients who did not initially possess one. Unfortunately it is often impossible to obtain good premorbid information. There is, however, one case report in the literature relevant to the MCMI where good early history was available (Neenan, Felkner, & Reich, 1986). In this case a patient who had normal socialization and interpersonal interaction at age 17 and then developed panic disorder. At that time he began to withdraw socially to reduce his anxiety. The panic disorder, as it often is, was a chronic condition and lasted until we tested him at age 42. At that point the MCMI diagnosed him as both avoidant and schizoid personality disorders. There was no family history of schizophrenia in this patient's family. Given the limitations of the case report method no firm conclusions can be drawn, but it is a finding of theoretical interest.

PERSONALITY AND THE OUTCOME OF FAMILY HISTORY IN THE ANXIETY DISORDERS

There is one study using the MCMI which examines how the presence of a personality disorder in probands affects the prevalence of psychiatric disorders in relatives, as measured by the family history method (Reich, 1988b). This study utilized psychiatric outpatient whose Axis I disorder was diagnosed by standardized psychiatric interviews. The family history method was a standardized method for diagnosing anxiety disorders and the DSM-III personality disorder clusters (Reich, 1988a). The probands were all diagnosed as having DSM-III panic disorder. Relatives of probands who had any MCMI personality disorder (compared to those who did not) had a significantly higher rate of panic disorder in relatives. Relatives of probands who had a Dramatic cluster personality disorder diagnosis or a borderline personality disorder diagnosis had a significantly higher rate of generalized anxiety disorder. Those relatives of probands who had any MCMI personality disorder also had significantly higher level of anxiety disorder in combination with a personality disorder.

Interestingly, the presence of a personality disorder in probands also affected the prevalence of depression and alcoholism in relatives of panic patients. Relatives of panic patients with Schizoid cluster, schizoid, borderline, dependent, avoidant, or passive-aggressive personality disorders had significantly higher rates of depression. Those relatives of probands with Schizoid cluster, histrionic, and passive-aggressive personality disorders had a significantly higher level of alcoholism. These results indicate that the presence of an MCMI personality disorder alters the family history of patients with panic disorder provide evidence for the instrument's validity.

Case Example

Mr. Z was a 40-year-old male who presented to the clinic in response to a newspaper advertisement soliciting subjects for a treatment trial for panic disorder. He was married and ran his own small retail establishment with the help of his wife. His panic attacks had begun at age 28 and since that time he had been limited to within a 2-mile radius of his home due to the fear that he would have a panic attack. He altered his life so that he would not have to go beyond that radius. Being an intelligent man with a quick wit he was always able to find plausible reasons for not going beyond his set radius. So successful was he at hiding his symptoms that his wife of 10 years was not aware of them, although she did claim to be exasperated at times with his behavior. At the time he presented to the clinic he was having about two spontaneous panic attacks a week. He would also have situational panic attacks when he periodically tried to go beyond his 2-mile radius. Between attacks he was not especially anxious and seemed to get along well with friends and customers.

On the MCMI his three top scales were dependent (above 85), avoidant (above 75) and anxiety (above 65). He related well and responded well to a combination of education and benzodiazepine treatment. His wife was also included in his therapy. After a time of continued gains he was able to function on a reduced dosage of benzodiazepines, sometimes using them for specific difficult situations. Having learned that panic attacks were not a physical danger he was also a bit less worried about them when they did occur. Being relatively well adjusted initially, the overall pattern of his life did not change greatly, but he was able to travel more and expand his social circle and he did become more involved in community events.

Conclusions

It is clear that the MCMI is a valuable and relatively unresearched aid to the research and treatment of the anxiety disorders. The personality scales seem to have some ability to distinguish between different anxiety disorders, predict outcome and family history. It is possible that the instrument could also be useful in examining "secondarily" induced personality disorders. The exact abilities and limitations of this instrument for the anxiety disorders will have to await further research.

REFERENCES

Millon, T. (1987). *Millon Clinical Multiaxial Inventory-II, Manual for the MCMI* (2nd ed.). Minneapolis: National Computer Systems.

Neenan, P., Felkner, J., & Reich, J. (1986). Schizoid personality traits developing secondary to panic disorder. *Journal of Nervous and Mental Disease, 174,* 483.

Reich, J. (1988a). A family history method for DSM-III anxiety and personality disorders. *Psychiatry Research, 26,* 131–139.

Reich, J. (1988b). DSM-III personality disorders and family history of mental illness. *Journal of Nervous and Mental Disease, 176,* 45–49.

Reich, J. (1988c). DSM-III personality disorders and the outcome of treated panic disorder, *American Journal of Psychiatry, 145,* 1149–1152.

Reich, J., & Green, A. I. (1991). Effect of personality on outcome of treatment. *Journal of Nervous and Mental Disease, 179,* 74–82.

Reich, J., & Noyes, R. (1987). A comparison of DSM-III personality disorders in acutely ill panic and depressed patients. *Journal of Anxiety Disorders, 1,* 123–131.

Reich, J., Noyes, R., Hirschfeld, R. P., Coryell, W., & O'Gorman, T. (1987). State effects on personality measures in depressed and panic patients. *American Journal of Psychiatry, 144,* 181–187.

Reich, J., Noyes, R., & Troughton, E. (1987a). Dependent personality disorder associated with phobic avoidance in patients with panic disorder. *American Journal of Psychiatry, 144,* 323–326.

Reich, J., Noyes, R., & Troughton, E. (1987b). Comparison of instruments to measure DSM-III, Axis II. In *Proceedings of the Millon Clinical Inventory Conference, 1986,* T. Millon (Ed.), Minnetonka, MN: National Computer Systems, pp. 223–235.

Reich, J., Noyes, R., & Yates, W. (1989). Alprazolam treatment of avoidant personality traits in social phobic patients. *Journal of Clinical Psychiatry, 50,* 91–95.

Reich, J. & Troughton, E. (1988a). A comparison of DSM-III personality disorders in recovered depressed and panic disorder patients. *Journal of Nervous and Mental Disease, 176,* 300–304.

Reich, J., & Troughton, E. (1988b). Frequency of DSM-III personality disorders in patients with panic disorder: Comparison with psychiatric and normal control subjects. *Psychiatry Research, 26,* 89–100.

III

CORRESPONDENCE TO DSM-III-R DISORDERS

11

The MCMI-II Personality Disorder Scales and Their Relationship to DSM-III-R Diagnosis

Thomas A. Widiger, Ph.D.
Elizabeth M. Corbitt, M.A.

One of the unique and perhaps most popular features of the MCMI and the MCMI-II are the personality disorder scales. The diagnosis and assessment of personality disorders has become of substantial clinical and theoretical interest due in large part to the placement of the personality disorders on a separate axis in the third edition of the American Psychiatric Association's (APA) Diagnostic and Statistical Manual of Mental Disorders (DSM-III; APA, 1980). The development of the MCMI was closely coordinated with the 1980 appearance of DSM-III (Millon, 1983a) and the popularity of the MCMI has been due in part to its provision of DSM-III personality disorder diagnoses.

This chapter reviews the validity of the MCMI and the more recent MCMI-II revision (hereafter, MCMI(-II) will refer to both the MCMI and the MCMI-II) as a measure of the DSM-III(-R) personality disorders. We begin with a brief discussion of the conceptual relationship between the MCMI(-II) and DSM-III (-R), followed by an overview of relevant validity and reliability research.

THE COORDINATION OF THE MCMI WITH THE DSM-III

The MCMI(-II) has been commended for being well-grounded in Millon's (1969, 1981, 1986) theory of personality psychopathology and for providing current DSM-III(-R) diagnoses (McCabe, 1984; Millon, 1983a, 1987; Wetzler, 1990). To the extent that the nomenclatures of Millon and the DSM-III(-R) are congruent, the MCMI(-II) could provide a valid assessment of both taxonomies. However, to the extent that they are not congruent it is questionable whether one instrument could assess both taxonomies with equal validity using the same scoring algorithms.

The first edition of the MCMI was published in 1977 as the Millon Multiaxial Clinical Inventory (Millon, 1977). "Each of the scales was constructed as an operational measure of a syndrome derived from a theory of personality and psychopathology" (Millon, 1977, p. 1). This theory posited eight basic personality syndromes derived from four reinforcement styles (dependent, independent, ambivalent, and detached) crossed with an activity versus passivity polarity: (a) asocial (passive-detached), (b) avoidant (active-detached), (c) submissive (passive-dependent), (d) gregarious (active-dependent), (e) egotistic or narcissistic (passive-independent), (f) aggressive (active-independent), (g) conforming (passive-ambivalent), and (h) negativistic (active-ambivalent). Millon (1969, 1981) also posited three severe variants of these eight syndromes:

1. cycloid (a more severe variant of the submissive and negativistic personality syndromes, although to some extent the conforming and gregarious as well);

2. schizoid (a more severe variant of the asocial and avoidant detached personality syndromes), and

3. paranoid (a more severe variant of the narcissistic and aggressive independent personality syndromes, although to some extent the conforming and negativistic personality syndromes as well).

"The three, more serious patterns of personality pathology are elaborations of one of the basic eight styles that develop under the pressure of persistent and unrelieved adversity . . . They are best understood as extensions and distortions that derive from, and are fully consonant with, the basic personality style" (Millon, 1977, p. 33).

The derivation and cross-validation studies for the MCMI were based on this taxonomy. In the original derivation study that sampled 682 patients (1972–1974), the clinicians were given narrative descriptions of each of Millon's (1969, 1977) pre-DSM-III personality syndromes. In the cross-validation study that sampled an additional 296 patients (1975–1976) these narrative descriptions were supplemented with criteria that Millon had written as initial drafts for the DSM-III personality disorders (Widiger, Williams, Spitzer, & Frances, 1985).

Millon was a consultant to the DSM-III Task Force and a member of the DSM-III Personality Disorders Advisory Committee (APA, 1980) and as such he had a considerable impact on the development of the DSM-III personality disorders (PDs). However, the final criteria sets for the PDs were not based on Millon's (1969, 1981) taxonomy. The decisions regarding which personality disorders to include and what criteria to use for their diagnosis were based on a variety of theoretical and empirical concerns (Frances, 1980; Gunderson, 1983).

For example, the antisocial PD criteria set was based primarily on the formulation of the antisocial personality disorder by Robins (1966), not on the formulation of the aggressive personality syndrome by Millon (1969, 1977).

Millon (1981) in fact took "strong exception to the narrow view promulgated in the DSM-III" (p. 182). Similarly, the DSM-III narcissistic PD was based on the psychoanalytic literature, particularly the work of Kohut (1971) and Kernberg (1970) (Frances, 1980; Gunderson, 1983), whereas Millon (1983b) indicated that his egotistic (narcissistic) personality syndrome "was not written within the framework of currently popular psychoanalytic authors, notably Kohut (1971) and Kernberg (1970), but rather derived from a social-learning developmental model (Millon, 1969)" (p. 812).

The DSM-III schizotypal PD was developed on the basis of consultations with Drs. Kety, Rosenthal, and Wender, and its initial draft was empirically evaluated and revised using case records diagnosed by these researchers as having borderline schizophrenia (Spitzer, Endicott, & Gibbon, 1979). Likewise, the DSM-III borderline PD was based on consultations with Drs. Gunderson, Kernberg, Rinsley, Sheehy, and Stone and evaluated empirically on the basis of cases diagnosed borderline by Drs. Kernberg and Stone (Frances, 1980; Spitzer et al., 1979). The only DSM-III PD that was based largely on Millon's theoretical model and taxonomy was the avoidant (Frances, 1980; Gunderson, 1983).

Widiger et al. (Widiger, Williams, Spitzer, & Frances, 1985) demonstrated empirically that the differences in the theoretical and empirical foundations for the taxonomies of Millon and the DSM-III were paralleled by substantial differences in the content of the items from the respective MCMI scales and DSM-III criteria sets for the antisocial and histrionic personality disorders (the nine other PDs were not assessed in this study). Widiger et al. (1985) suggested, therefore, that "one should be cautious in one's interpretation of the MCMI as a measure of DSM-III disorders" (p. 377).

The algorithms used in scoring the MCMI, however, were subsequently revised to be more congruent with the DSM-III nomenclature (Millon, 1983a). In addition, it is conceivable that the MCMI could provide valid assessments of the DSM-III PD diagnoses despite substantial differences in the content of the respective MCMI scales and DSM-III criteria sets. There does not need to be a one-to-one correspondence in content to provide valid assessments (Millon, 1985).

CONVERGENT VALIDITY FOR DSM-III PERSONALITY DISORDERS

Table 11.1 presents the correlations reported from five studies of the MCMI PD scales with the respective scales from the MMPI personality disorder scales developed by Morey, Waugh, and Blashfield (1985). The findings are rather consistent. The only substantial variability occurs for the paranoid PD scale. For example, Morey and LeVine (1988) obtained a correlation of .69 in a sample of 61 outpatients and 15 inpatients (72% female), whereas McCann (1989) obtained

TABLE 11.1
Correlation of MCMI PD Scales with MMPI PD Scales

MCMI Scale	S & M[a]	D & W[b]	M[c]	M & L[d]	G & F[e] M	F
Paranoid	.33*	.44***	.08	.69***	–	–
Schizoid	.64*	.35**	.67***	.68***	.68	.61
Schizotypal	.41*	.51***	.74***	.78***	–	–
Antisocial	.30*	.14	.15	.25	.30	-.07
Borderline	.55*	.28*	.42**	.54***	–	–
Histrionic	.61*	.66***	.68***	.71***	-.20	-.34
Narcissistic	.66*	.55***	.78***	.55***	.53	.18
Avoidant	.62*	.65***	.82***	.76***	.49	.65
Dependent	.52*	.68***	.50***	.68***	.15	.50
Compulsive	-.38*	-.42**	-.30*	-.31**	.02	.07
Pass-Agg	.51*	.50***	.57***	.48***	.19	.36

[a]Streiner and Miller (1988); n = 74. Specific significance levels were not given; all correlations were significant at least at the .05 level.
[b]Dubro and Wetzler (1989).
[c]McCann (1989); n = 47 (26 M, 21 F).
[d]Morey and LeVine (1988); n = 76.
[e]Greene and Farr (1987); n = 79 (55 M, 24 F). No significance levels were given.
*p < .05; **p < .01; ***p < .001.

a correlation of only .08 in a sample of 4 outpatients and 43 inpatients (45% female). There is no clear explanation for this inconsistency, although it could reflect in part differences in the demographic characteristics of the respective samples (discussed further below).

Substantial convergent validity is evident for the histrionic and avoidant scales (with correlations above .60 across four of the five studies) and good convergent validity for the schizoid, schizotypal, narcissistic, dependent, and passive-aggressive scales (with correlations above .50 for at least three of the studies). Weak convergent validity is evident for the borderline PD scale, with correlations ranging from .28 (Dubro & Wetzler, 1989) to .55 (Streiner & Miller, 1988). All of the correlations for the borderline scale were statistically significant, but the proportion of shared variance was never greater than 30%. The convergent validity for the antisocial scale was consistently poor, with correlations ranging from −.07 (Greene & Farr, 1987) to only .30 (Streiner & Miller, 1988). The lowest correlation obtained in any single study usually concerned the antisocial scale. Finally, a particularly unusual finding is the negative correlation for the compulsive PD scale that was obtained in four of the five studies. This negative correlation was never substantial (ranging from −.30 to −.42) but it is striking to consistently obtain a significant negative correlation for two scales that purportedly assess the same construct.

The explanation for the weak findings for the borderline, antisocial, and compulsive scales is not readily apparent. Either the MCMI or the MMPI (or both) could be providing a poor measurement of the respective construct.

Streiner and Miller (1988) interpreted the weak correlations as indicating inadequacies with the MMPI. This is a reasonable interpretation, given the absence of any supportive validity data for the MMPI PD scales at the time the Streiner and Miller study was completed (other than the internal consistency data reported by Morey et al., 1985). The MCMI PD scales did at least have some supportive data published in the test manual and elsewhere. Morey and LeVine (1988), however, took the opposite interpretation. Their weakest findings were obtained for the antisocial, compulsive, and passive-aggressive scales and they noted that "interestingly, for each of these three disorders there is reason to expect that the MCMI scale may differ from the corresponding DSM-III constructs" (p. 341).

Some clarification can be obtained by considering the convergent validity coefficients of the MCMI PD scales with additional instruments assessing the DSM-III personality disorders. Table 11.2 presents correlations of the MCMI PD scales with the respective scales from two semistructured interviews (Hogg, Jackson, Rudd, & Edwards, 1990; Nazikian, Rudd, Edwards, & Jackson, 1990; Reich, Noyes, & Troughton, 1987; Torgersen & Alneas, 1990; Widiger & Freiman, 1988), clinicians' ratings (Millon, 1983a; Piersma, 1987), and a self-report questionnaire (Reich et al., 1987). The findings presented in Table 11.2

TABLE 11.2
Correlation of MCMI with Other Personality Disorder Measures

MCMI Scale	SIDP[a] (r)	SIDP[b] (r)	SIDP[c] (r)	SIDP[d] (r)	PDQ[d] (r)	Clin[e] (k)	PIQ[f] (r)	Clin[g] (k)
PRN	.22**	.28	.03	.29	.30	–	.08	.59
SZD	.39**	.20	.47*	.40	.28	–	.02	.62
STY	.37**	.15	.39*	.31	.39	–	.33*	.60
ANT	–	.30	.23	.23	.15	–	.28+	.47
BDL	.32**	.80**	.33+	.32	.47	.25	.51**	.59
HST	.20**	.22	.26	.05	.15	-.09	.01	.59
NAR	.18**	.14	.34+	.04	.47	–	.21	.57
AVD	.42**	.31	.60**	.53	.68	–	.53**	.71
DEP	.38**	.38+	.21	.51	.53	.27	.64**	.76
CPS	-.05	.15	-.04	-.29	-.47	-.09	-.32+	.35
PAG	.14**	.50**	.17	.28	.59	–	.15	.56

Note. PRN = paranoid, SZD = schizoid, STY = schizotypal, ANT = antisocial, BDI = borderline, HST = histrionic, NAR = narcissistic, AVD = avoidant, DEP = dependent, CPS = compulsive, PAG = passive-aggressive.
[a]Torgersen and Alnaes (1990); $n = 298$; SIDP = Structured Clinical Interview for DSM-III Personality Disorders.
[b]Nazikian, Rudd, Edwards, and Jackson (1990); $n = 31$ (15 M, 16 F).
[c]Hogg, Jackson, Rudd, and Edwards (1990); $n = 40$ (32 M, 8 F).
[d]Reich, Noyes, and Troughton (1987); $n = 128$ (SIDP), $n = 121$ (PDQ). No significance levels were given; PDQ = Personality Diagnostic Questionnaire.
[e]Piersma (1987); $n = 151$ (54 M, 97 F). K = kappa for agreement between MCMI and clinician diagnoses; no significance levels were given.
[f]Widiger and Frieman (1988); PIQ = Personality Interview Questions.
[g]Millon (1983a); $n = 256$.
+ $p < .05$; * $p < .01$; ** $p < .001$.

are less consistent than those provided in Table 11.1. This is due in part to the variability in the assessment instruments. Some studies have reported weak convergent validity for semistructured interview and self-report inventory assessments of the personality disorders (e.g., Skodol, Oldham, Rosnick, Kellman, & Hyler, in press), and it is not surprising that the correlations of the respective MCMI scales would not always be substantial and would at times be inconsistent across a variety of assessment instruments.

However, the first four columns of Table 11.2 concern the correlations of the MCMI with only one instrument: the Semi-structured Interview for the DSM-III Personality Disorders (SIDP: Stangl, Pfohl, Zimmerman, Bowers, & Corenthal, 1985). Two of these reports came from the same research program (i.e., Hogg et al., 1990, and Nazikian et al., 1990), but substantially different results were obtained for the borderline, avoidant, and passive-aggressive scales. Nazikian et al. obtained a substantial correlation for the borderline scale but not for the avoidant, whereas Hogg et al. obtained a substantial correlation for the avoidant scale but not for the borderline. One possible explanation for this inconsistency is that 52% of the subjects in Nazikian et al. were female whereas only 20% were female in Hogg et al. Most borderline patients will be female (Widiger & Frances, 1989), and it is possible that research findings for the borderline personality disorder will be attenuated or at least distorted when only a small proportion of the sample is female. Likewise, findings with respect to the avoidant scale may be attenuated or distorted when the sample is not predominated by male subjects. This speculation receives some support in the MMPI findings reported separately for male and female subjects by Greene and Farr (1987) presented in Table 11.1. The correlations for the dependent and histrionic scales were higher for the female subjects than for the male subjects, and the correlation for the antisocial scale was higher for the male than for the female subjects, paralleling differences in the sex ratios for these personality disorders (APA, 1987). Greene and Farr, however, did not replicate this trend for the avoidant scale, nor did it occur for the compulsive.

Another explanation for the inconsistency is the inherent instability of a semistructured interview. The administration and scoring of the SIDP can vary substantially across studies, but the administration and scoring of the MCMI and the MMPI will be essentially constant. The weak convergent validity coefficients provided in Table 11.2 that are inconsistent with the convergence of the MCMI and the MMPI reported in Table 11.1 could be due in part to unstable and idiosyncratic administration of a semistructured clinical interview.

Six of the seven studies, however, did report good convergent validity coefficients for the avoidant PD scale. It is perhaps no coincidence that the best results are obtained for this scale, given that the DSM-III formulation of the avoidant diagnosis was based closely on Millon's (1969, 1981) taxonomy. Most of the studies also reported significant correlations for the borderline scale.

If one excludes the Millon (1983a) findings obtained from the test manual (discussed below), it is apparent that most of the studies reported weak convergent validity for (a) the antisocial scale, with correlations ranging from .15 (Reich et al., 1987) to .30 (Nazikian et al., 1990); (b) the paranoid scale, with correlations ranging from .03 (Hogg et al., 1990) to .30 (Reich et al., 1987); and (c) the histrionic scale, with correlations ranging from −.09 (Piersma, 1987) to .26 (Hogg et al., 1990). The antisocial and histrionic personality disorders were the two DSM-III diagnoses highlighted by Widiger et al. (1985) as being substantially different in content from the aggressive and gregarious personality syndromes of Millon (1981), respectively.

The results provided in Table 11.2 also replicate for the most part the negative correlation for the compulsive scale reported in Table 11.1. Three of the studies obtained moderate negative correlations, with the compulsive PD assessed by the Personality Diagnostic Questionnaire (Reich et al., 1987), the SIDP semistructured interview (Reich et al., 1987), and the Personality Interview Questions semistructured interview (Widiger & Freiman, 1988). The other studies reported an absence of any significant correlations for the MCMI compulsive scale.

Table 11.2 also provides convergent validity data from the test manual (Millon, 1983a). These convergent validity values are kappa coefficients we calculated on the basis of hit rate data provided in Table V:8 (Millon, 1983a, p. 59). Millon reported true and false positive rates, base rates, and total percent of correct classifications for a cross-validation sample of 256 patients (obtained from over 40 psychiatrists, psychologists, and social workers who provided the criterion diagnoses for each of the personality syndromes as described in Millon, 1983a). We used these data to derive a kappa value for the agreement between the diagnoses provided by the MCMI and the clinicians. The results are typically higher than has been obtained by the other studies summarized in Table 11.2, but they are also lower than one might have expected given the substantial agreement rates reported in Table V:8 of the test manual (e.g., overall rate of agreement ranged from 77% to 93%). Percent of agreement will typically be much higher than kappa because the latter will control for the chance capitalization on extreme base rates. The rank order of the kappa values, however, is consistent with the findings obtained in the other studies. For example, the agreement for the avoidant scale was among the highest, and the agreement for the antisocial and compulsive scales was poor (kappa values of only .47 and .35, respectively).

Summary

The results overall provided consistent and strong support for the convergent validity of the MCMI avoidant scale. There was also (inconsistent) support for the schizoid, schizotypal, narcissistic, borderline, dependent, passive-aggressive, and histrionic scales (e.g., the MCMI obtained good convergent validity for the histrionic scale when the MMPI was used as the criterion, but this was not replicated with the semistructured interviews, the clinician ratings, or the

Personality Diagnostic Questionnaire). The support for the paranoid scale was weak, the support for the antisocial scale was poor, and the MCMI compulsive scale appears to be measuring something that is almost opposite to the DSM-III compulsive personality disorder.

The results for the compulsive scale are perhaps the most interesting. The MCMI compulsive scale has correlated negatively with most other PD scales (McCann, 1989; Morey & LeVine, 1988) and it may be providing a measure of ego strength, self-discipline, emotional control, and adjustment rather than a personality disorder (Costa & McCrae, 1990; Joffe & Regan, 1988). It is clearly not assessing the DSM-III construct of a compulsive personality disorder.

The results for the antisocial scale also suggest a lack of congruence between the MCMI and the DSM-III. As we indicated earlier, Millon (1981) was critical of the DSM-III formulation of the antisocial personality disorder and it appears that his emphasis on the traits of hostile affectivity, assertive self-image, interpersonal vindictiveness, hyperthymic fearlessness, and malevolent projection (Millon, 1977, 1981) do not agree well with the DSM-III emphasis on a pattern of continuous and chronic violation of the rights of others, exploitation, delinquency, and criminality (APA, 1980). The MCMI scale may in fact provide a more useful and informative assessment of psychopathy than the DSM-III (Widiger et al., 1985) but it does not provide a valid assessment of the DSM-III antisocial personality disorder diagnosis.

MCMI-II

The research considered earlier was based on the MCMI. Millon has revised the MCMI in response to this research and in anticipation of the appearance of DSM-III-R in 1987 (APA, 1987; Millon, 1987). Specifically, two new PD scales were added (self-defeating and sadistic) to provide an assessment of these respective additions to the appendix of DSM-III-R, 45 items were revised and/or replaced, items were given weights (of 1, 2, or 3) in line with their presumed strength of association with the respective construct assessed by each scale, and moderator scales were added to correct for artifactual elevations due to depressed mood, exaggeration tendencies, and other factors (Millon, 1987).

We are aware of only one published study that has concerned the convergent validity of the MCMI-II PD scales. McCann (1991) provided the correlations between the respective PD scales from the MCMI-II and the MMPI. Table 11.3 presents these results, along with the MMPI findings provided previously in Table 11.1 from McCann (1989). It is useful to compare these two sets of findings since they involve the same external validator (MMPI PD scales) obtained by the same researcher using a similar sample of subjects (McCann, 1989, involved 47 patients, 91% of whom were inpatients; McCann, 1991, involved 80 inpatients).

It is evident from Table 3 that the convergent validity coefficients have in-

TABLE 11.3
Correlation of MCMI and MCMI-II With MMPI and Clinician Diagnoses

PD Scale		MMPI[a] (r)	Clinician[b] (k)
Paranoid	MCMI	.08	.59
	MCMI-II	.50	.56
Schizoid	MCMI	.67	.62
	MCMI-II	.73	.65
Schizotypal	MCMI	.74	.60
	MCMI-II	.86	.58
Antisocial	MCMI	.15	.47
	MCMI-II	.57	.72
Borderline	MCMI	.42	.59
	MCMI-II	.68	.78
Histrionic	MCMI	.68	.59
	MCMI-II	.74	.61
Narcissistic	MCMI	.78	.57
	MCMI-II	.65	.66
Avoidant	MCMI	.82	.71
	MCMI-II	.87	.72
Dependent	MCMI	.50	.76
	MCMI-II	.56	.69
Compulsive	MCMI	-.30	.35
	MCMI-II	-.04	.63
Passive-Aggressive	MCMI	.57	.56
	MCMI-II	.70	.60

Note. PD = personality disorder.
[a]MCMI data from McCann (1989) and MCMI-II data from McCann (1991); r = Pearson r correlations between MCMI (-II) and MMPI personality disorder scales.
[b]MCMI data from Millon (1983a) and MCMI-II data from Millon (1987); K = kappa for agreement between MCMI (-II) and clinician diagnoses.

creased for all of the scales, with the exception of the narcissistic (which decreased from .78 to .65). The correlations for the paranoid and antisocial scales increased substantially (from .08 to .50, and from .15 to .57, respectively). These results suggest that the MCMI-II does provide a better measure of the DSM-III(-R) than was provided by the MCMI (Millon, 1985). Only one of the convergent validity coefficients was below .50 (i.e., the compulsive), and five are at least .70. This is as good if not better than has been obtained with other PD instruments (e.g., Hyler, Skodol, Kellman, Oldham, & Rosnick, 1990; Skodol et al., in press). The findings should be considered as only preliminary until further replication, but they are at least encouraging.

Table 11.3 also presents a comparison of kappa values we calculated on the basis of the hit rate data presented in the respective test manuals of the MCMI (Table V:8 from Millon, 1983a) and the MCMI-II (Table 3–14 from Millon, 1987). The kappa values for the agreement between the MCMI-II and clinicians' diagnoses are again appreciably lower than the agreement percentages presented in the MCMI-II test manual (which varied from 88% to 97%) due to the correction for a capitalization on chance, but they also demonstrate an improvement for the antisocial, compulsive, and borderline scales. The lowest kappa values were obtained for the paranoid and schizotypal scales.

MCMI, MCMI-II, and the Five-Factor Model of Personality

A useful means by which to interpret the revisions to the MCMI is to compare the respective correlations of the MCMI and the MCMI-II to an independent variable. Table 11.4 presents the correlations (from Costa & McCrae, 1990) of the MCMI and the MCMI-II PD scales with the NEO-PI scales for the 5-factor model of personality that includes the dimensions of neuroticism, extraversion (vs. introversion), openness to experience, agreeableness (vs. antagonism), and conscientiousness (Costa & McCrae, 1985). These dimensions are said to represent the fundamental dimensions of personality (Digman, 1990) and the correlations of the MCMI(-II) to the NEO-PI are quite helpful in understanding the effects of the revision.

For example, the MCMI compulsive scale correlated negatively with neuroticism and openness, and positively with conscientiousness. Conscientiousness is a basic dimension of personality characterized by the traits of being organized, hardworking, reliable, neat, scrupulous, self-disciplined, punctual, and ambitious (Costa & McCrae, 1985). Widiger and Trull (in press) suggest that the compulsive personality disorder is essentially a maladaptive and extreme variant of conscientiousness, an hypothesis verified by Wiggins and Pincus (1989) and consistent with the findings of Costa and McCrae (1990). The negative correlation of the MCMI with openness was not predicted by Widiger and Trull, but it is consistent with a compulsive personality disorder as persons low on openness tend to be conventional, rigid, and narrow in their interests. Neuroticism concerns adjustment versus emotional instability; persons low in neuroticism tend to be calm, relaxed, and secure. The negative correlation of the MCMI compulsive scale with neuroticism is inconsistent with the DSM-III formulation of the compulsive personality disorder, and it may explain the negative correlations obtained by the MCMI compulsive scale with various other indices of personality dysfunction (e.g., Tables 11.1 and 11.2). The MCMI-II revision of the compulsive scale appears to be substantial, eliminating the negative correlation with neuroticism and essentially confining the relationship of the compulsive scale to conscientiousness.

Table 11.4 also presents the respective correlations for the MMPI PD scales

TABLE 11.4

Correlation of MCMI-II, and MMPI to NEO-PI Factors[a]

| | NEO-PI Factor | | | | |
Inventory	N	E	O	A	C
Paranoid					
MCMI	-.08	-.02	-.04	-.27***	.15*
MCMI-II	.04	.24	.12	-.07	.02
MMPI	.36**	-.02	-.09	-.31***	-.13
Schizoid					
MCMI	.04	-.64***	-.08	-.04	-.07
MCMI-II	-.14	-.49***	.04	.10	.14
MMPI	.16**	-.62***	.06	-.12	.14*
Schizotypical					
MCMI	.43***	-.46***	-.19**	.11	-.14
MCMI-II	.39**	-.34**	-.07	.06	.01
MMPI	.46***	.48***	.00	-.15*	.04
Antisocial					
MCMI	-.27***	.12	.22**	-.49***	.17*
MCMI-II	.15	.21	.08	-.42***	-.40***
MMPI	.13*	.07	.18**	-.35***	-.42***
Borderline					
MCMI	.52***	-.22**	-.10	.14*	-.10
MCMI-II	.46***	-.09	-.16	-.22	-.22
MMPI	.48***	.19**	.09	-.21***	-.32***
Histrionic					
MCMI	.00	.60***	.20**	-.02	-.21**
MCMI-II	.02	.57***	.03	-.19	-.39**
MMPI	-.17**	.65***	.15*	.00	-.22***
Narcissistic					
MCMI	-.28***	.47***	.27***	-.30***	.10
MCMI-II	-.22	.42***	.17	-.31*	-.24
MMPI	-.28***	.56***	.07	-.18**	.01
Avoidant					
MCMI	.44***	-.53***	-.11	.03	-.07
MCMI-II	.36**	-.32**	-.11	.05	.03
MMPI	.52***	-.54***	-.03	-.02	-.02
Dependent					
MCMI	.37**	-.06	-.36***	.38***	-.10
MCMI-II	.20	.09	-.26*	.34**	-.04
MMPI	.50***	-.30***	-.10	.22***	-.22***
Compulsive					
MCMI	-.39***	-.09	-.19**	.09	.38***
MCMI-II	-.05	-.03	-.11	.15	.52***
MMPI	.50***	-.16**	-.07	-.15*	-.06
Passive-Aggressive					
MCMI	.50***	-.07	.12	-.04	-.17*
MCMI-II	.53***	.01	-.14	-.20	-.23
MMPI	.39***	-.17**	-.02	-.16**	-.33***

Note. MCMI = Millon Clinical Multiaxial Inventory; MMPI = Minnesota Multiphasic Personality Inventory; NEO-PI = NEO Personality Inventory; N = Neuroticism; E = Extraversion; O = Openess to Experience; A = Agreeableness; C = Conscientiousness.

N = 207 for MCMI, 62 for MCMI-II, and 274 for MMPI.

[a]Results obtained from Costa and McCrae (1990). Personality disorders and the five-factor model of personality. *Journal of Personality Disorders, 4,* 362-371.

*p < .05; **p < .01; ***p < .001.

(also from Costa & McCrae, 1990) and these findings are particularly instructive for the compulsive scale. The most substantial correlation for the MMPI compulsive scale was a positive correlation with neuroticism (with much smaller positive correlations with introversion and antagonism). In other words, whereas the MCMI compulsive scale correlated negatively with neuroticism, the MMPI compulsive correlated positively with neuroticism. This inverse relationship to a fundamental dimension of personality dysfunction would explain for the most part the negative correlation of the MCMI with the MMPI. It is also evident from Table 11.4, however, that the MCMI-II and MMPI compulsive scales still fail to be congruent (they correlated only −.04 in McCann, 1991). The MMPI compulsive scale is essentially a measure of neuroticism, whereas the MCMI-II compulsive scale is essentially a measure of conscientiousness. To the extent that one conceptualizes the compulsive personality disorder as a maladaptive and extreme variant of conscientiousness (Widiger & Trull, in press) the MCMI-II is much more likely than the MMPI to provide a valid assessment of compulsive personality disorder traits.

Neuroticism includes facets of impulsivity, hostility, vulnerability, trait depression, trait anxiety, and self-consciousness (Costa & McCrae, 1985). Widiger and Trull (in press) suggest that the borderline personality disorder is essentially extreme neuroticism, with the most dysfunctional cases having elevations on all of the facets. This formulation is consistent with the findings of Wiggins and Pincus (1989) and Table 11.4. The MCMI, however, also obtained a positive correlation with introversion and agreeableness. Widiger and Trull suggested that to the extent to which borderline PD does involve other dimensions of personality, they would most likely be extraversion (with facets of excitement-seeking and emotionality) rather than introversion, and antagonism (irritable, uncooperative, manipulative, and vengeful) rather than agreeableness (helpful, forgiving, and good-natured). These predictions are consistent with the findings obtained for the MMPI (see Table 11.4) but not for the MCMI. The MCMI-II revision though is more consistent with this formulation and with the MMPI. The positive correlations with introversion and agreeableness have been eliminated and the MCMI-II now obtains a positive correlation with antagonism.

Persons low in conscientiousness tend to be aimless, unreliable, lax, negligent, and hedonistic (Costa & McCrae, 1985). This would clearly be more consistent with an antisocial personality disorder than the conscientiousness traits of being reliable, scrupulous, and punctual. The MCMI antisocial scale, however, obtained a significant positive correlation with conscientiousness whereas the MMPI obtained a negative correlation. The MCMI antisocial scale also obtained a positive correlation with openness. Persons high on openness tend to be curious, creative, original, imaginative, and untraditional (Costa & McCrae, 1985). It is conceivable that a proportion of antisocial persons would be characterized by openness (manifested in part by social rebellion) but openness to experience is not an integral facet of the antisocial personality disorder. Both the

MMPI and the MCMI also obtained substantial positive correlations with antagonism. Antisocial persons are likely to be rude, uncooperative, ruthless, manipulative, irritable, and cynical (Widiger & Trull, in press). The MCMI-II revision of the antisocial scale reversed the correlation with conscientiousness (from positive to negative) and eliminated the positive correlation with openness. The emphasis of the MCMI-II and the MMPI are now both on low conscientiousness and high antagonism.

The NEO-PI findings for the rest of the MCMI and MCMI-II scales are largely consistent. One curious inconsistency, however, occurs for the paranoid scale. The MCMI paranoid scale correlated with antagonism and conscientiousness. The MMPI paranoid scale correlated with neuroticism, antagonism, and low conscientiousness. The MCMI-II revision does not appear to be appreciably closer to the MMPI. The positive correlation with conscientiousness has been eliminated but so has the correlation with antagonism. The highest correlation for the MCMI-II paranoid scale is with extraversion, which is not at all consistent with the paranoid personality disorder (Widiger & Trull, in press). It is also worth noting again here that the lowest level of agreement between the MCMI-II and clinician diagnoses reported in the test manual occurred with the paranoid scale (kappa = .56; see Table 11.3), and the second lowest correlation with the respective MMPI scale reported by McCann (1991) also concerned the paranoid scale (r = .50). These results would suggest that the MCMI-II paranoid scale does warrant future attention and caution in interpretation.

MCMI-II Self-Defeating and Sadistic Scales

The MCMI-II also includes two new scales for the self-defeating and sadistic personality disorders that were included in an appendix to DSM-III-R for proposed diagnoses needing further study (Widiger, Frances, Spitzer, & Williams, 1988). The self-defeating scale was derived in large part from items that had previously been contained in the MCMI passive-aggressive scale, and the sadistic scale was derived in large part from items from the MCMI antisocial scale (Millon, 1987).

There has not yet, however, been any published research on the convergent validity of these scales with an independent measure of these personality disorders other than the data reported in the test manual. Based on the data provided in Table 3–14 of Millon (1987), we calculated that the self-defeating scale obtained a kappa of .56 with respect to clinicians' assessments of this PD, and the sadistic scale obtained a kappa of .69. The kappa value of .56 is the lowest for the MCMI-II PD scales (see Table 11.3). Costa and McCrae (1990) also reported that the MCMI-II self-defeating scale correlated only with neuroticism (r = .45), and the sadistic scale correlated only with antagonism (r = .46). The results for the sadistic scale are consistent with expectations (Widiger & Trull, in press), but the findings for the self-defeating scale suggest little distinction from the borderline scale (see Table 11.4). McCann (1991) as well reported a correlation of .88 between the MCMI-II borderline and self-defeating scales. The correlations of the MCMI-II self-defeating scale with other MMPI PD scales were also substantial and suggested a lack of specificity (e.g., .77 with dependent, .69 with avoidant, .66 with passive-aggressive, .66 with schizotypal, .56 with paranoid, .54 with compulsive, .50 with borderline, .40 with schizoid, and −.59 with narcissistic).

The validity of the sadistic and self-defeating scales, however, may be a moot issue. Neither PD diagnosis is likely to receive formal recognition in DSM-IV, which is scheduled to appear in 1993 (Frances et al., 1991). Neither may even be included in the appendix for proposed diagnoses needing further study (demotion is particularly likely for the sadistic). However, DSM-IV will likely include in this appendix a diagnosis of depressive personality disorder (Phillips, Gunderson, Hirschfeld, & Smith, 1990). It is equally likely then that the MCMI-II will be revised in anticipation of these forthcoming changes to the DSM-III-R.

RELIABILITY AND STATE EFFECTS

Fundamental to the validity of an assessment of a DSM-III-R personality disorder is temporal stability. A variety of studies have indicated that the MCMI(-II) PD scales have higher test-retest reliabilities than the MCMI scales that assess other clinical syndromes, such as mood and anxiety disorders, that are less chronic and are more responsive to treatment (McMahon, Flynn, & Davidson, 1985; Millon, 1983a, 1987; Murphy, Greenblatt, Mozdzierz, & Trimakas, 1990; Overholser, 1990; Piersma, 1986). This is particularly impressive given the overlap of the personality disorder and other clinical syndrome scales. For example, the MCMI-II borderline scale shares 37% of its items with the dysthymia scale and 44% with the major depression scale (Millon, 1987).

One qualification, however, is that these findings were based for the most part on the correlation in subjects' scale scores across time. A test-retest correlation indicates the extent to which the subjects maintained their relative position with respect to the group mean, not the extent to which the subjects maintained the same elevation on the respective PD scale (Libb et al., 1990). If all subjects' borderline PD scale scores decrease by 20 (e.g., a change in each case from the presence to the absence of a borderline personality disorder) the test-retest correlation would be perfect ($r = 1.0$) despite the absence of any stability in the borderline PD diagnoses. In other words, a test-retest correlation could be as high as 1.0 despite the fact that none of the subjects who were given a borderline diagnosis at Time 1 were given this diagnosis at Time 2.

There is reason to be concerned that such a phenomenon could occur with the MCMI(-II) PD scales. Piersma (1987) demonstrated with the MCMI that most PD scale scores decrease substantially during hospitalization. For example, 25%

of his 151 patients were diagnosed with borderline PD on the basis of an MCMI administered at the time of admission and only 7.3% at discharge; 12% were diagnosed with schizotypal personality disorder at admission and only 4% at discharge. Test-retest kappa (which considers the change in diagnosis) was only .11 for the borderline diagnosis, .09 for compulsive, .01 for passive-aggressive, and .27 for schizotypal. It is conceivable that personality functioning will improve to some extent during hospitalization, but it is unlikely that a brief hospitalization would have such a substantial effect. Piersma (1989) subsequently reported similar findings with the MCMI-II. Significant decreases were obtained for the schizoid, avoidant, dependent, passive-aggressive, self-defeating, schizotypal, borderline, and paranoid scales (and a significant increase for the histrionic and narcissistic scales). The highest mean obtained for any scale at admission was 80 (for the dependent scale); at discharge the highest mean was 68 (for the dependent and avoidant scales). Piersma (1989) concluded "quite clearly that the MCMI-II is not able to measure long-term personality characteristics ('trait' characteristics) independent of symptomatology ('state' characteristics)" (p. 91).

Self-report assessment of maladaptive personality traits can be distorted substantially by depression and anxiety (Widiger & Frances, 1987). Persons who are depressed tend to describe themselves as being more dependent, introverted, helpless, pessimistic, and vulnerable than they would prior to or subsequent to the occurrence of depression. The findings of Piersma (1987, 1989) suggest that the MCMI(-II) PD scales are subject to this distortion. Similar findings have been reported by Joffe and Regan (1988) and Libb et al. (1990). Joffe and Regan, for example, compared MCMI PD scores during and after an episode of major depression for 42 subjects. During their depression 84% obtained base rate scores above 74 for the passive-aggressive scale; only 19% when they were in remission. Similar decreases were obtained for the schizotypal (from 84% to 19%), borderline (69% to 17%), dependent (81% to 41%), avoidant (74% to 29%), and schizoid (57% to 21%) scales. Joffe and Regan also noted that there was a significant relationship between the MCMI borderline scale and a semi-structured interview assessment of borderline personality disorder during the remission of depression ($r = .40$, $p < .01$) but not when the subjects were depressed ($r = .24$, $p > .05$). Joffe and Regan (1988) also reported a significant increase in the narcissistic, histrionic, antisocial, and compulsive scales after the remission of depression. They concluded that their study "strongly challenges the validity and clinical utility of the MCMI in the diagnosis of personality disorders" (p. 284).

Libb et al. (1990) likewise reported significant changes in the MCMI PD scores for 28 patients before and after 12 weeks of pharmacologic treatment for depression. Significant decreases were obtained for the schizoid, avoidant, passive-aggressive, and borderline scales. Significant increases were obtained for the narcissistic and compulsive scales. Fifteen of the 28 subjects (54%) obtained scores above 84 on the passive-aggressive scale during their depression, whereas only 3 (11%) after treatment. Eleven subjects obtained scores above 84 on the borderline scale during their depression; only 3 did so after treatment. Libb et al. concluded that "only 4 of the 11 personality scales may be considered stable in our sample of depressed outpatients: Dependent, Histrionic, Antisocial, and Paranoid" (p. 215).

The confusion of affective and personality disorder symptomatology is particularly evident in a study by Choca, Bresolin, Okenek, and Ostrow (1988). Choca et al. administered the MCMI to 270 adult outpatients with major affective disorder to assess the convergent validity of "four MCMI affective scales" (p. 97). One of the four "affective scales" was the borderline personality disorder scale, which Choca et al. interpreted as measuring "mainly affective instability" (p. 97) rather than borderline personality disorder. The borderline scale successfully discriminated unipolar from bipolar mood disorder and was particularly useful in assessing current depressed mood. Choca et al. concluded that the borderline scale (along with the dysthymic, hypomanic, and psychotic depression scales) provided "an accurate indication of the overall mood state of the patient at the time the inventory is administered. As such, the data confirmed the convergent validity of the scales for assessing current mood state" (p. 102).

In sum, it appears that the scores on the MCMI(-II) PD scales can be distorted by the current mood and/or anxious state of the subject. The borderline, passive-aggressive, avoidant, schizoid, and schizotypal scales are particularly likely to be elevated by a depressed and/or anxious mood, while the narcissistic and compulsive scales may be diminished. The inflation of PD scales is not particularly surprising but the depression of the narcissistic and compulsive scales may be counterintuitive. However, the narcissistic scale includes items that assess self-worth and confidence and the compulsive scale includes items that assess emotional control. It is then understandable that scores on these scales could be diminished by a depressed and/or anxious mood (Joffe & Regan, 1988).

MCMI-II Correction Scales. The MCMI-II includes additional corrections for state depression and anxiety. The avoidant, self-defeating, and borderline scales are corrected downward for elevations on the anxiety and/or dysthymia scales (Millon, 1987). Only one of the above studies used the MCMI-II (Piersma, 1989) and these findings appear to have been based on uncorrected scores. It will be of particular interest in future studies to determine whether there is in fact an adequate adjustment to the avoidant, self-defeating, and borderline scales, whether downward adjustments should also be made to the passive-aggressive, schizoid, and schizotypal scales, and whether upward adjustments should be made to the narcissistic and compulsive scales. In the meantime, clinicians are advised to be very cautious when interpreting the results for these PD scales when their patient is either depressed and/or anxious.

Research on these (and other) correction scales, however, will be hindered by the inherent complexity they provide to the scoring of the MCMI-II. It is suggested that it takes about one-half hour to handscore an MCMI-II and this would appear to be no exaggeration. The first step in hand scoring the MCMI-II is to obtain a raw score for each of the 25 scales. Each raw score is obtained by summing the response weights (ranging from 1–3) for each item on the scale endorsed. Next, the Raw X scale score (a disclosure level correction) is calculated using the raw scores of the basic personality syndrome scales (scales 1–8B), with the following formula:

$$
\begin{aligned}
\text{Raw X Scale Score} = & \ [(\text{sum of scales 4 and 8A}) \times 1.5) \\
& + [(\text{sum of scales 1, 2, 3, and 8B}) \times 1.6] \\
& + (\text{sum of scales 5, 6A, 6B, and 7}).
\end{aligned}
$$

The *initial* base rate (BR) score for each scale is found in a table (using the raw score) provided for each gender in appendices to the *Hand Scoring Guide* (Millon, 1990). The initial BR scores are then submitted to a total of six adjustments.

First, the initial BR score for each scale is corrected using one of two values determined from the Raw X score. One correction value is used for the 10 basic personality syndrome scales (1–8B); the other is used for the three severe personality pathology scales (i.e., the borderline, paranoid, and schizotypal scales). These values are found in two tables in the *Hand Scoring Guide* (Millon, 1990).

Three scales—2 (avoidant), 8B (self-defeating), and C (borderline)—are next adjusted for depression and anxiety. This correction considers the patient's scores on scales D (dysthymia) and A (anxiety), the setting in which the patient is seen, and the duration of the patient's "Axis I" (clinical syndrome) episode. For illustrative purposes, we use a fictional numerical example in calculating the depression/anxiety (DA) adjustment for the C (borderline) scale, as follows:

1. a figure called *DAadjust* is computed using the BR scores on scales D and A; for example, if D = 95 and A = 100, DAadjust = $[(95 - 85) + (100 - 85)]$ = 25. (Note: If D < 85, this adjustment is not done, and if A < 85, the A portion of the formula is omitted);

2. the correct combination of setting (inpatient or noninpatient) and Axis I episode duration is determined and the appropriate instructions are followed. For example, for an inpatient with an Axis I duration of 1 to 4 weeks, the appropriate correction for the C scale would be: .75 $\times$ (DAadjust with a maximum of 15) = .75 $\times$ 15 = 11.25, which is rounded to 11. (The number 15 is used instead of 25 because 15 is the maximum value to be used in this calculation.) Finally, the result (11) is subtracted from the borderline BR score to produce the BR Score after DA adjustment.

The next correction for the borderline scale would be the desirability/debasement (DD) adjustment, which is calculated using the BR scores for the Y (desirability) and Z (debasement) scales using the following formula: DD $= (Y - Z)/10$. This figure is rounded to the nearest whole number and added (to a maximum of $+/-10$) to the borderline BR score.

Next, the denial/complaint (DC) adjustment is made, but only if certain basic personality syndrome scores are elevated in relation to others. The correction is done in two parts, and each part must be checked separately for applicability. The first adjustment is added if scale 4 (histrionic) or scale 5 (narcissistic) currently has the highest BR score of the 10 basic personality syndrome scales and/or if scale 7 (compulsive) currently has one of the two highest BR scores of these scales. The second adjustment is subtracted if scale 8B (self-defeating) has the highest current BR score of the 10 basic personality syndrome scales and/or if scale 2 (avoidant) has one of the two highest current BR scores of these scales.

It is unlikely that a research program could efficiently handscore 50–100 MCMI-II answer sheets. The National Computer Systems does provide a discount for the computer scoring for research purposes. The discount is substantial, but the computer scoring does not provide the raw, Raw X, DA adjustment, DD adjustment, and DC adjustment scores. Only the final BR score would be provided. One would then be unable to analyze the effectiveness of the various corrections.

The authors and publishers of the MCMI-II appear to be somewhere between a rock and a hard place. The inclusion of the various corrections for depression, anxiety, setting, denial, and exaggeration might be necessary to provide valid assessments, but their inclusion complicates the scoring of the MCMI-II to the point that handscoring becomes impractical. The only apparent solution is to provide all of the scores in the computer report for research purposes. This would represent an additional expense for the National Computer Systems but it would appear to be a reasonable and forthright provision to encourage and support the validation of the MCMI-II.

CONCLUSIONS

There are currently a variety of self-report instruments for the assessment of the DSM-III(-R) personality disorders. Two for which there are published research are the MMPI PD scales (Morey et al., 1985) and the Personality Diagnostic Questionnaire-Revised (Hyler et al., 1990). A variety of others are currently being developed. Our review of the research on the MCMI(-II) would suggest that it is unlikely that any will clearly provide a more valid and/or a more reliable assessment than the MCMI-II. There are limitations to the MCMI-II (particularly the barriers to research), but the MCMI-II does appear to represent an improvement over the MCMI. The issues with respect to the effects of state depression and anxiety are substantial, but they apply to all other self-report instruments and the MCMI-II at least includes a variety of moderating and correction scales to address these concerns. It is regrettable that it has been so costly for independent researchers to assess the validity and reliability of the MCMI(-II) (Widiger, 1985), but it is likely that the MCMI-II will continue to be one of the more popular and useful self-report inventories for the assessment of personality disorder pathology.

REFERENCES

American Psychiatric Association. (1980). *Diagnostic and statistical manual of mental disorders* (3rd ed.). Washington, DC: Author.

American Psychiatric Association. (1987). *Diagnostic and statistical manual of mental disorders* (3rd ed., rev. ed.). Washington, DC: Author.

Choca, J., Bresolin, L., Okonek, A., & Ostrow, D. (1988). Validity of the Millon Clinical Multiaxial Inventory in the assessment of affective disorders. *Journal of Personality Assessment, 52*, 96–105.

Costa, P. T., & McCrae, R. R. (1985). *The NEO Personality Inventory manual.* Odessa, FL: Psychological Assessment Resources.

Costa, P. T., & McCrae, R. R. (1990). Personality disorders and the five-factor model of personality. *Journal of Personality Disorders, 4*, 362–371.

Digman, J. M. (1990). Personality structured: Emergence of the five-factor model. *Annual Review of Psychology, 41*, 417–440.

Dubro, A. F., & Wetzler, S. (1989). An external validity study of the MMPI personality disorder scales. *Journal of Clinical Psychology, 45*, 570–575.

Frances, A. J. (1980). The DSM-III personality disorders section: A commentary. *American Journal of Psychiatry, 137*, 1050–1054.

Frances, A. J., Widiger, T. A., First, M., Pincus, H. A., Tilly, S. M., Miele, G. M., & Davis, W. W. (1991). DSM-IV: Toward a more empirical diagnostic system. *Canadian Psychology.*

Greene, R. L., & Farr, S. P. (1987, September). *Concordance among the MCMI and MMPI personality disorder scales.* Paper presented at the 95th Annual Meeting of the American Psychological Association, New York.

Gunderson, J. G. (1983). DSM-III diagnosis of personality disorders. In J. Frosch (Ed.), *Current perspectives on personality disorder diagnosis* (pp. 20–39). Washington, DC: American Psychiatric Press.

Hogg, B., Jackson, H. J., Rudd, R. P., & Edwards, J. (1990). Diagnosing personality disorders in recent-onset schizophrenia. *Journal of Nervous and Mental Disease, 178*, 194–199.

Hyler, S. E., Skodol, A. E., Kellman, H. D., Oldham, J. M., & Rosnick, L. (1990). Validity of the Personality Diagnostic Questionnaire-Revised: Comparison with two structured interviews. *American Journal of Psychiatry, 147*, 1043–1048.

Joffe, R. T., & Regan, J. J. (1988). Personality and depression. *Journal of Psychiatric Research, 22*, 279–286.

Kernberg, O. F. (1970). A psychoanalytic classification of character pathology. *Journal of the American Psychoanalytic Association, 18*, 800–822.

Kohut, H. (1971). *The analysis of the self.* New York: International Universities Press.

Libb, J. W., Stankovic, S., Sokol, R., Freeman, A., Houck, C., & Switzer, P. (1990). Stability of the MCMI among depressed psychiatric outpatients. *Journal of Personality Assessment, 55*, 209–218.

McCabe, S. (1984). Millon Clinical Multiaxial Inventory. In D. Keyser & R. Sweetland (Eds.), *Test critiques* (Vol. 1, pp. 455–465). Kansas City, KA: Westport.

McCann, J. T. (1989). MMPI personality disorder scales and the MCMI: Concurrent validity. *Journal of Clinical Psychology, 45*, 365–369.

McCann, J. T. (1991). Convergent and discriminant validity of the MCMI-II personality disorder scales. *Psychological Assessment: A Journal of Consulting and Clinical Psychology, 3,* 9–18.

McMahon, R. C., Flynn, P. M., & Davidson, R. S. (1985). Stability of the personality and symptom scales of the Millon Clinical Multiaxial Inventory. *Journal of Personality Assessment, 49,* 231–234.

Millon, T. (1969). *Modern psychopathology.* Philadelphia, PA: Saunders.

Millon, T. (1977). *Millon Multiaxial Clinical Inventory manual.* Minneapolis, MN: National Computer Systems.

Millon, T. (1981). *Disorders of personality. DSM-III: Axis II.* New York: Wiley.

Millon, T. (1983a). *Millon Clinical Multiaxial Inventory manual* (3rd ed.). Minneapolis, MN: National Computer Systems.

Millon, T. (1983b). The DSM-III: An insider's perspective. *American Psychologist, 38,* 804–814.

Millon, T. (1985). The MCMI provides a good assessment of DSM-III disorders: The MCMI-II will prove even better. *Journal of Personality Assessment, 49,* 379–391.

Millon, T. (1986). Personality prototypes and their diagnostic criteria. In T. Millon & G. Klerman (Eds.), *Contemporary directions in psychopathology* (pp. 671–712). New York: Guilford.

Millon, T. (1987). *Manual for the MCMI-II* (2nd ed.). Minneapolis, MN: National Computer Systems.

Millon, T. (1990). *MCMI-II: User's guide for hand-scoring.* Minneapolis, MN: National Computer Systems.

Morey, L. C., & LeVine, D. J. (1988). A multitrait-multimethod examination of Minnesota Multiphasic Personality Inventory (MMPI) and Millon Clinical Multiaxial Inventory (MCMI). *Journal of Psychopathology and Behavioral Assessment, 10,* 333–344.

Morey, L. C., Waugh, M. H., & Blashfield, R. K. (1985). MMPI scales for DSM-III personality disorders: Their derivation and correlates. *Journal of Personality Assessment, 49,* 245–251.

Murphy, T. J., Greenblatt, R. L., Mozdzierz, G. J., & Trimakas, K. A. (1990). Stability of the Millon Clinical Multiaxial Inventory among psychiatric inpatients. *Journal of Psychopathology and Behavioral Assessment, 12,* 143–150. '

Nazikian, H., Rudd, R. P., Edwards, J., & Jackson, H. J. (1990). Personality disorder assessments for psychiatric inpatients. *Australian and New Zealand Journal of Psychiatry, 24,* 37–46.

Overholser, J. C. (1990). Retest reliability of the Millon Clinical Multiaxial Inventory. *Journal of Personality Assessment, 55,* 202–208.

Phillips, K. A., Gunderson, J. G., Hirschfeld, R. M., & Smith, L. E. (1990). The depressive personality. *American Journal of Psychiatry, 147,* 830–837.

Piersma, H. L. (1986). The stability of the Millon Clinical Multiaxial Inventory for psychiatric inpatients. *Journal of Personality Assessment, 50,* 193–197.

Piersma, H. L. (1987). The MCMI as a measure of DSM-III Axis II diagnoses: An empirical comparison. *Journal of Clinical Psychology, 43,* 478–483.

Piersma, H. L. (1989). The MCMI-II as a treatment outcome measure for psychiatric inpatients. *Journal of Clinical Psychology, 45,* 87–93.

Reich, J., Noyes, R., & Troughton, E. (1987). Lack of agreement between instruments assessing DSM III personality disorders. In C. Green (Ed.), *Conference on the Millon clinical inventories* (pp. 223–234). Minnetonka, MN: National Computer Systems.

Robins, L. N. (1966). *Deviant children grown up.* Baltimore, MD: Williams & Wilkins.

Skodol, A. E., Oldham, J. M., Rosnick, L., Kellman, H. D., & Hyler, S. E. (in press). Diagnosis of DSM-III-R personality disorders: A comparison of two structured interviews. *Methods in Psychiatric Research.*

Spitzer, R. L., Endicott, J., & Gibbon, M. (1979). Crossing the border into borderline personality and borderline schizophrenia. *Archives of General Psychiatry, 36,* 17–24.

Stangl, D., Pfohl, B., Zimmerman, M., Bowers, W., & Corenthal, C. (1985). A structured interview for the DSM-III personality disorders. *Archives of General Psychiatry, 42,* 591–596.

Streiner, D. L., & Miller, H. R. (1988). Validity of MMPI scales for DSM-III personality disorders: What are they measuring? *Journal of Personality Disorders, 2,* 238–242.

Torgersen, S., & Alnaes, R. (1990). The relationship between the MCMI personality scales and DSM-III, Axis II. *Journal of Personality Assessment, 55,* 698–707.

Wetzler, S. (1990). The Millon Clinical Multiaxial Inventory (MCMI): A review. *Journal of Personality Assessment, 55,* 445–464.

Widiger, T. A. (1985). Review of Millon Clinical Multiaxial Inventory. In J. V. Mitchell (Ed.), *The ninth mental measurements yearbook* (Vol. 1, pp. 986–988). Lincoln, NE: Buros Institute of Mental Measurements.

Widiger, T. A., & Frances, A. J. (1987). Interviews and inventories for the measurement of personality disorders. *Clinical Psychology Review, 7,* 49–75.

Widiger, T. A., & Frances, A. J. (1989). Epidemiology, diagnosis, and comorbidity of borderline personality disorder. In A. Tasman, R. Hales, & A. Frances (Eds.), *Review of psychiatry* (Vol. 8, pp. 8–24). Washington, DC: American Psychiatric Press.

Widiger, T. A., Frances, A. J., Spitzer, R. L., & Williams, J. B. W. (1988). The DSM-III-R personality disorders: An overview. *American Journal of Psychiatry, 145,* 786–795.

Widiger, T. A., & Freiman, K. (1988, November). *Personality Interview Questions-II: Reliability and methodological issues.* Paper presented at the National Institute of Mental Health Workshop on Assessment of Personality Disorders, Bethesda, MD.

Widiger, T. A., Williams, J. B. W., Spitzer, R. L., & Frances, A. J. (1985). The MCMI as a measure of DSM-III. *Journal of Personality Assessment, 49,* 366–378.

Widiger, T. A., & Trull, T. J. (in press). Personality and psychopathology: An application of the five-factor model. *Journal of Personality.*

Wiggins, J. S., & Pincus, A. L. (1989). Conceptions of personality disorders and dimensions of personality. *Psychological Assessment: A Journal of Consulting and Clinical Psychology, 1,* 305–316.

12

The MCMI as a Predictor of DSM-III Diagnostic Categories: A Review of Empirical Research

Harry L. Piersma, Ph.D., ABPP

The diagnostic congruence between the Millon Clinical Multiaxial Inventory (MCMI; Millon, 1983) and the Diagnostic and Statistical Manual of Mental Disorders (DSM-III; American Psychiatric Association, 1980) has generated considerable controversy since the inception of the MCMI. Several debates have centered around how consonant Millon's taxonomy (Millon, 1981) is with the DSM-III taxonomy. Widiger, Williams, Spitzer and Frances (1985) have argued that the congruence is only partial for several of the MCMI scales. They also noted that there had been little empirical research to validate the congruence between the MCMI and DSM-III.

Since Widiger et al.'s 1985 article, however, numerous studies have evaluated the MCMI and DSM-III congruence. This chapter is a critical assessment of the existing research. First, the congruence between the MCMI and Axis I diagnoses is examined, followed by a review of how well the MCMI has functioned as a predictor of Axis II disorders. Next, critical methodological issues are highlighted, followed by recommendations for more constructive paradigms for future work. Finally, additional problems in researching the MCMI-II (Millon, 1987) and DSM-III-R (American Psychiatric Association, 1987) are briefly discussed.

MCMI AND AXIS I DISORDERS

The following section is a review of selected studies evaluating the MCMI as a predictor of Axis I disorders. This review is not exhaustive, but highlights characteristic findings for DSM-III diagnostic categories.

Depression and Anxiety

Wetzler, Kahn, Strauman, and Dubro (1989) examined the MCMI Dysthymia (D) and Psychotic Depression (CC) scales regarding how well they identified 48 patients diagnosed by attending psychiatrists as having a major depression. For this depressed sample and a general psychiatric comparison group, they found the D scale to have a sensitivity of .71 and a specificity of .70. The CC scale, however, had a sensitivity of only .04, although the specificity was .97. Choca, Bresolin, Okonek, and Ostrow (1988) evaluated 270 adult patients on an affective disorders unit. Each patient was administered a 1- to 2-hour semistructured diagnostic interview, and consensual DSM-III diagnoses were reached by a multidisciplinary diagnostic team. For unipolar depressed patients, the sensitivity of the D scale was .87, while it was .20 for the CC scale. Goldberg, Shaw, and Segal (1987) administered the MCMI, the Hamilton Rating Scale, and the Beck Depression Inventory to 95 psychiatric outpatients. The CC scale had a sensitivity of .18 to clinician's diagnoses of major depression. The authors noted that both the D and CC scales correlated more highly to the Beck than to the Hamilton, which they attributed to the fact that both MCMI scales lack the somatic and vegetative items that are a significant component of the Hamilton. Finally, Piersma (1987a) examined the performance of the D and CC scales in relation to DSM-III diagnoses given by attending psychiatrists at a private psychiatric hospital. He found that the CC scale identified very few patients diagnosed as having a major depression, at either BR > 74 or BR > 84. Also, the computerized diagnoses generated by the MCMI interpretive report frequently predicted the diagnosis of generalized anxiety disorder, although this diagnosis was given very infrequently by clinicians.

Hypomania and Bipolar Disorder

DeWolf, Larson, and Ryan (1985) administered the MCMI to 48 inpatients who had a bipolar diagnosis. These patients were tested prior to the initiation of chemotherapy, and 45 of them were in the manic phase of the bipolar disorder. Only 13 (27%) were identified by the MCMI computerized report (BR > 74 on the Hypomania or N scale). Choca et al. (1988) noted that the N scale identified 56% of patients who were manic when they completed testing. They also noted that the specificity of this scale for unipolar depressed patients was very high, that is, the N scale was almost never significantly elevated for clinically depressed patients.

Drug Abuse

Calsyn, Saxon, and Daisy (1990) administered the MCMI to 75 White male veterans undergoing treatment for opioid or cocaine dependence. Approximately 39% were correctly identified (BR > 74) by the Drug Abuse (T) scale. However, they noted that the specificity of the scale was very high for psychiatric controls.

Marsh, Stile, Stoughton, and Trout-Landen (1988) evaluated 163 patients participating in a methadone maintenance program and found that 49% had BR > 74 on the T scale. They believed that this relatively low specificity could be partially attributed to the fact that only 5 of the 46 items on the T scale specifically concern substance use. In a study that examined both alcohol and drug abuse symptomatology among psychiatric inpatients, Bryer, Martines, and Dignan (1990) found that the T scale (BR > 74) identified 49% of those patients who had either (a) a substance abuse diagnosis, or (b) other information in the medical record indicating substance abuse difficulties.

Alcohol Abuse

McMahon, Gersch, and Davidson (1989) divided 256 male alcoholics into continuous and episodic groups, finding mean BR scores >90 on the B scale for each group. Sensitivity or specificity statistics for the B scale were not reported. In the Bryer et al. (1990) study, the B scale correctly classified 43% of psychiatric inpatients having either an alcohol abuse/dependence diagnosis or problem (BR > 74). Miller and Streiner (1990) classified individuals as alcoholic based either on discharge diagnosis or interviews done with the Diagnostic Interview Schedule (DIS; Robins, Helzer, Croughan, Williams, & Spitzer, 1981). They compared the B scale with the MacAndrew Alcoholism Scale (MAC; Mac-Andrew, 1965) and found the MAC to have a greater sensitivity than the B scale for alcoholics. However, in nonalcoholic samples, the specificity of the B scale exceeded that of the MAC. They concluded that the B scale did not evidence the degree of diagnostic efficiency reported in the MCMI manual (Millon, 1983).

Schizophrenia

Relatively little research has evaluated the diagnostic efficiency of the MCMI in relation to schizophrenic disorders. Patrick (1988) reported that the sensitivity of the Psychotic Thinking (SS) scale was only .07 for a sample of 103 psychiatric inpatients. However, it was not clear from this study which schizophrenic subtypes were used to calculate specificity indices. Sexton, McIlwraith, Barnes, and Dunn (1987) developed factor scores for both the MCMI and MMPI-168 for 136 adult psychiatric inpatients. They found the MCMI to be more accurate in predicting affective disorders than schizophrenic disorders.

Conclusions—Axis I Research

The following conclusions appear warranted on the basis of previous studies evaluating the congruence between the MCMI and DSM-III:

   1. The Psychotic Depression (CC) scale is not a very good measure of severe depressive symptomatology, either of a psychotic or nonpsychotic nature. There

seems to have been conceptual confusion in the development of this scale, in that even though it is named *Psychotic* Depression, there are no items having to do with actual psychotic symptoms. On the other hand, if this scale was developed to measure the DSM-III construct of major depression, more items having to do with vegetative or somatic depressive symptoms should have been included. At any rate, the preponderance of studies have shown the CC scale to be much less sensitive to the depressive diagnoses and symptoms than the D scale.

2. In general, the Alcohol Abuse(B), Drug Abuse(T), and Hypomania(N) scales have not shown very high sensitivity compared to DSM-III diagnostic categories, particularly for homogeneous diagnostic groupings. However, for heterogeneous psychiatric patient samples, the specificity of each of these scales has been quite high. In other words, these scales often fail to identify individuals who truly do have the disorder. However, the scales rarely make the mistake of categorizing individuals as having the disorder when they do not give evidence of it.

3. Relatively little work has been done concerning the MCMI and schizophrenic/other psychotic diagnostic categories. What little has been done suggests that the MCMI is more helpful in diagnosing affective disorders than schizophrenic disorders.

MCMI AND AXIS II DISORDERS

The majority of Axis II–MCMI studies have fallen into one of two categories. The first category consists of studies that compare the MCMI to Axis II diagnoses given by clinicians in routine or standard clinical practice. This most commonly means that the clinician's diagnosis is based on a diagnostic interview and any other collateral information available at that time. The second category includes studies comparing the MCMI to diagnoses which were made on the basis of structured interviews specifically designed for Axis II disorders.

MCMI and Standard Clinical Practice Axis II Diagnoses

Piersma (1987b) evaluated the MCMI–Axis II correspondence for 151 psychiatric inpatients. At discharge, 61 of 151 patients (40%) received an Axis II diagnosis from their attending psychiatrist. However, 148 patients (98%) received an Axis II diagnosis at both admission and discharge on the MCMI computerized report. Agreement was relatively low between clinicians and the MCMI regarding the diagnosis of specific categories of personality disorder. Agreement was highest in regard to the diagnosis of dependent personality. Interestingly, the admission and discharge MCMI Axis II diagnoses were in agreement for only 27% of patients. Repko and Cooper (1985) evaluated 100 workman's compensation cases and also found that the MCMI predicted Axis II disorders much more frequently than did clinicians. Wetzler and Dubro (1990) found that for 41 patients and 74 inpatients, 41 (36%) received an Axis II diagnosis from the attending psychiatrist. Using the psychiatrist diagnosis as the gold standard, they found relatively little agreement between the MCMI and psychiatrists for either diagnoses of specific personality disorders or clusters of diagnoses. They also found that the MCMI predicted Axis II diagnoses much more frequently than did clinicians.

MCMI and Structured Interview Axis II Diagnoses

Dubro, Wetzler, and Kahn (1988) compared MCMI personality scales with diagnoses obtained by the Structured Interview for DSM-III Personality Disorders (SIDP; Pfohl, Stangl, & Zimmerman, 1983). They found that 61% of the psychiatric patients they interviewed met the SIDP criteria for a personality disorder, while only 5% of a medical control group received a personality disorder diagnosis. They found the MCMI to be very sensitive to the diagnosis of any personality disorder (.96), although the specificity was only .48. For clusters of personality disorders, the MCMI was moderately sensitive and specific. Widiger and Sanderson (1987) examined 53 inpatients at a state mental hospital, after excluding any patients with the diagnosis of schizophrenia, major depression, or a chronic mental disorder. All patients were administered the Personality Interview Questions (PIQ), which is a semistructured interview. On this basis, patients were placed in one or more of the following categories: antisocial, passive-aggressive, avoidant, and dependent. They found that the MCMI was a better predictor of the dependent/avoidant categories than the antisocial/passive-aggressive categories. They postulated that one reason for this finding was that Millon's dependent/avoidant formulations are more consonant with the DSM-III than are his formulations for antisocial/passive-aggressive disorders. Finally, Torgersen and Alnaes (1990) examined the MCMI in relation to the Structured Interview for the DSM-III Personality Disorders (SIDP) in a sample of 272 outpatients at the University of Oslo. They reported good correspondence between the MCMI and SIDP for the avoidant and dependent disorders, fairly good correspondence for the schizotypal, histrionic, borderline, narcissistic, and paranoid scales, and no correspondence for the schizoid, passive-aggressive, and compulsive scales. Interestingly, they found that the passive-aggressive scale was highly positively correlated with personality disorders in general, while the compulsive scale was negatively correlated with most personality disorders.

Conclusions—Axis II Research

1. Whatever MCMI standard is used (BR > 74, B > 84, or computerized diagnostic predictions), the MCMI diagnoses more personality disorders than do clinicians operating according to standard clinical practice, with standard clinical

practice representing diagnoses which are based on unstructured interviews and collateral information. One explanatory factor for this finding may be that in routine clinical practice, clinicians are more focused on obtaining Axis I diagnoses, since these diagnoses are most relevant to immediate treatment concerns.

2. The majority of evidence is supportive of Wetzler's (1990) contention, that the diagnostic efficiency of the MCMI for Axis II disorders has been greater for studies in which the MCMI is evaluated against structured interviews than studies in which it has been compared against unstructured interviews. If one grants that structured interviews are more reliable than unstructured interviews, then the MCMI may be, in Wetzler's words, ". . . a better Axis II diagnostician than is the typical practitioner" (Wetzler, 1990, p. 457).

3. Overall, the MCMI seems to be most efficient in diagnosing dependent and avoidant disorders, whether the "gold standard" is either structured or unstructured interviews. This finding would support Widiger and Sanderson's (1987) contention that Millon's typology for personality disorders is most consistent with the DSM-III nosology for the dependent and avoidant categories.

METHODOLOGICAL ISSUES

The following section lists methodological issues and problems in previous research evaluating the MCMI as a predictor of DSM-III diagnoses.

1. *Against what standard should MCMI findings be compared?* Probably the most glaring methodological limitation in past research is that many studies have used "standard clinical practice" or chart reviews as the diagnostic standard against which the MCMI is compared. In many instances, researchers have assumed that the chart diagnoses are a reliable and valid standard against which to evaluate the MCMI. Of course, such assumptions are quite suspect. For example, during the DSM-III field trials (APA, 1980) evaluators based diagnoses on standard clinical practice. For these trials, the Kappa coefficient for Axis II diagnoses was .62. However, this coefficient represents agreement between clinicians as to whether there was *any* personality disorder present. Reliability estimates for specific disorders was much lower. Thus, a diagnostic standard of routine clinical practice is not likely to provide the most valid criterion against which to judge the MCMI.

2. *What should the MCMI standard be?* One source of confusion in interpreting previous studies is the fact that researchers use different standards to determine whether or not the MCMI "diagnoses" a personality disorder. Thus, some have used BR > 74 as the standard, some have used BR > 84 as the standard, and some have used the diagnostic predictions generated by the computerized interpretive. Occasionally, researchers have not made it clear which MCMI standard they were using.

3. *How does one handle the issue of multiple diagnoses?* Frequently, patients will have several personality or syndrome scales above the clinically significant cut-off point, whether it be BR74 or BR84. Multiple elevations are consistent with Millon's theoretical framework, which postulates the intercorrelation of differing personality traits and styles. In this way, the MCMI is an instrument designed to alert the clinician to as many diagnostic considerations as possible. However, in clinical practice, the tendency of most practitioners is to condense diagnostic possibilities. For example, it is likely that if the typical patient met criteria for both a dysthymic disorder and a generalized anxiety disorder, the clinician would list only the dysthymic disorder on Axis I.

4. *How are state and trait characteristics best measured?* One recurring problem in MCMI research concerns the point in the treatment process when MCMI's are most appropriately administered. Even though the goal of the MCMI was to measure state factors as independently of trait factors as possible, this ideal can never be obtained (cf. Piersma, 1986 for a discussion of personality and syndrome scale differences observed for psychiatric inpatients who were tested at admission and discharge). The validity of the MCMI for predicting Axis II disorders is likely to be compromised when patients are tested at a point of acute situational stress, such as when patients are tested shortly following admission to the hospital. However, for Axis I disorders, concurrent validity would likely be maximized by testing patients at the time they are experiencing the most severe psychiatric symptoms.

5. *How is MCMI data most meaningfully reported?* Most researchers have typically reported MCMI data as mean BR scores, often with associated tests of statistical significance. However, this method has no relevance to the sensitivity or specificity of individual MCMI scales. The diagnostic efficiency of the MCMI can only be evaluated if each study includes information concerning the proportion of patients correctly identified at BR > 74 or BR > 84.

SUGGESTED PARADIGMS FOR FUTURE STUDIES

Given the methodological problems in past MCMI research, what changes could most improve the quality of future research?

1. There is no doubt that the preferred methodology for future studies is to evaluate the MCMI against diagnostic standards which are based on structured interviews. A good proportion of MCMI studies have used routine clinical diagnostic practice as the gold standard against which the MCMI is compared. Given the much lesser reliability of unstructured interviews compared to structured interviews, it hardly seems fair to criticize the MCMI because it does not coincide with a criterion that itself is highly unreliable.

2. In many instances, the optimal point in time for MCMI administration will

differ for Axis I and Axis II studies. For Axis I, MCMI syndrome scale performance is most validly assessed when patients are the most symptomatic. For outpatients, this would most likely be at the time of the initial session. For inpatients, this would be at the time of admission or shortly thereafter. For Axis II, MCMI data would be most comparable to other diagnostic standards if testing were done when the patient is relatively symptom-free. Thus, Axis II studies would be best carried out when patients were ready to terminate treatment, or possibly at midcourse in the treatment process.

3. Even though the preferable methodology is to compare the MCMI with structured diagnostic interviews, many researchers simply do not have the personnel or financial resources to utilize structured interviews. However, if routine clinical diagnostic practice is going to be the standard against which the MCMI is evaluated, there are ways in which the methodological limitations can be at least partially addressed. For example, in such studies it would be wise to have two clinicians conduct independent diagnostic interviews. In this way, the diagnostic reliability between the two clinicians could be determined. It would be informative to determine if the reliability between clinicians exceeds the reliabilities between each individual clinician and the MCMI.

4. Finally, the problem of multiple MCMI diagnoses must be addressed. One method for partially controlling this variable would be for clinicians, either in structured or unstructured interviews, to rate patients as *yes* or *no* for meeting DSM-III categories. For example, two clinicians might see a sample of patients and rate each individual according to whether he/she met the criteria for an anxiety disorder, a somatoform disorder, or a dysthymic disorder. These ratings could then be assessed for reliability between the clinicians, and also for how well their clinical ratings compared to the BR cut-off scores for the anxiety, somatoform, and dysthymia scales. For Axis II, the clinicians could rate whether the individual met the criteria for each of the DSM-III personality disorders, and then compare this information against BR scores on the MCMI personality scales.

THE MCMI-II—FURTHER CONSIDERATIONS

This article has focused entirely on studies involving DSM-III and MCMI comparisons. Of course, the DSM-III-R (APA, 1987) is the current diagnostic standard, and the MCMI-II (Millon, 1987) became available several years ago. One major methodological concern in future research will be that while almost all clinicians use the nomenclature of the DSM-III-R, many continue to use the MCMI rather than the MCMI-II. This will make comparisons between the two even more problematic than past comparisons between the MCMI and DSM-III. Although handscoring keys have now become available for the MCMI-II, handscoring time will average three times longer than was the case for the MCMI.

This fact will discourage many researchers from using the MCMI-II in diagnostic studies. Thus, many clinicians and researchers are likely to continue to use the MCMI even though they use the updated diagnostic criteria of the DSM-III-R. Finally, for those who do study the MCMI-II *versus* the DSM-III-R, Millon (1987) has noted that the diagnostic possibilities generated by the computerized report are more tied to configural relationships between scales than was the case for the MCMI. Thus, researchers might most validly evaluate the MCMI-II's diagnostic accuracy by looking at the computerized diagnoses, rather than BR cut-off scores.

REFERENCES

American Psychiatric Association. (1980). *Diagnostic and statistical manual of mental disorders* (3rd ed.). Washington, DC: Author.

American Psychiatric Association. (1987). *Diagnostic and statistical manual of mental disorders* (3rd rev. ed.). Washington, DC: Author.

Bryer, J. B., Martines, K. A., & Dignan, M. A. (1990). Millon Clinical Multiaxial Inventory alcohol abuse and drug abuse scales and the identification of substance abuse patients. *Journal of Consulting and Clinical Psychology, 2,* 438–441.

Calsyn, D. A., Saxon, A. J., & Daisy, F. (1990). Validity of the MCMI Drug Abuse Scale with drug abusing and psychiatric samples. *Journal of Clinical Psychology, 46,* 244–246.

Choca, J., Bresolin, L., Okonek, A., & Ostrow, D. (1988). Validity of the Millon Clinical Multiaxial Inventory in the assessment of affective disorders. *Journal of Personality Disorders, 52,* 96–105.

DeWolf, A., Larson, J. K., & Ryan, J. (1985). Diagnostic accuracy of the Millon test computer reports for bipolar affective disorders. *Journal of Psychopathology and Behavioral Assessment, 7,* 185–189.

Dubro, A., Wetzler, S., & Kahn, M. (1988). A comparison of three self-report questionnaires for the diagnosis of DSM-III personality disorders. *Journal of Personality Disorders, 2,* 256–266.

Goldberg, J., Shaw, B., & Segal, Z. (1987). Concurrent validity of the Millon Clinical Multiaxial Inventory Depression Scales. *Journal of Consulting and Clinical Psychology, 50,* 554–567.

MacAndrew, C. (1965). The differentiation of male alcoholic outpatients from nonalcoholic psychiatric outpatients by means of the MMPI. *Quarterly Journal of Studies on Alcohol, 26,* 238–246.

Marsh, D. T., Stile, S. A., Stoughton, N. L., & Trout-Landen, B. L. (1988). Psychopathology of opiate addiction: Comparative data from the MMPI and MCMI. *American Journal of Drug and Alcohol Abuse, 14,* 17–27.

McMahon, R. C., Gersh, D., & Davidson, R. S. (1989). Personality and symptom characteristics of continuous *vs* episodic drinkers. *Journal of Clinical Psychology, 45,* 161–168.

Miller, H. R., & Streiner, D. L. (1990). Using the Millon Clinical Multiaxial Inventory's Scale B and the MacAndrew Alcoholism Scale to identify alcoholics with concurrent psychiatric diagnoses. *Journal of Personality Assessment, 54,* 736–746.

Millon, T. (1981). *Disorders of personality. DSM-III: Axis II.* New York: Wiley.

Millon, T. (1983). *Millon Clinical Multiaxial Inventory Manual* (3rd ed.). Minneapolis: National Computer Systems.

Millon, T. (1987). *Manual for the MCMI-II* (2nd ed.). Minneapolis, MN: National Computer Systems.

Patrick, J. (1988). Concordance of the MCMI and MMPI in the diagnosis of three DSM-III Axis I disorders. *Journal of Clinical Psychology, 44,* 186–190.

Pfohl, B., Stangl, D., & Zimmerman, M. (1983). *Structured interview for the DSM-III personality disorders (SIDP)*. Unpublished manual. Iowa City: University of Iowa.

Piersma, H. L. (1986). The Millon Clinical Multiaxial Inventory (MCMI) as a treatment outcome measure for psychiatric inpatients. *Journal of Clinical Psychology, 42*, 493–499.

Piersma, H. L. (1987a). MCMI computer-generated diagnoses: How do they compare to clinician judgment? *Journal of Psychopathology and Behavioral Assessment, 9*, 305–312.

Piersma, H. L. (1987b). The MCMI as a measure of DSM-III Axis II diagnoses: An empirical comparison. *Journal of Clinical Psychology, 43*, 478–483.

Repko, G. R., & Cooper, R. (1985). The diagnosis of personality disorder: A comparison of MMPI profile, Millon inventory, and clinical judgment in a worker's compensation population. *Journal of Clinical Psychology, 41*, 867–881.

Robins, L. N., Helzer, J. E., Croughan, J., Williams, J. B. W., & Spitzer, R. L. (1981). *NIMH Diagnostic Interview Schedule: Version III*. Bethesda, MD: National Institute of Mental Health.

Sexton, D., McIlwraith, R., Barnes, G., & Dunn, R. (1987). Comparison of MCMI and MMPI-168 as psychiatric inpatient screening inventories. *Journal of Personality Assessment, 51*, 388–398.

Torgersen, S., & Alnaes, R. (1990). The relationship between the MCMI personality scales and DSM-III, Axis II. *Journal of Personality Assessment, 55*, 698–707.

Wetzler, S. (1990). The Millon Clinical Multiaxial Inventory (MCMI): A review. *Journal of Personality Assessment, 55*, 445–464.

Wetzler, S., & Dubro, A. (1990). The diagnosis of personality disorders by the MCMI. *Journal of Nervous and Mental Diseases, 178*, 261–263.

Wetzler, S., Kahn, R., Strauman, T., & Dubro, A. (1989). The diagnosis of major depression by self-report. *Journal of Personality Assessment, 53*, 22–30.

Widiger, T. A., & Sanderson, C. (1987). The convergent and discriminant validity of the MCMI as a measure of the DSM-III personality disorders. *Journal of Personality Assessment, 51*, 228–242.

Widiger, T., Williams, J., Spitzer, R., & Frances, A. (1985). The MCMI as a measure of DSM-III. *Journal of Personality Assessment, 49*, 366–378.

13 Computer-Assisted Interpretation of the MCMI-II

Kevin L. Moreland, Ph.D.

This chapter discusses, in some detail, the system for computer-assisted interpretation of the MCMI-II developed by Professor Millon and distributed by National Computer Systems' Professional Assessment Services Division (cf. Millon, 1987; National Computer Systems, 1991). Although other computer-assisted test interpretation (CATI) systems for the MCMI-II exist, I have chosen not to deal with them for two reasons. First, those systems are not very well documented. Second, they appear to operate like less sophisticated versions of Millon's system. In particular, Millon's system relies heavily on his updated biopsychosocial theory (Millon, 1986a, 1986b) in addition to the empirical data available on the MCMI and MCMI-II. Other systems, on the other hand, appear to make far less use of Millon's theory. Thus, at this writing, my judgment is that one can readily evaluate the likely utility of other MCMI-II CATI systems by examining the empirical data presented in the MCMI-II manual (Millon, 1987).[1]

The first section of the chapter describes the content of the computer-generated interpretive reports. The second describes the development and functioning of Millon's CATI system. Because no empirical studies of the MCMI-II CATI system have been published, I then review the empirical studies of Millon's CATI system for the MCMI (cf. Millon, 1983). This review includes my judgment about the degree to which those findings are likely to generalize to the MCMI-II CATI. The chapter concludes with tips on optimal use of the CATI system.

---

[1]At this writing (mid 1991) only a handful of empirical studies of the MCMI-II have been published outside the test manual.

CONTENT OF MILLON'S CATI FOR THE MCMI-II

The first page of Millon's CATI (see Fig. 13.1) presents a histogram-like profile of the MCMI-II base rate (*BR*) scores along with demographic information about the client. The two paragraphs that kick off the second page are boilerplate. They caution the user about the limitations that should always be kept in mind in using these reports. (Similar boilerplate paragraphs begin all the major sections of the CATI.) The next paragraph describes the demographic characteristics of the instant client and specific situational characteristics that should be kept in mind when using the specific report at hand. A comment is then made about the reliability and validity of the report. That is, any response biases and other distortions apparent in the client's responses to the MCMI-II are described. Then the report-proper begins.

The case-specific clinical narrative begins with up to a page-and-a-half of narrative describing the client's personality pattern and level of DSM-III-R Axis II impairment. This section of the report relies heavily on Millon's (1986a, 1986b) updated biopsychosocial theory. Millon's theory fleshes out the descriptive, mainly behavioral descriptions of the Axis II disorders found in DSM-III-R. Unlike the DSM-III-R, Millon systematically addresses the client's likely behavior, mood/affect, cognitive style and content, interpersonal conduct, and self-image. Reading this section of the sample report you will note that it is distinctly psychodynamic.

The next section of the report, which may be up to a page in length, presents narrative descriptions of the Axis I disorders that appear to be troubling the client. These descriptions are frequently enhanced by the inclusion of relevant inferences based on the configuration of Axis II scales. Thus, for example, the paragraph on alcoholism in the sample report does not simply report that the client is likely to be experiencing alcohol-related problems. In addition it says, "Anxious, lonely, and socially apprehensive, she finds drinking to be a useful lubricant that reduces her tensions and fears, provides brief moments of enhanced self-esteem, and enables quick resolution of the psychic pain to which she is routinely exposed." These inferences about the functions alcohol serves for the client are clearly based on her high score on the Avoidant scale (cf. McMahon & Davidson, 1985, 1986) and perhaps her high scores on the Self-Defeating and Borderline scales too. The Axis I paragraphs are presented in order of the salience of each disorder for the client. So, in the sample report, the client's score of 96*BR* on the Alcohol Dependence scale earns that disorder precedence over Dysthymic Disorder (77*BR*).

"Noteworthy [item] Responses" are presented following the Axis I narrative. Noteworthy Responses are presented in four categories: Health Preoccupation, Interpersonal Alienation, Emotional Dyscontrol, and Self-Destructive Potential. The Noteworthy Responses supplement the scale-derived inferences nicely because the four categories of items cut across the scales rather than paralleling

MILLON CLINICAL MULTIAXIAL INVENTORY-II
FOR PROFESSIONAL USE ONLY

ID NUMBER = SAMPLE   VALID REPORT
PERSONALITY CODE = 2 8B ** 5 3 * 1 8A 6B 6A 4 + 7 " -   // C ** - * //
SYNDROME CODE = B ** D * // - ** - * //
DEMOGRAPHIC = 00010518/OP/F/32/W/N/ G1/P/JO/LO/30081/01/01/30150/ 331 0002

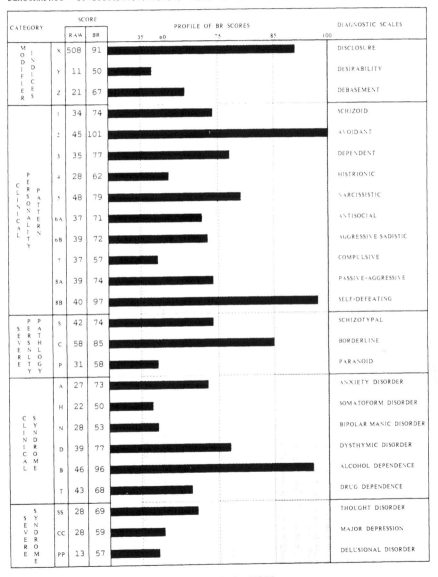

CATEGORY		SCORE		PROFILE OF BR SCORES	DIAGNOSTIC SCALES
		RAW	BR	35 60 75 85 100	
MODIFIER INDICES	X	508	91		DISCLOSURE
	Y	11	50		DESIRABILITY
	Z	21	67		DEBASEMENT
CLINICAL PERSONALITY PATTERN	1	34	74		SCHIZOID
	2	45	101		AVOIDANT
	3	35	77		DEPENDENT
	4	28	62		HISTRIONIC
	5	48	79		NARCISSISTIC
	6A	37	71		ANTISOCIAL
	6B	39	72		AGGRESSIVE SADISTIC
	7	37	57		COMPULSIVE
	8A	39	74		PASSIVE-AGGRESSIVE
	8B	40	97		SELF-DEFEATING
SEVERE PERSONALITY PATHOLOGY	S	42	74		SCHIZOTYPAL
	C	58	85		BORDERLINE
	P	31	58		PARANOID
CLINICAL SYNDROME	A	27	73		ANXIETY DISORDER
	H	22	50		SOMATOFORM DISORDER
	N	28	53		BIPOLAR MANIC DISORDER
	D	39	77		DYSTHYMIC DISORDER
	B	46	96		ALCOHOL DEPENDENCE
	T	43	68		DRUG DEPENDENCE
SEVERE SYNDROME	SS	28	69		THOUGHT DISORDER
	CC	28	59		MAJOR DEPRESSION
	PP	13	57		DELUSIONAL DISORDER

Please see reverse side for NOTE

FIG. 13.1

MCMI reports are normed on patients who were in the early phases of
assessment or psychotherapy because of emotional discomforts or social
difficulties. Respondents who do not fit this normative population or
who have inappropriately taken the MCMI for nonclinical purposes may
have distorted reports. To optimize clinical utility, the report
highlights pathological characteristics and dynamics rather than
strengths and positive attributes. This focus should be kept in mind
by the referring clinician reading the report.

Based on theoretical inferences and probabilistic data from actuarial
research, the MCMI report cannot be judged definitive. It must be
viewed as only one facet of a comprehensive psychological assessment,
and should be evaluated in conjunction with additional clinical data
(e.g., current life circumstances, observed behavior, biographic
history, interview responses, and information from other tests). To
avoid its misconstrual or misuse, the report should be evaluated by
mental health clinicians trained in recognizing the strengths and
limitations of psychological test data. Given its limited data base
and pathologic focus, the report should not be shown to patients or
their relatives.

INTERPRETIVE CONSIDERATIONS

In addition to the preceding considerations, the interpretive
narrative should be evaluated in light of the following demographic
and situational factors. This 32 year old single white woman with a
graduate/professional school education, currently seen professionally
as an outpatient, reports her most recent problems as Job/School/Work
and Loneliness; difficulties appear to have taken the form of an Axis
I disorder within a period of less than one week.

The response style of this patient showed no unusual test-taking
attitude that would distort MCMI results.

AXIS II: PERSONALITY PATTERNS

The following pertains to those enduring and pervasive
characterological traits that underlie this woman's personal and
interpersonal difficulties. Rather than focus on her more marked but
essentially transitory symptoms, this section concentrates on her
habitual, maladaptive methods of relating, behaving, thinking, and
feeling.

Evidence of a moderate level of pathology exists in the overall
personality structure of this woman. She likely has a checkered
history of disappointments in her personal and family relationships.
Deficits in her social attainments may be notable, as well as a
tendency to precipitate self-defeating vicious circles. Earlier hopes
may have resulted in frustrating setbacks, and efforts to achieve a
consistent niche in life may have failed. Although she usually is
able to function on a satisfactory ambulatory basis, she may
experience periods of marked emotional, cognitive, or behavioral
dysfunction.

The emotions of this troubled woman are characterized by pervasive
apprehensiveness, intense and variable moods, prolonged periods of
dejection and self-deprecation, and episodes of withdrawn isolation or
unpredictable anger. A long-standing expectancy that others will be
rejecting or disparaging precipitates profound gloom one time,
self-defeating and self-abnegating behaviors the next, and irrational
negativism another. Vacillation in mood is exhibited among desires
for affection, self-destructive acts, fear, and a general numbness of
feeling. Despite her longing for warmth and acceptance, she withdraws
to maintain a safe distance from close psychological involvements.
Retreating defensively, she not only becomes remote from her much
needed and desired sources of support but also impulsively seeks
self-sabotaging pursuits. A surface apathy may characterize her
efforts to conceal her excess sensitivity. Behind this front of
restraint may be intense contrary feelings that break through in
displays of temper toward those whom she sees as being unsupportive,
critical, and disapproving. The little security that she possesses,

FIG. 13.1
(*Continued*)

however, is threatened when these resentments are expressed.
Therefore, to protect against further loss, she attempts to conceal
or resist expressing anger, albeit unsuccessfully.

Also notable are times of contrition when she may engage in expiatory
self-damaging acts and suicidal gestures. Thus, when she is not
withdrawn and drifting aimlessly in peripheral social roles, she
behaves in an unpredictable manner, impulsively seeking troublesome
situations. Innumerable wrangles and disappointments with others
occur as she vacillates among self-denial, sullen passivity,
self-destructive activities, and explosive anger. Frequently, these
behaviors are interspersed with genuine expressions of guilt and
contrition that are then mixed with feelings of being misunderstood,
unappreciated, and demeaned by others. Not atypically, she
intentionally provokes condemnations through her behaviors, and then
accuses others of having mistreated her.

Deprived of a sense of self-worth, this woman cannot help but
painfully contemplate the pitiful and futile state of her identity. A
tendency toward extreme introspection compounds her identity problem.
The alienation that she feels from others is paralleled by feelings of
alienation from herself, adding to undercurrents of tension, sadness,
and anger.

She has learned to expect ridicule and derision. She can detect the
most minute traces of disinterest expressed by others and makes the
molehill of a minor slight into a mountain of personal contempt and
condemnation. Life has taught her that good things do not last and
that overtures of affection end in disappointment and rejection.
Anticipating disillusionment, she undermines potentially positive
opportunities with impulsive hostility. A cyclical variation may be
observed as her efforts at constraint are followed by impulsive
outbursts that, in turn, are followed by remorse and regret. These
erratic emotions are not only intrinsically distressing but also upset
her limited capacity to cope with everyday tasks. Unable to orient
her emotions and thoughts logically, she may drift occasionally into
personal irrelevancies and autistic asides. Her inability to
communicate ideas and feelings in a relevant social manner further
alienates her from others.

AXIS I: CLINICAL SYNDROMES

The features and dynamics of the following distinctive Axis I clinical
syndromes are worthy of description and analysis. They may arise in
response to external precipitants, but are likely to reflect and
accentuate enduring and pervasive aspects of this woman's basic
personality makeup.

Alcoholism is a major problem for this troubled woman. Anxious,
lonely, and socially apprehensive, she finds drinking to be a useful
lubricant that reduces her tensions and fears, provides brief moments
of enhanced self-esteem, and enables quick resolution of the psychic
pain to which she is routinely exposed. By dislodging preoccupations
with her aggrieved status in life, alcohol serves to undo her deep
sense of alienation and isolation. Alcohol briefly bolsters her
depleted feelings of self-worth and erases the pressing awareness of
her troubled existence by providing an illusory respite from anguish
and frustrations.

Clinical features of dysthymia are an integral part of this depressed
woman's characterological makeup. Not only when she is notably
downhearted and blue is her sorrowful and disconsolate demeanor
apparent, for feelings of dejection and self-defeating attitudes are
intrinsic to her life. She routinely voices concerns over her social
adequacy and personal worthiness, makes repeated self-deprecatory and
guilt-ridden comments about her failures and unattractiveness, and
regularly complains about her inability to do things right. Although
she reports being aggrieved and mistreated by others, she also claims
to deserve the anguish and abuse she receives, an admittance
consistent with her self-image as an unworthy and undeserving person.

FIG. 13.1
(Continued)

In consonance with her unconscious dynamics, she not only may tolerate relationships that aggravate her misery but also may precipitate conditions and events that perpetuate it.

NOTEWORTHY RESPONSES

The following statements were answered by the patient in the direction noted in the parentheses. These items suggest specific problem areas that may deserve further inquiry on the part of the clinician.

HEALTH PREOCCUPATION

29. I have a hard time keeping my balance when walking (T).
33. I feel weak and tired much of the time (T).
71. I feel tired all the time (T).

INTERPERSONAL ALIENATION

13. I have little interest in making friends (T).
47. I'm so quiet and withdrawn, most people don't even know I exist (T).
49. I am a quiet and fearful person (T).
83. A long time ago, I decided it's best to have little to do with people (T).
141. I am very ill-at-ease with members of the opposite sex (T).

EMOTIONAL DYSCONTROL

5. In the last few weeks I begin to cry even when the slightest of things goes wrong (T).
43. My own "bad temper" has been a big cause of my troubles (T).
67. Lately, I feel jumpy and under terrible strain, but I don't know why (T).
151. People have said in the past that I became too interested and too excited about too many things (T).
167. Lately, I have gone all to pieces (T).

SELF-DESTRUCTIVE POTENTIAL

59. I have given serious thought recently to doing away with myself (T).
79. Serious thoughts of suicide have occurred to me for many years (T).
115. Sometimes I feel like I must do something to hurt myself or someone else (T).

PARALLEL DSM-III-R MULTIAXIAL DIAGNOSES

Although the diagnostic criteria utilized in the MCMI-II differ somewhat from those in the DSM-III-R, there are sufficient parallels to recommend consideration of the following assignments. More definitive judgments should draw on biographic, observation, and interview data in addition to self-report inventories such as the MCMI-II.

AXIS I: CLINICAL SYNDROME

The major complaints and behaviors of the patient parallel the following Axis I diagnoses, listed in order of their clinical significance and salience.

305.00 Alcohol Abuse
300.40 Dysthymia

AXIS II: PERSONALITY DISORDERS

A deeply ingrained and pervasive pattern of maladaptive functioning underlies the Axis I clinical syndromal picture. The following personality diagnoses represent the most salient features that characterize this patient.

FIG. 13.1
(*Continued*)

Personality configuration composed of the following:

301.82 Avoidant Personality Disorder

301.90 Personality Disorder NOS (Self-defeating Personality Disorder)

301.83 Borderline Personality Disorder

Course: The major personality features described previously reflect long term or chronic traits that are likely to have persisted for several years prior to the present assessment.

The clinical syndromes described previously tend to be relatively transient, waxing and waning in their prominence and intensity depending on the presence of environmental stress.

AXIS IV: PSYCHOSOCIAL STRESSORS STATEMENTS

In completing the MCMI-II, this individual identified the following factors that may be complicating or exacerbating their present emotional state. They are listed in order of importance as indicated by the client. This information should be viewed as a guide for further investigation by the clinician.

Work Problems; Social/Personal Difficulties

PROGNOSTIC AND THERAPEUTIC IMPLICATIONS

The possibility of a current alcohol or drug abuse disorder or both should be carefully considered. If verified, appropriate behavioral management or group therapeutic programs should be implemented.

Once the patient has been adequately stabilized, attention may be directed toward the long-term goals suggested in the following paragraphs.

Because she tends to demean her self-worth and to mistrust others, this woman is unlikely to sustain a consistent therapeutic relationship. Maneuvers designed to test the sincerity of the therapist will probably be evident. Since she fears facing her feelings of unworthiness and senses that her coping defenses are weak, she may withdraw from treatment before any real gains are made. Efforts to explore the contradictions in her feelings and attitudes may result in a seesaw struggle, with periods of temporary progress followed by retrogression. Genuine gains will require slow, laborious work and a building of trust by enhancing her shaky sense of self-worth.

The potential gains of therapy not only may fail to motivate this patient but also may serve as a deterrent. Therapy may reawaken what she views as false hopes; that is, it may remind her of the dangers and humiliations she experienced when she tendered her affections to others but received rejection in return. Now that she has found a modest level of comfort by distancing herself from others, she would rather let matters stand and maintain the level of adjustment to which she has become accustomed.

At the cognitive-behavioral level, therapeutic attention may be carefully directed to her hesitancy, suspiciousness, and self-deprecating attitudes, behaviors that evoked humiliation, contempt, and derogation in the past. Efforts to press her to reduce her sensitivity to rebuff and her fearful style may only reinforce her aversive inclinations.

Another realm worthy of attention is associated with her extensive scanning of the environment, by which she actually increases the likelihood that she will encounter what she wishes to avoid. Her exquisite antennae pick up and transform what most people overlook. In effect, her hypersensitivity backfires by becoming an instrument that brings to awareness, time and again, the very pain she wishes to escape. Her vigilance and self-demeaning comments intensify rather than diminish her anguish.

FIG. 13.1
(Continued)

```
ID NUMBER: SAMPLE              DATE: 29-MAR-88                 PAGE:  6

  Analytic procedures can be useful in reconstructing unconscious
  anxieties and mechanisms that pervade all aspects of her behavior.
  Family techniques can be employed to moderate destructive patterns of
  communication that contribute to or intensify her social problems.  In
  addition, group therapy may assist her in learning new attitudes and
  skills in a more benign and accepting social setting than she normally
  encounters.
```

FIG. 13.1

them. For example, many psychiatric diagnoses are characterized by increased suicide risk and, of course, a client may be at risk for suicide even if he or she manifests a syndrome not usually associated with increased suicide risk. Indeed, many suicides could not have been assigned any psychiatric diagnosis! It is thus essential that the clinician's attention be drawn to any item responses suggesting potential for suicide.

The Noteworthy Responses are followed by a section indicating the most likely DSM-III-R diagnoses on axes I and II, and the Axis IV Psychosocial Stressors reported by the client. There is also a boilerplate statement describing the likely course of the client's Axis I and Axis II problems. The CATI concludes with a 1 to 1½ page description of the prognostic and therapeutic implications of client's responses to the MCMI-II. These comments are derived from the understanding of the client arrived at through the lens of Millon's biopsychosocial theory. Specific psychotherapeutic maneuvers that are likely to be successful are described and psychotherapeutic modalities likely to be optimal for dealing with the client's various problems are recommended.

DEVELOPMENT AND FUNCTIONING OF MILLON'S CATI SYSTEM FOR THE MCMI-II

Millon (1987) has described his CATI system for the MCMI-II as: ". . . similar in content to those developed for the MMPI (Butcher, 1969). [It] summarize[s] in a comprehensive report those characteristics derived from a theory of psychopathology which are found to correlate empirically with specific profile patterns" (p. 214). More specifically, he has detailed its development and functioning as follows.

Several conditions will cause an MCMI-II protocol to be declared invalid: omission or double-marking 12 or more items; a raw score of 2 or higher on the Validity scale; or extreme scores (<145 or >590) on the Disclosure Level scale. If one of these three conditions obtains, a statement to that effect is generated and the CATI is terminated. Otherwise, a rationally-derived interpretation of the configuration of the Disclosure Level, Desirability, and Debasement scales is presented.

Selection of interpretive classifications, similar to MMPI code types, was guided by Millon's updated biopsychosocial theory (Millon, 1986a, 1986b) and the multiaxial diagnostic system of the DSM-III-R. Clinical judgment data from the MCMI-II development project were examined to find which of the test profiles proved to be "mixed types" that were significant variants of the basic prototypes provided by the biopsychosocial theory and the DSM-III-R. All the empirical profile types that were consistent with theoretical or DSM-III-R formulations were selected to define interpretive classifications. The interpretive classifications were in some instances defined with reference to the MCMI-II Aggressive/Sadistic and Self-Defeating scales even though those classifications are included in the DSM-III-R only for research purposes.

The interpretive data base was composed of quantitative clinical ratings of descriptive paragraphs developed to characterize the MCMI scales (cf. Millon, 1983, pp. 40–41) and descriptive phrases developed to describe clients with high scores on the MCMI-II Axis II scales (Millon, 1987, pp. 178–182). The most frequent and clinically descriptive combinations of these descriptions formed the major portion of the output narrative. Theory-based behavioral inferences were used to synthesize and augment the empirical descriptors where advantageous.

Thus, Millon's MCMI-II interpretive system can be best described as a mixed empirical-theoretical system. As noted in the preceding section, the system relies most heavily on theory for those statements generated by combinations of the MCMI-II's Axis II scales.

Millon's CATI system handles the 22-scale MCMI-II profile by dividing it into several sections. First, the most elevated scales among the ten basic[2] Axis II scales are used to select Axis II narrative paragraphs, as well as Prognostic and Therapeutic Implications paragraphs. The most common configurations of those scales can be found in Table 4-1 of the MCMI-II manual (Millon, 1987, p. 210). If scores on all those scales are below $60BR$ no paragraphs are chosen because the profile is too low and too flat to discriminate the instant client from others with emotional disorders. A statement to that effect is printed and the CATI is terminated. If some of the ten scores are higher than $59BR$ and none is higher than $74BR$, up to the three most highly elevated scales are used to choose the interpretive paragraphs. An analogous rule applies if at least one scale is in the $75BR—84BR$ range. If one scale is greater than $84BR$ and the others are less than $75BR$ the highest scale defines the initial set of Axis II and Prognostic and Treatment Implications paragraphs. These same elevation rules are used to interpret the configuration of scores on the Paranoid, Schizoid, and Schizotypal scales.

The configuration of elevated scores on the Paranoid, Schizoid, and Schizotypal scales serves to modify the interpretative paragraphs initially chosen on the basis of the configuration of the ten basic scales. The most common configurations of those three scales with the 10 basic scales can be found in Table 4-2 of the MCMI-II manual (Millon, 1987, p. 211). An elevation between $60BR$ and $74BR$ on at least one of those three scales also generates the suggestion that the client's personality malfunctioning is probably chronic and moderately severe. If one or more of those scales is $85BR$ or higher the client's personality malfunctioning is said to likely be chronic and severe.

The interpretive rules that are applied to generate the Axis I narrative statements are somewhat different from the rules applied to the Axis II scales. Elevations between $60BR$ and $74BR$ are interpreted only for the six scales Millon calls the moderately severe clinical syndromes.[3] Elevations in that range are interpreted only if none of those six scales is $75BR$ or higher. The final three Axis I scales, Thought Disorder, Major Depression, and Delusional Disorder, are never interpreted unless they exceed $74BR$. The CATI system chooses up to three of the nine Axis I scales which are interpreted in scale-by-scale fashion. As noted in the preceding section, the Axis I interpretive paragraphs are typically modified by

---

[2] Including Aggressive/Sadistic and Self-Defeating but excluding Paranoid, Schizoid, and Schizotypal.

[3] Including the following MCMI-II scales: Anxiety Disorder, Somatoform Disorder, Bipolar: Manic Disorder, Dysthymic Disorder, Alcohol Dependence, and Drug Dependence.

comments based on the Axis II scales. Those modifications may be empirically grounded, but they are most likely based on Millon's biopsychosocial theory. The most common combinations of Axis I scale elevations and configurations on the 10 basic Axis II scales are presented in Table 4-3 in the MCMI-II manual (Millon, 1987, p. 211).

The Parallel DSM-III-R Multiaxial Diagnoses include straightforward renderings of up to three Axis I diagnoses and three Axis II diagnoses chosen using the same rules used to select the narrative paragraphs. An elevation on the Thought Disorder scale suggests a diagnosis of schizophrenia. Obviously, the MCMI-II alone, and hence the CATI, cannot address all possible Axis I diagnoses. At present, the MCMI-II cannot address distinctions within some of the major categories. The MCMI-II, for example, does not address the rather subtle distinction between Hypochodriasis and Somatization Disorder. It also does not address some of the very low base rate disorders such as the Dissociative Disorders. Naturally, the MCMI-II alone also cannot suggest Organic Mental Syndromes. The Axis IV Psychosocial Stressors are the Major Problems the client reported in the demographic section of the MCMI-II answer sheet.

EMPIRICAL EVALUATION OF MILLON'S CATI SYSTEM FOR THE MCMI

Unfortunately, no studies of Millon's CATI system for the MCMI-II have been published at the time of this writing. Given this absence of published research, it seems sensible to discuss studies of Millon's CATI system for the MCMI. The logic of the two CATI systems is nearly identical. The empirical interpretive data base for the MCMI-II is superior to the data base that was available at the time the MCMI interpretive system was developed. A comparison of the MCMI and MCMI-II is beyond the scope of this chapter; however, it is my judgment that the MCMI-II is at least as good an instrument as the MCMI. Thus, it makes sense to assert that Millon's CATI system for the MCMI-II is at least as good as his MCMI CATI system. In some instances, noted below, there is reason to believe that the MCMI-II interpretive system is superior to the MCMI interpretive system.

Organization and Clarity, Accuracy, and Utility of Millon's CATIs for the MCMI

Three researchers used similar methods to investigate users' opinions about Millon's CATIs for the MCMI. Green (1982) surveyed 23 mental health practitioners' reactions to a total of 100 specific reports, about two-thirds from outpatient settings and the rest from inpatient settings. Jolosky (1985) reported 92

TABLE 13.1
Organization and Clarity of Millon's CATIs for the MCMI Across Three Studies

Report Organization and Clarity	Excellent	Good	Adequate	Poor
Organization	64 (51)	24 (39)	11 (8)	0 (2)
Intelligibility and clarity	58 (38)	29 (42)	12 (12)	1 (8)
Internal consistency	44 (29)	44 (38)	9 (15)	3 (18)

Note. MCMI values are unweighted average percentages.

practitioner's reactions to their cumulative experience with the CATI system.[4] Siddall (1986) questioned 10 clinicians about 660 CATIs they had used as aids in diagnosis and treatment planning for court-referred polydrug abusers. Table 13.1 presents the average ratings of the CATIs' organization and clarity across these three studies. For purposes of rough comparison the table also includes, in parentheses, parallel data Green (1982) obtained for the MMPI CATI developed by noted MMPI expert Raymond Fowler and published by the Roche Psychiatric Service Institute (Fowler, 1966). At the time Green collected her data the Roche CATI system was almost certainly the most widely used CATI system in the United States and the rest of the world (cf. Moreland, 1987). The MCMI reports compared favorably with the Roche reports when it came to organization, clarity, and internal consistency. In these respects I believe that MCMI-II CATIs compare favorably to the most popular CATIs currently available for the MMPI-2.

Green and Siddall also asked clinicians to rate the accuracy of Millon's MCMI CATIs along several dimensions. Table 13.2 presents the average ratings of the CATIs' accuracy across these two studies. Green's results for Roche MMPI CATIs are again presented in parentheses for purposes of rough comparison. Again, the MCMI CATIs compared favorably with the Roche MMPI CATIs. The degree to which the CATI system for the MCMI-II might improve upon the ratings presented in Table 13.2 is, for most of the dimensions, difficult to estimate. Two of the categories that fare poorest in Table 13.2 are probably exceptions to that uncertainty. In validating the MCMI-II Millon attended to self-image and thought processes in a much more systematic manner than he did in the validation of the MCMI (cf. Millon, 1987, pp. 180–181). Therefore, it seems reasonable to suppose that the CATI system for the MCMI-II is more accurate than the MCMI CATI system when it comes to self-image and thought processes.

Table 13.3 presents the average results of the Green, Jolosky, and Siddall studies when it comes to the utility of the MCMI CATI system. These results are

---

[4]No data are available on the work settings or clientele of Jolosky's respondents. However, my experience working for National Computer Systems from 1982 to 1988 leads me to believe that a large majority worked mainly with mental health outpatients.

TABLE 13.2
Accuracy of Millon's CATIs for the MCMI Across Two Studies

Report Accuracy	Excellent	Good	Adequate	Poor
Personality traits and behavior	57 (17)	28 (37)	12 (26)	3 (20)
Interpersonal attitudes and relationships	42 (34)	43 (27)	12 (23)	3 (16)
Affective tone and moods	40 (41)	44 (30)	12 (22)	4 (7)
Primary symptoms and complaints	32 (31)	46 (37)	16 (14)	6 (18)
Stress or conflict areas	27 (18)	40 (22)	28 (47)	5 (13)
Coping styles	26 (14)	55 (27)	16 (34)	3 (25)
Self-image	21 (3)	45 (19)	27 (39)	7 (39)
Severity of disturbance	21 (24)	24 (28)	44 (37)	11 (11)
Thought processes	11 (21)	35 (15)	44 (46)	10 (18)

Note. MCMI values are unweighted average percentages.

important because it is perfectly possible for the CATIs to be highly accurate and still be of absolutely no use in client management and treatment. Green's results for Roche MMPI CATIs are presented in parentheses for purposes of rough comparison. The bottom line appears to be that the clinicians found the CATIs useful in their practical dealings with clients. There is no reason to suppose that studies of the MCMI-II CATIs will not yield similar results.

Methodological Problems: The Barnum Effect

One question has cast a large shadow of uncertainty over the results of most studies of the accuracy of computer-assisted personality test interpretations. This is the question of the degree to which CATIs are rated accurate not because they are pointed descriptions of the individual in question, but because they are full of glittering generalities (Moreland, 1985). Describing this problem, Paul Meehl (1956) suggested "that we adopt the phrase *Barnum Effect* to stigmatize those pseudo successful clinical procedures in which patient descriptions from tests are

TABLE 13.3
Utility of Millon's CATIs for the MCMI Across Three Studies

Report Utility	Substantial	Moderate	Minimal	None
Confirmation of Knowledge	60 (32)	32 (42)	6 (17)	2 (9)
Addition of relevant information	49 (13)	34 (41)	13 (24)	4 (22)
Clarification of case	41 (20)	43 (32)	11 (21)	5 (27)
Helpful in treatment[a]	33 (18)	43 (30)	19 (35)	5 (17)
Inclusion of trivial Information	4 (10)	8 (19)	57 (37)	31 (34)
Inclusion of misleading information	4 (10)	13 (14)	47 (42)	36 (34)
Exclusion of important information	7 (27)	12 (14)	64 (43)	16 (16)

Note. Values are unweighted average percentages.
[a]Rated, from left to right, excellent, good, adequate, and poor.

made to fit the patient largely or wholly by virtue of their triviality; and in which any nontrivial, but perhaps erroneous, inferences are hidden in a context of assertions or denials which carry high confidence simply because of the population base rates, regardless of the test's validity" (p. 266).

Dr. Millon, his colleagues, and his students were concerned about the problems posed by the Barnum Effect and first tackled them when Millon developed his CATI system for the MCMI. Several of the ratings of report utility presented in Table 13.3 (i.e., addition of relevant information, clarification of case, helpful in treatment, and inclusion of trivial information) cast some light on this issue. Those results suggest that the Barnum Effect had minimal effect on the clinicians' ratings of the MCMI CATIs' accuracy. There have been other, more sophisticated, efforts to evaluate the impact of the Barnum Effect. Green (1982), for example, attempted to control for this confound in two ways. She compared MCMI CATIs with two different MMPI CATIs on the same clients. She also reported a pilot study (see Sandberg, 1987, below) that attempted to directly determine the impact of the Barnum Effect on ratings of the MCMI CATIs. The results of those more sophisticated studies are consistent with the conclusion that ratings of the MCMI CATIs' accuracy reflect more than the influence of the Barnum Effect. However, given humans' well-known shortcomings as information processors, including a notorious capacity for self-deception, it should come as no surprise that the results of the more sophisticated studies are less favorable than those reported earlier. Knowledge of the impact of the Barnum Effect is, in my judgment, indispensable in judging the degree to which results presented in Table 13.2 support the use of Millon's CATIs for the MCMI (and, presumably, the MCMI-II). Thus, three more rather sophisticated studies that attempted to control for the Barnum Effect are presented here in some detail.

Sandberg (1987) presented a useful analogue study of Millon's CATI system for the MCMI. He first asked 34 students in clinical, counseling, or behavioral medicine doctoral programs to describe the personality characteristics and clinical symptoms of two patients. The students were then asked to complete MCMI protocols as they believed those two patients would. Subsequently the students were asked to rate two MCMI reports along the dimensions employed by Green (1982). The students were led to believe that they were rating a computer-generated narrative report for one of their role-played patients and a clinician-generated narrative report for the other. In fact, both reports were computer-generated. One was based on the MCMI responses they gave while role-playing one patient (genuine reports); the other was based on the MCMI responses given by another one of the role-playing students (fake reports).

Sandberg found that, contrary to the fears of CATI critics (e.g., Matarazzo, 1986), belief that reports were computer-generated, as opposed to clinician-generated, did not give the former a spurious air of accuracy. The students rated the real reports better all-around than the fake reports. In terms of accuracy, the real reports averaged about 3.8 on a 5-point scale, whereas the fake reports averaged only about 2.8 (estimated from Fig. 2 in Sandberg, 1987). The differences on the individual accuracy dimensions were statistically significant except for Primary Symptoms and Complaints ($p < .057$). The genuine reports were also rated more useful than the fake reports (3.8 vs. 3.0 estimated from Figs. 1 and 3, where high scores indicate greater utility). The differences on the individual utility dimensions were all statistically significant.

This study supports the usefulness of Millon's CATI for the MCMI, but it is not above criticism. First of all, it may be much easier to generate accurate and apparently useful reports for role-played, prototypical patients than it is to do the same for the complex and often puzzling patients one commonly encounters in clinical practice. It may also have been especially easy for students from Dr. Millon's university, who presumably were steeped in his biopsychosocial theory (Millon, 1969) which guided the development of the MCMI and the CATI system, to role-play on the MCMI and identify reports based on that role-playing. Finally, Snyder, Widiger, and Hoover (1990) would contend that good or bad ratings on one part of a report may have predisposed the students to give similar ratings to other parts of those reports.

Gualtieri, Gonzales, and Baldwin (1987) asked 175 alcoholics in a halfway house to respond to the MCMI according to one of four sets of instructions: (1) as honestly as possible, (2) based on behavior when drinking, (3) based on behavior when sober, or (4) based on behavior over the year preceding testing. They expected that CATIs based on "behavior when drinking" protocols would exaggerate and distort the alcoholics' actual disturbance at the time of testing. Twenty-four alcoholism rehabilitation counselors rated the accuracy of reports for their patients in seven different areas. Ratings were made on a 7-point scale with higher ratings indicating greater accuracy. Neither the scores on the MCMI scales nor the accuracy ratings of the CATIs differed as a function of the instructions. The average of the ratings for six different parts of the reports (5.01) was in excellent agreement with the counselors' single ratings of the "overall accuracy" of the reports (5.09).

As the authors themselves pointed out, their failure to find significant differences among their experimental conditions makes the unequivocal interpretation of their results impossible. Maybe the MCMI and the CATI system are robust in the face of these different instructional sets. On the other hand, it may be that alcoholics cannot describe themselves accurately regardless of the instructions. And it may be that the CATI system is filled with glittering generalities irrespective of these instructional sets. Still, considered together with the results of the other studies reviewed here, it seems most appropriate to view Gualtieri et al.'s results as supporting the utility of Millon's MCMI CATI system.

My colleague Julie Onstad and I conducted a study we thought controlled effectively for the Barnum Effect (Moreland & Onstad, 1987). We had eight clinicians rate the accuracy of 99 genuine MCMI CATIs, 78 of which were from outpatients. We also had the clinicians rate 99 MCMI CATIs matched on the basis of sex, but otherwise selected at random. The clinicians did not know which report was which at the time they completed their ratings. In fact, they did not know one of the reports was selected at random. They were led to believe that one report was generated using the usual interpretive rules another report was generated according to a set of experimental interpretive rules. This study has been severely criticized, first by Cash, Mikulka, and Brown (1989), and then by Snyder et al. (1990). The most damaging criticism, in my view, is Snyder et al.'s claim that a Halo Effect artificially inflated our ratings of the genuine CATIs' accuracy. Godfrey (nee Onstad) and I have replied to these critiques elsewhere (Moreland & Godfrey, 1989, 1991). We feel that some of the criticisms were justified but feel that they do not vitiate our basic conclusion that the genuine MCMI CATIs were significantly more accurate than those selected at random. (We encourage you to read the relevant articles and decide for yourself.)

The genuine CATIs had a mean accuracy rating of 2.90 on a five-point scale (SD = 1.57, Median = 3, Mode = 4) while their random counterparts had a mean accuracy rating of 1.96 (SD = 1.55, Median = 2, Mode = 1) (Moreland & Godfrey, 1991). We also found that the individual sections of the genuine reports were, with two exceptions, rated as significantly more accurate than their random counterparts. The differences between the genuine and random CATIs when it came to the sections on Axis IV psychosocial stressors and severity were in the right direction, but they were not statistically significant.

Axis I Diagnostic Accuracy of Millon's CATI for the MCMI

Two studies examined the accuracy of the diagnostic suggestions offered by Millon's CATIs for the MCMI using formal, clinical diagnosis as the criterion. DeWolfe, Larson, and Ryan (1985) studied 48 patients with a discharge DSM-III diagnosis of Bipolar Affective Disorder (Manic). The hit rate for the CATI was 27% in this study. This result suggests a problem with the MCMI and its CATI that may generalize to the MCMI-II and its CATI. The subjects used in the construction and norming of the MCMI (and the MCMI-II) were over-whelmingly outpatients (cf. Millon, 1983, p. 10; Millon, 1987, p. 106) whereas DeWolfe et al.'s subjects were all inpatients. Moreover, only four percent of the MCMI construction sample (and a similar proportion of the MCMI-II normative sample) were bipolar (manic) patients (Millon, 1983, p. 16). Base rate scores, by their very nature, are sensitive to the prevalence of disorders within a population (cf. Baldessarini, Finklestein, & Arana, 1983). And bipolar patients are undoubt-edly more common in inpatient settings. Thus, as Millon (1987, p. 65) himself suggested "use of a more appropriate cutting line, that is, one suited to the prevalence of bipolar disorders in this patient population" should lead to more accurate diagnosis of this disorder. Support for this hypothesis is provided by a study by Piersma (1987).

Piersma (1987) examined the diagnostic accuracy of the MCMI CATI in a sample of 151 patients with anxiety disorders and depressive disorders in his psychiatric hospital setting. He found that the CATI overdiagnosed anxiety disorders. Anxiety disorders were the second most common Axis I diagnosis in the samples used in the construction and norming of the MCMI, accounting for 24% of the construction sample (Millon, 1983, p. 16). It seems very unlikely that anxiety disorders are that prevalent in Piersma's inpatient setting. On the other hand, the CATI underdiagnosed depressive disorders. Depressive disorders account for the vast majority of the Axis I diagnoses in Piersma's setting (personal communication). Dysthymia was the most common Axis I disorder among the patients used to construct and norm the MCMI (26%) but Major Depression, the depressive disorder most likely to be found in inpatient settings, accounted for only 3% of those samples. Prevalence rates for these disorders for the MCMI-II norm sample were very similar to those of the MCMI construction and norming samples (cf. Millon, 1987, p. 175).

The relatively poor performance of Millon's MCMI CATI system in the DeWolfe et al. (1985) and Piersma (1987) studies suggests that the performance of the CATI system deteriorates when used in settings very different from those in which most of the MCMI construction and norming subjects were tested. Presumably this will be true of the MCMI-II CATI system too. In this vein, it is worthwhile to note that most of the clients tested in the (favorable) studies of entire MCMI CATIs reported above were—like most of those used in MCMI construction and norming, and MCMI-II norming—outpatients.

The Bottom Line

In my view the foregoing results support the use of MCMI-II CATIs in settings where the prevalence of disorders is similar to their prevalence in the MCMI-II norm sample. In practice, I think this means that the CATIs are most likely to be accurate if used with outpatients. More about this follows.

TIPS ON OPTIMAL USE OF MILLON'S MCMI-II CATIS

Optimal Populations

Given the immediately preceding discussion, it will come as no surprise that I recommend you carefully consider the characteristics of the client you have in front of you before choosing to use Millon's CATI for the MCMI-II or, indeed, the MCMI-II itself. The more unlike the subjects used to develop, norm, and validate the MCMI-II your client is, the less likely the MCMI-II and Dr. Millon's CATI will help you. I know this is a Barnum statement that is true of any test and any CATI, but I feel constrained to make it here because over the years I have observed a lot of well-meaning attempts to use square tests for round clinical purposes. We all have our favorite broad-bandwidth tests that we reach for instinctively when confronted with a wide variety of clinical problems. On the other hand, I must also point out that in many instances in which the MCMI-II is less than optimal there will be no good alternative measure available. In such circumstances I recommend especially cautious use of the MCMI-II and the CATI.

Perusal of the characteristics of the MCMI-II norm sample (Millon, 1987, p. 106) suggests some groups with which the MCMI-II and Millon's CATI may be less useful than with other groups. Older clients, particularly gerontological patients, constitute such a group. Only 6.1% of the MCMI-II norm sample were over 55 years-of-age. The MMPI-2 may shortly become—at least until more research is done on the MCMI-II—a better alternative with this population. Many data were collected on elderly subjects during the research project that led to the revision of the MMPI, but most have not yet been published. The nature of the relationship between racial/ethnic group membership and psychopathology is controversial. Some contend that the apparently higher rates of psychopathology among American ethnic minorities is a manifestation of bigotry while others believe them to be veridical (cf. Dahlstrom, Lachar, & Dahlstrom, 1986). Dahlstrom and his colleagues concluded, on the basis of an exhaustive review of the literature and 10 year's worth of original research, that the use of MMPI norms based on caucasian subjects with American minority clients does not bias the results against those minority clients. Given the similarities between the two instruments, these results suggest that the fact that the MCMI-II norm sample was 88% caucasian (vs. 85% of the United States population in the 1980 census and the census bureau's projections for 1995 [cf. Bureau of the Census, 1984]) will not adversely impact its use with ethnic minority clients. A more conservative approach would be to use the MMPI-2 with ethnic minority clients until more data are available on the usefulness of the MCMI-II with those clients.

As noted earlier, the subjects used to norm the MCMI-II were overwhelmingly outpatients: 82% to be exact. The norm subjects also reported the kind of "Major Problems" one would expect from an outpatient group. Thirty-one percent reported marital or family problems, 17% problems with school or work, and 16% problems with self-confidence. On the other hand, only 4% and 2% reported major problems with alcohol or drugs, respectively. The distribution of disorders within a representative subsample of the norm sample are, unsurprisingly, what one would expect in an outpatient setting (Millon, 1987, pp. 174–175). For example, 29% of the norm subjects suffered from dysthymia and 23% from anxiety disorders, whereas only 3% were in the schizophrenic spectrum and only 9% suffered from mania or Major Depression. I interpret all these data as supporting my contention that Millon's CATIs (and the MCMI-II itself) are more likely to be useful with outpatients than with inpatients. I also believe that, assuming (for the sake of argument) equal *accuracy* with inpatients and outpatients, the CATIs are likely to be most *useful* with outpatients. In my opinion, the major value of the CATIs lies in their descriptions of personality patterns and recommendations for psychotherapy. I know of no other instrument or CATI system that seems better suited to these tasks, Alex Caldwell's awesome expertise with the MMPI notwithstanding. I believe that these descriptions are much more likely to be helpful in treating outpatients with personality disorders, clients with what we used to call neurotics, and in efforts to keep the more seriously disturbed in the community than in treating patients hospitalized in the throes of a florid psychotic episode. The MMPI-2, with its enormous interpretive data base consisting mainly of data collected in inpatient settings (cf. Greene, 1991) and several empirically studied CATI systems (cf. Eyde, Kowal, & Fishburne, 1991), is more likely to be useful with inpatients.

Scores Near Cutoffs

Once one has made the decision to use Millon's CATI for the MCMI-II there are several conditions, implicit in the functioning of the CATI system, that call for particularly circumspect use of the CATIs. One of these is the situation in which a number of scale scores hover near one of the cutoffs of 60*BR*, 75*BR,* and 85*BR*. When several scores are near a cutoff the CATI system must make a psychometrically arbitrary (i.e., insupportable in view of the standard error of the difference between scale scores) decision about which scale to interpret. Obviously, this increases the likelihood that the CATI will be inaccurate or, at least, incomplete.

Undifferentiated Profiles

One may encounter undifferentiated profiles in spite of Professor Millon's extensive efforts to minimize that eventuality. Two types of undifferentiated profiles are most likely. Several scales may be highly elevated and not very different from each other. Or, the profile may be relatively flat and undifferentiated. In either case the implication is the same as when several scores are near cutoffs: The CATI system must arbitrarily choose which scales to interpret.

Unusual Configurations of the Ten Basic Scales

Both the theory undergirding the MCMI-II and its psychometric properties make unusual configurations of the ten basic Axis II scales unlikely. However, they do sometimes occur. In those cases Millon had to rely less on empirical data and coherent theory, and more on his clinical acumen to develop interpretive statements. Dr. Millon would be the first one to admit that the former are more secure bases for interpretation than the latter.

Low Base Rate Phenomena

Finally, just as with any clinical tool, one should be particularly careful when using the MCMI-II CATI to search for evidence of phenomena that are unusual among one's clients. Suicidal intent, being relatively unusual even in clinical settings, is the classic example of a low base rate phenomenon, but others can be found. Indeed, this takes us full circle because I began this section by indicating that, if one uses the CATI with populations very different from the ones employed in its development, low base rate phenomena (as far as the CATI system is concerned) will abound.

CODA

Obviously I am a proponent of computer-assisted test interpretation—otherwise I would not have written this chapter. I am more than that. At the risk of being kicked out of my profession (I have already been branded a heretic a time or two), I will go on record as believing that, given the same information, *CATIs developed by widely recognized experts who have devoted a major portion of their career to the instrument and CATI system in question* are virtually always more accurate than test interpretations written by us workaday clinicians. I would be very surprised to discover that *any* clinician, given the same information, could out-perform Professor Millon's CATI for the MCMI-II. These statements are actually not as radical as they may appear at first blush. The phrase "given the same information" gives me wiggle room. Important wiggle room.

It goes without saying that a clinician will always have information about a client that is not employed in the MCMI-II CATI system. The data in Table 13.3 indicate that such extra information will often dovetail nicely with the CATI. At times that extra information will provide a context that allows you to improve upon the CATI. For example, I encountered a situation in which the CATI suggested that schizophrenia was the most salient Axis I diagnosis and Bipolar: Manic was not on the list, that score being above 74*BR* but only the fourth highest Axis I scale behind Drug Dependence and Alcohol Dependence in addition to Thought Disorder. On interview, I found no evidence of a personal or family history of schizophrenia. Instead, I unearthed a history of favorable response to lithium and a young sister who had an episode of severe depression. These data suggested that the patient was, in fact, suffering from bipolar disorder. I concluded that the apparent CATI "miss" was due to the difficulty distinguishing a schizophrenic episode characterized by positive symptoms from acute mania on the basis of symptoms alone (this patient had psychotic symptoms), and to the tendency of bipolar patients (like this one) to misuse substances. Even if extra information does not suggest a way to improve upon the CATI per se, it helps one decide which of the CATI statements (perhaps all of them!) are most likely to be correct. In other words, the CATI is just a tool in your clinical tool kit, not a modern psychodiagnostic mechanic. CATIs are not, even in the eyes of enthusiastic proponents like me, replacements for clinical acumen. CATIs are powerful tools, but it is up to you to use those tools wisely.

REFERENCES

Baldessarini, R. J., Finklestein, S., & Arana, G. W. (1983). The predictive power of diagnostic tests and the effect of prevalence of illness. *Archives of General Psychiatry, 40*, 569–573.

Bureau of the Census (1984). *Projections of the population of the United States by age, sex, and race: 1983 to 2080: May 1984*. Population report series P-20, no. 148. Washington, DC: Author.

Butcher, J. N. (1969). *MMPI: Research developments and clinical applications*. New York: McGraw-Hill.

Cash, T. F., Mikulka, P. J., & Brown, T. A. (1989). Validity of Millon's computerized interpretation system for the MCMI: Comment on Moreland and Onstad. *Journal of Consulting and Clinical Psychology, 57*, 311–312.

Dahlstrom, W. G., Lachar, D., & Dahlstrom, L. E. (1986). *MMPI patterns of American minorities*. Minneapolis: University of Minnesota Press.

DeWolfe, A., Larson, J. K., & Ryan, J. J. (1985). Diagnostic accuracy of the Millon test computer reports for bipolar affective disorders. *Journal of Psychopathology and Behavioral Assessment, 7*, 185–189.

Eyde, L. D., Kowal, D. M., & Fishburne, F. J., Jr. (1991). The validity of computer-based interpretations of the MMPI. In T. B. Gutkin & S. J. Wise (Eds.), *The computer and the decision-making process* (pp. 75–123). Hillsdale, NJ: Lawrence Erlbaum Associates.

Fowler, R. D. (1966). *The MMPI notebook: A guide to the clinical use of the automated MMPI*. Nutley, NJ: Roche Psychiatric Service Institute.

Green, C. J. (1982). The diagnostic accuracy and utility of MMPI and MCMI computer interpretive reports. *Journal of Personality Assessment, 46*, 359–365.

Greene, R. L. (1991). *The MMPI/MMPI-2: An interpretive manual* (2nd ed.). Framingham, MA: Allyn & Bacon.

Gualtieri, J., Gonzales, E., & Baldwin, N. (1987). The accuracy of MCMI computerized narratives for alcoholics. In C. J. Green (Ed.), *Conference on the Millon clinical inventories (MCMI, MBHI, MAPI)* (pp. 263–268). Minneapolis, MN: National Computer Systems.

Jolosky, T. (1985). Millon user survey report. *Noteworthy Responses, 1(2)*, 2–3. (Available from National Computer Systems, P. O. Box 1416, Minneapolis, MN 55440.)

Matarazzo, J. D. (1986). Computerized clinical psychological test interpretations: Unvalidated plus all mean and no sigma. *American Psychologist, 41*, 14–24.

McMahon, R. C., & Davidson, R. S. (1985). Transient versus enduring depression among alcoholics in inpatient treatment. *Journal of Psychopathology and Behavioral Assessment, 7*, 317–328.

McMahon, R. C., & Davidson, R. S. (1986). An examination of depressed vs. nondepressed alcoholics in inpatient treatment. *Journal of Clinical Psychology, 42*, 177–184.

Meehl, P. E. (1956). Wanted a good cookbook. *American Psychologist, 11*, 263–272.

Millon (1969). *Modern psychopathology*. Philadelphia: Saunders.

Millon, T. (1983). *Millon Clinical Multiaxial Inventory manual* (3rd ed.). Minneapolis, MN: National Computer Systems.

Millon, T. (1986a). A theoretical derivation of pathological personalities. In T. Millon & G. L. Klerman (Eds.), *Contemporary directions in psychopathology: Toward the DSM-IV* (pp. 639–670). New York: Guilford.

Millon, T. (1986b). Personality prototypes and their diagnostic criteria. In T. Millon & G. L.

Klerman (Eds.), *Contemporary directions in psychopathology: Toward the DSM-IV* (pp. 671–672). New York: Guilford.

Millon, T. (1987). *Manual for the MCMI-II* (2nd ed.). Minneapolis, MN: National Computer Systems.

Moreland, K. L. (1985). Validation of computer-based test interpretations: Problems and prospects. *Journal of Consulting and Clinical Psychology, 53,* 816–825.

Moreland, K. L. (1987). Computerized psychological assessment: What's available. In J. N. Butcher (Ed.), *Computerized psychological assessment: A practitioner's guide* (pp. 26–49). New York: Basic Books.

Moreland, K. L., & Godfrey, J. O. (1989). Yes, our study could have been better: Reply to Cash, Mikulka, and Brown. *Journal of Consulting and Clinical Psychology, 57,* 313–314.

Moreland, K. L., & Godfrey, J. O. (1991). *Improving computer-assisted test interpretations: Comments on Snyder, Widiger, and Hoover.* Manuscript submitted for publication.

Moreland, K. L., & Onstad, J. A. (1987). Validity of Millon's computerized interpretation for the MCMI: A controlled study. *Journal of Consulting and Clinical Psychology, 55,* 113–114.

National Computer Systems (1991). *Professional Assessment Services 1991 catalog.* Minneapolis: Author.

Piersma, H. L. (1987). Millon Clinical Multiaxial Inventory (MCMI) computer-generated diagnoses: How do they compare to clinical judgment? *Journal of Psychopathology and Behavioral Assessment, 9,* 305–312.

Sandberg, M. (1987). Is the ostensive accuracy of computer interpretive reports a result of the Barnum Effect? A study of the MCMI. In C. J. Green (Ed.), *Conference on the Millon clinical inventories (MCMI, MBHI, MAPI)* (pp. 155–164). Minneapolis, MN: National Computer Systems.

Siddall, J. W. (1986). Use of the MCMI with substance abusers. *Noteworthy Responses, 2(2),* 1–3. (Available from National Computer Systems, P. O. Box 1416, Minneapolis, MN 55440.)

Snyder, D. K., Widiger, T. A., & Hoover, D. W. (1990). Methodological considerations in validating computer-based test interpretations: Controlling response bias. *Psychological Assessment: A Journal of Consulting and Clinical Psychology, 2,* 470–477.

IV NEW DEVELOPMENTS

14 Special Scales for the MCMI: Theory, Development, and Utility

Paul Retzlaff, Ph.D.

This chapter presents the potential use of special scales for the MCMI. To that end, the chapter includes the various approaches to scale development, the presentation of two sets of special scales, research uses of these scales, and, finally, the clinical use of these scales.

APPROACHES TO SPECIAL SCALE CONSTRUCTION

There are basically four different ways to construct psychometric scales. They include domain theory technique, content analysis, empirical item selection, and factor analytic methods. A case is made that for the development of initial scales for new tests the domain theory technique is the best method. Second, for special additional scale development from item pools in existing tests, that variants of domain theory and factor analytic techniques are probably the best methods.

Domain theory test construction (Nunnally, 1978) allows the use of both expert opinion and statistical methodology thus assuring both clinical reality and psychometric reliability. In this method, as in the development of both MCMI-I and MCMI-II, domains of personality or psychopathology are identified as the initial construction phase. The authors decide that Antisocial and Psychosis, for example, are areas of interest. At this point, the domains are fleshed out in paragraph form to better describe what the domain is and isn't. Next, experts write items that are consistent with the individual domains. Judges then screen items for awkwardness, poor grammar, sexist language, and other obvious issues. As an additional expert judge screen, items are sorted by naive clinicians into domains to determine if items which were written by the experts survive

237

further clinical content screen. The preceding allows for a fairly thorough clinical content saturation and ensures that domains and items have "real world" applicability.

The final stages of domain theory construction ensure psychometric integrity and reliability. The initial pools of items for each domain are given to a large number of representative subjects. At this point each item is correlated with the total score for that scale to determine which items are most representative of that domain and which saturate that variable the best. Items with the highest item-total correlations are retained for the final scale. Usually, at least 12 items are required and 20 are usually sufficient to ensure high internal consistency (reliability). Additionally, some domains may not have survived due to poor domain definition or poor items. At this point a set of scales have been developed which are highly reliable but not necessarily valid. Further clinical samples are recruited to administer the final scales and additional validity measures such as other tests or diagnostic criteria. This last step allows for the determination of validity estimates of the final scales but may show that, while a scale is highly reliable, it is not particularly valid.

The use of domain theory construction technique assures highly reliable scales, thus hopefully maximizing validity. The alternative is to have scales with low reliability which can never be highly valid. Having said this, it is apparent that special additional scales tapping domains not originally included cannot be constructed in this manner from existing tests, and, as such, cannot be as reliable or valid as scales built from scratch. This is a caveat that must be kept in mind throughout any discussion of special scale construction. However, the use of item-total correlations is a key element that can be modified in some cases to develop special scales.

The second method of scale construction, often used particularly for special additional scales, is the analysis of content. This method is the simplest and usually the poorest. In essence, the face validity of an item drives its inclusion in a scale. If an item sounds like something an alcoholic, for example, would endorse, it is included. This method, however, is restricted to the available items in the pool and there may simply be no good alcohol abuse items. Further, it is common for the expert judges to be relatively few in number and not naive to the underlying theory. Therefore, many of these scales are rather idiosyncratic.

The next method is often referred to as "dustbowl empiricism." Here, all available items are correlated with some outside criteria such as alcohol abuse. Items that correlate highly with the variable are included in the scale and those that show low correlation are excluded regardless of their face validity or domain relevance. In large part, the MMPI was constructed in this manner. Because items are placed in a scale based upon their relationship to the outside variable rather than their relationship to one another, reliabilities are often low. Although initial empirical methods result in good initial validity estimates, cross validation often suffers a great deal. And inasmuch as the scale has a low reliability, it cannot hope to improve these poor cross validation validities. All of these problems are exacerbated when low base-rate phenomena are being predicted, such as suicide or prison escape.

Finally, factor analytic methods are often used for scale construction. Pools of items are subjected to factor analysis and scales are derived as a function of the item-factor loadings. This method allows the relationships among items to determine the kind and number of domains. Reliabilities are often high because item-factor loadings are akin to item-total loadings. The problems inherent in this method often include the lack of attention to initial domain conceptualization and item generation. Further, domains are driven by statistical properties rather than clinical needs. For example, item factor analyses of both the MCMI-I and MCMI-II reveal a "Crying" factor composed of three items with "crying," "tears," and "cry" content. While these items do indeed define a domain statistically, they are only relevant clinically for the syndrome of depression. Finally, the use of items in factor analysis is highly problematic, due to items inherent low reliabilities. Factor structures are often unstable and overly driven by the specific populations. A population with many schizotypals may provide a schizotypal scale but a general clinical or normal population will not reveal a schizotypal factor due to the heterogeneity of schizotypy. The use of factor analysis at a scale level, however, is more promising, stable, and clinically relevant.

SPECIAL SCALES FOR THE MCMI-I

The MCMI is a broad-spectrum test of psychopathology based upon Millon's (1969, 1981, 1983, 1987) theory of personality and designed to be consistent with DSM-III (and -R) categories. Its properties are well described elsewhere in this book.

Despite its overall excellent operating characteristics, (Gibertini, Brandenburg, & Retzlaff, 1986) the MCMI is beset by a few structural problems that can make interpretation of the scale scores difficult. Among the most bothersome of these problems is the tendency for MCMI profiles to "float." One reason MCMI profiles may show many high scores, among which the clinician would like to distinguish, is that the scales of the MCMI share a large percentage of their items. This extensive item-overlap causes a "built-in" correlational structure among the scales of the inventory and makes it difficult for the individual scales to vary independently (Retzlaff & Gibertini, 1987). Users of the MCMI have found that, because of extensive item overlap across scales, differential diagnosis is sometimes difficult.

Although the MCMI has been shown to be useful in a number of contexts, its reliance on extensive item overlap to provide the dual attributes of comprehensiveness and brevity has added a measure of confusion to multiscale elevation interpretations. When scales share items, several scales may be elevated for a particular patient due to: (a) the endorsement of that core of items common to the scales, (b) the endorsement of each of the individual scales' core items, or (c) both of these cases operating. Obviously, the first situation is an artifact which disturbs the straightforward interpretation of the profile in general and the differentiation of the second situation in particular. For example, if a patient has elevations on both the Schizoid and Avoidant scales, the clinician does not know whether this joint elevation is due to the endorsement of the social withdrawal items common to both scales or is due to the existence of primary schizoid *and* primary avoidant personality features. Central to the resolution of this issue is an understanding of the primary items within scales and the factor structures within the MCMI and an operationalization of these concepts into scales for use by clinicians. This chapter provides special additional scales that are simpler at both scale and test levels.

Attributes and Prototypes

A personality attribute is the characteristic defining behavior pattern of a given trait complex. For example, the taxon "schizoid," as measured by the MCMI schizoid scale, is a complex of behaviors, cognitions, and affects, which includes: social isolation, idiosyncratic thought, bland affect and deficits in emotional responsiveness, apathy, and deficits in perception of common social mores and interpersonal cues. This taxon maps (both theoretically as well as operationally) onto the MCMI scales of schizoid, avoidant, psychotic depression, psychotic delusion, psychotic thinking, and schizotypal. The characteristic defining behavioral pattern of the schizoid taxon (i.e., its primary personality attribute) is the tendency toward social withdrawal with a concomitant inability to adequately respond to common interpersonal cues and situations. Thus, the personality attribute "schizoid" is a simplex of behaviors involving only extreme social peripheralizing. Note that some personality and clinical syndrome taxa share the same defining behavior pattern, differing more in secondary characteristics than in primary. Consider, for example, the differences between avoidant and schizoid: both share the primary attribute of social withdrawal but differ in secondary attributes (e.g., bland affect as opposed to anxious affect). For this reason, there may be no avoidant simplex as it is not distinguishable from Schizoid at the level of personality attributes. Attention to the pattern of personality attributes may help tease out the underlying dynamics in an otherwise difficult to interpret MCMI profile.

Clinical prototypes are analogous to personality attributes in that they are defined as the core symptoms comprising a clinical syndrome. A prototype is an idealized patient: one who has the bare essentials of the disorder in question and nothing else. The disorder of dysthymia, for example, may contain chronic depressed mood, sleep disturbance, pervasive guilt, anxiety, and a sense of hopelessness. The clinical prototype of depression is a simplex of pervasive dysphoria and attendant psychophysical complaints. Clinical Syndrome and Personality Attribute prototypes can help the clinician focus on specific disturbances in the patient's overall clinical picture.

Factors

Personality factors are not discrete attributes but major tendencies. Factors can give a broad picture of the patient's general orientation towards sociality, assertiveness, and emotional expression. They are also important as they are driven by the MCMI at a scale level and as such are highly reliable and stable.

Retzlaff and Gibertini (1987) reasoned that, due to the item-overlap among MCMI scales, the clinicians in the item sorting stage of the MCMI construction made operational distinctions among the items on the basis of a number of clinical categories that was fewer than the number of scales. In order to discover the number and type of clinical categories that were actually guiding the sorting of items for the eight basic personality scales, they factored the item-overlap matrix and five subject samples. The samples included three of their own, Millon's original sample, and a fifth independent sample. The six coefficient matrices produced three highly stable factors suggesting that the item-overlap determined the factor structure regardless of population specific variance. The three factors present in the MCMI personality scales are Aloof/Social, Submissive/Aggressive, and Labile/Restrained.

These factors are remarkably consistent with the thoughts of the Advisory Committee on Personality Disorders for DSM-III (and -R). Widiger, Frances, Spitzer, and Williams (1988) have suggested these very dimensions as potentially underlying DSM-III type personality disorders. They have considered the addition of such dimensional factors to DSM-III, specifically "to include dimensions of affiliation (introversion–extroversion) and power (dominance–submission) and basic clinical spectra (degree of affective dyscontrol, cognitive-perceptual aberrations, and anxiety)."

From a broader clinical perspective, all areas of pathology tapped by the MCMI must be analyzed. To determine the structure of all 20 scales of the test, Gibertini and Retzlaff (1988) performed factor analyses of the interscale item-overlap coefficients and four subject samples in a manner similar to above. When these matrices were factored, five orthogonal factors were found which were termed Clinical Convergence factors: Detached, Submissive, Suspicious, High Social Energy, and General Distress.

The purpose of this work was to develop scales that operationalize (a) the core attributes of the personality scales, (b) the core prototypical items from the clinical scales, (c) the personality factors, and (d) the clinical convergence factors for use by clinicians and researchers.

Scale Development

Three diverse general and specialty groups were included to assure gener- alizability. Sample 1 consisted of 253 male and female outpatients from private, military, and VA mental health clinics. Their mean age was 31 with a range of 18 to 66. Sample 2 consisted of 185 primarily male inpatient alcoholics (mean age 28, range 19 to 59) taking part in a 28-day alcohol rehabilitation program. And, sample 3 consisted of 184 male and female Air Force basic trainees (mean age 19, range 18 to 26) who were referred to a mental hygiene clinic for evaluation of personality disorders and/or distress.

A variation of domain theory test construction was developed for the attribute and prototype scales. The Non-overlapping Personality Attribute Scales were found by correlating the keyed items of the original 11 MCMI personality scales with the raw scores for those scales. The items that had the highest item-total correlations for each scale were retained. Items were examined across scales and across samples. Although items are keyed on several scales, items were only retained on the scale with the highest item-total correlations. For example, if an item correlated .7 with Schizoid, .5 with Avoidant, and .4 with Schizotypal, it was only included in the Schizoid scale. Further, item-total correlations had to be high and stable across all three samples.

A number of scales were eliminated for psychometric reasons. Avoidant was eliminated due to its vast item-overlap with Schizoid. Narcissism contained too few items and had very low reliability. Finally, Schizotypal also contained too few unique items and overlapped too greatly with Schizoid.

The Non-overlapping Clinical Prototype Scales were found in a similar man- ner as the nonoverlapping personality attribute scales. The items of the 9 original MCMI clinical syndrome scales were correlated with the raw scores for the scales and the above general selection criteria were again used. It was found that there were very few unique and psychometrically sound items for the clinical scales. As such, it was necessary to combine scales to achieve sufficient items with Alcohol and Drug Abuse collapsed as well as the psychotic scales. There- fore, only five scales survived the development hurdles. These included Anxiety, Mania, Depression, Substance abuse, and Psychotic potential.

The Personality Factor Scales were derived by correlating the 175 MCMI items with the three Personality Factor scores. Generally, items with the highest item-factor correlations were included in each of these three scales. Again, items had to have high item-total correlations across all three samples.

The five Clinical Convergence Scales were arrived at through a scale con- struction protocol that was designed to exemplify the underlying assumptions of the clinician item sorting in the MCMI construction. The two MCMI scales which loaded highest on each Clinical Convergence factor were used as marker scales. Items which were contained in both marker scales were used as "seed clusters." The 175 MCMI items were correlated with the five "seed clusters" and, generally, the items with the highest item-"seed cluster" correlations were included in each of these five scales.

General guidelines were used for all four sets of scales. Specifically, items from the 175-item pool were added to the scales if they met most of the following criteria:

1. the item correlated more highly with the scale/factor/cluster under consideration than with any other scale/factor/cluster and the correlations with all other scales/factors/clusters in the set of scales were low;

2. the item's correlation was consistent across the three subject samples;

3. item content fit the scale/factor/cluster;

4. the item had not already been added to another scale in the set;

5. the item's inclusion added significantly to the scale's alpha across all three samples.

The Special Scales

The final scales and number of items per scale are presented in Table 14.1. Scale item keys are in Tables 14.2 to 14.5.*

Most scales have sufficient items as assessed by a priori "rules of thumb." Only Compulsive and Submissive with 10 items are potentially problematic but Submissive's reliabilities of .71 to .80 are strong. Compulsive's, with .60 to .70, are more difficult. Other reliabilities are seen as excellent with the nonoverlapping personality scales ranging from .60 to .93 across the three samples with only one scale on one sample with a reliability below .70. The Nonoverlapping clinical scales had reliabilities between .62 and .94, again with only one scale on one sample below .70. For the Personality Factor Scales .78 to .95 are found and the Clinical Convergence Scales are between .71 and .96.

The nonoverlapping personality special scales generally have their highest correlations with the regular MCMI scale of the same name. Schizoid, however, shares loadings with Avoidant, Antisocial with Passive-aggressive and Drug Abuse, Borderline with Avoidant, Passive-aggressive, Anxiety, and Dysthymia, and, finally, Paranoid with Psychotic thinking. The nonoverlapping clinical special scales also generally load as expected. Anxiety, though, includes Passive-aggressive, Depression includes Anxiety and Psychotic potential includes Avoidant. These covariances make clinical sense but also point to a large distress factor within the test items.

The personality factor special scales show the aloof factor to be weighted at one end by Schizoid, Avoidant, and Schizotypal with the other end being Histrionic. The Submissive factor is bipolar with Dependent at one extreme and

---

Editor's Note: The reader who is interested in detailed psychometric properties and raw score conversion tables for these scales are invited to write Dr. Retzlaff for this information.

TABLE 14.1
Special Scales and the Number of Items per Scale

Scale	Number of Items
Nonoverlapping Personality Scales	
Schizoid	19
Dependent	15
Histrionic	13
Antisocial	11
Compulsive	10
Passive-Aggressive	12
Borderline	16
Paranoid	11
Nonoverlapping Clinical Scales	
Anxiety	12
Mania	13
Depression	16
Substance abuse	13
Psychotic potential	20
Personality Factor Scales	
Aloof	18
Submissive	17
Labile	22
Clinical Convergence Scales	
Detached	14
Submissive	10
Suspicious	14
High social energy	14
General distress	39

Antisocial/Narcissistic at the other. The Labile personality scale has Avoidant, Passive-Aggressive, and Borderline at one end with Compulsive at the other end of the bipolar dimension. The clinical convergence factor scales show similar structures across the entire MCMI set of variables. Notably, the Suspicious scale loads nicely on Paranoid and Psychotic Delusion. The Social scale has high positive correlations with Histrionic and Narcissistic indicating the high degree of sociability in narcissism as measured by the MCMI.

Interpretation of the Special Scales

An analysis of the item content, factor structures, and MCMI scale correlations suggest the following interpretations for the special scales:

Nonoverlapping Personality Attribute Scales

Schizoid: Social withdrawal. High scorers express discomfort in social situations and a strong preference to remain peripheral. They display a pervasive inadequacy in perception of social cues.

Dependent: Passive dependency. High scorers express strong needs for guidance and approval from others. They can become panicky if nurturing figures show disapproval or threaten to withdraw support.

Histrionic: High energy, social stimulus seeking. High scorers display dramatic affects and high gregariousness. They consider themselves fun-loving and social but can be insensitive to the needs of others.

Antisocial: Bold aggressiveness with hostile demeanor. High scorers perceive others as hostile or inadequate. They can be condescending, combative, and violent.

Compulsive: Meticulous and fastidious. High scorers are very concerned with maintaining an ordered, well-controlled, and proper presentation in all areas. They are intolerant of ambiguity and gravitate towards highly structured, predictable social positions.

Passive-Aggressive: Chronic agitation with frequent lapses of control of emotional expression. High scorers feel continual conflict and pressure in demanding social situations and are unable to identify workable assertive responses.

Borderline: Chronic and pervasive affective/cognitive distress. High scorers will complain of dysphoria, anxiety, self-deprecatory cognitions, and wildly

TABLE 14.2
Items for Nonoverlapping Personality Scales

Scale

Schizoid
True: 3, 8, 13, 19, 37, 47, 49, 55, 63, 76, 83, 91, 101, 102, 120, 150, 158, 171
False: 60

Dependent
True: 7, 10, 25, 31, 42, 65, 77, 78, 106, 130, 133, 145, 162, 168, 173
False: 0

Histrionic
True: 6, 14, 20, 28, 48, 74, 85, 111, 125, 137, 154, 165, 170
False: 0

Antisocial
True: 1, 9, 24, 41, 43, 110, 123, 142, 147, 148, 172
False: 0

Compulsive
True: 61, 88, 126, 138, 149, 153, 159
False: 54, 56, 92

Passive-Aggressive
True: 12, 22, 26, 45, 50, 51, 58, 66, 95, 107, 121, 156
False: 0

Borderline
True: 2, 27, 67, 79, 82, 96, 97, 99, 108, 109, 112, 115, 132, 134, 136, 167
False: 0

Suspicious
True: 16, 38, 64, 80, 85, 98, 100, 127, 131, 135, 164
False: 0

TABLE 14.3
Items for Nonoverlapping Clinical Scales

Scale

Anxiety
True: 18, 44, 51, 67, 73, 109, 112, 114, 117, 121, 167, 158
False: 0

Mania
True: 11, 23, 46, 57, 81, 93, 104, 116, 131, 139, 151, 163, 174
False: 0

Depression
True: 27, 33, 36, 45, 53, 54, 59, 71, 72, 76, 96, 97, 99, 108, 132, 136
False: 0

Substance Abuse
True: 17, 35, 70, 87, 95, 105, 110, 119, 140, 157, 175
False: 52, 122

Psychosis
True: 3, 8, 13, 19, 37, 47, 55, 77, 83, 85, 98, 100, 101, 102, 115, 120, 124, 127, 160, 164
False: 0

---

vacillating opinions of significant others. They experience intense mood states which seem unconnected to external events.

Paranoid: Ruminative suspiciousness. High scorers experience intense worry over the security of their physical/social boundaries. They maintain a hypervigilant mistrust of the motives and behavior of others but rarely form clear impressions of the type of harm they feel they must guard against.

Nonoverlapping Clinical Prototype Scales

Anxiety: Sensations attending physiological arousal: muscle tension, agitation, gastrointestinal symptoms, cold hands and feet, sweating. High scorers will complain of a pervasive inability to relax or feel comfortable.

TABLE 14.4
Items for Personality Factor Scales

Scale

Aloof
True: 3, 8, 13, 19, 37, 47, 49, 55, 83, 101, 150, 158, 171
False: 6, 14, 60, 125, 137

Submissive
True: 7, 10, 25, 31, 42, 65, 78, 106, 130, 133, 145, 162
False: 4, 24, 30, 84, 103

Labile
True: 5, 18, 26, 27, 45, 50, 51, 53, 54, 56, 58, 71, 72, 76, 96, 98, 99, 107, 109, 114, 132, 167
False: 0

TABLE 14.5
Items for Clinical Convergence Scales

Scale

Detached
True: 3, 7, 8, 19, 37, 47, 55, 83, 101, 102, 120, 141, 160
False: 125

Submissive
True: 31, 42, 65, 77, 78, 106, 130, 145, 173
False: 4

Suspicious
True: 15, 21, 80, 84, 85, 89, 100, 123, 126, 131, 135, 138, 146, 164
False: 0

Hi Social
True: 6, 14, 28, 60, 74, 86, 111, 137, 165, 166, 170
False: 51, 158, 171

Borderline Stress
True: 2, 5, 9, 18, 26, 27, 29, 33, 36, 43, 44, 45, 50, 53, 54, 56, 58, 59, 67, 71, 73, 76, 79, 82,
       96, 97, 99, 108, 109, 112, 114, 115, 117, 121, 132, 136, 156, 162, 167
False: 0

Mania: Extremely high energy. High scorers manifest signs of intense arousal with agitation or euphoria. They may exhibit pressured speech, flight of ideas, and/or grandiosity.

Depression: Intense dysphoria. High scorers complain of downwardly spiraling mood states: sadness, emptiness, hopelessness, preoccupation with escape or suicide.

Substance Abuse: Primary substance abuse or addiction. High scorers admit to significant problems with alcohol or drugs.

Psychotic Potential: Tenuous reality contact. High scorers are likely to be prepsychotic, psychotic, or postpsychotic. They admit to high levels of suspiciousness, derealization, alienation, and affective disturbance.

Personality Factor Scales

Aloof/Social: Strong propensity to avoid social contact. High scorers will exhibit a generalized tendency to remain socially peripheral and aloof. Low scorers will exhibit a tendency to affiliate and enjoy the company of others.

Submissive/Aggressive: Strong propensity to yield to others. High scorers complain of being used and abused by others but are unable to envision themselves as autonomous. Low scorers vehemently defend their autonomy and may be unable to admit to dependency needs.

Labile/Restrained: Strong emotional responsivity. High scorers feel out of control of their affective responses. They complain of intense and vacillating moods. Low scorers rarely express affectivity; they may feel out of touch with the world of emotions.

Clinical Convergence Scales

Detached: Social withdrawal with idiosyncratic thought process. High scorers are socially awkward and prefer isolation. They harbor fears of rejection and prefer to believe they do not need social contact.

Submissive: Extremely yielding. High scorers depend on the nurturance of others to a degree that they tolerate considerable discomfort to secure it.

Suspicious: Vigilant mistrust with confident and condescending demeanor. High scorers are convinced that others covet what they possess. They see the world as threatening but manageable in that they remain confident in their ability to thwart the nefarious designs of others.

High Social Energy: Extremely gregarious. High scorers are very energetic and demand attention/stimulation from others. They are prone to dramatic displays of affect which are usually short-lived and shallow.

Generalized Distress: Chronic and pervasive dysphoria, anxiety, agitation, and rumination. High scorers feel stressed, fatigued, and tense in reaction to an acute or chronic psychosocial stressor.

USE OF THE SPECIAL SCALES

Eight narrow personality scales, five simplex clinical scales, three factor based personality scales, and five broader psychopathology scales have been presented, which have high reliabilities across several populations and have high and appropriate validity estimates against the MCMI itself.

These scales combine the clinical wisdom of the MCMI construction procedures with the psychometric information on endorsement patterns provided by several diverse samples. The new scales should allow clinicians and researchers to better utilize the MCMI test data and clarify elevated profiles through a better understanding of the common elements of the scales.

RESEARCH USE OF THE SPECIAL SCALES

The original need for special scales for the MCMI came out of work by Butters, Retzlaff, and Gibertini (1986). That work attempted to use the MCMI to predict clinician recommendations in an Air Force clinic. Essentially, highly distressed basic trainees were sent to a psychologist in order to determine if separation from the service were indicated. The first multivariate computer runs used a discriminant function analysis to predict group membership on the basis of the regular MCMI scales. A problem developed in that only one variable would enter the equations. The scales of the test seemed to be so intercorrelated that little variance remained after the first variable entered. The tests were factor analyzed to a four factor solution to make more independent variables. Using these four factors in a discriminant function analysis allowed for all four to be included and resulted in more predicted variance. It became apparent that in some situations with some samples, the regular MCMI scales do not perform well in multivariate work.

Along another line, Gibertini, Baile, Scott, Endicott, and Ross (in press) have used the personality factor scales in their work with cancer patients. Although there have been many theories involving cancer personalities, little psychometrically sound work is available. This research group assessed head and neck cancer patients during initial presentations to an oncology department at a major southeastern cancer hospital. Medical workup, after the MCMI was given, revealed those having malignant growths versus those having benign tumors. The 25 patients identified as having benign growths were higher on the Labile personality factor (mean = 63 percentile) than the malignant group. This latter group of 46 patients had a mean percentile level of 51. In this case, the personality factor scales do a very reliable job of measuring fundamental personality features that transcend an individual test or research design.

Adams and Clopton (1990) were interested in Mormon missionaries and their satisfaction with their mission work. These authors chose the nonoverlapping Compulsive scale and the Submissive personality factor scale along with the MMPI Denial scale to assess the personality characteristics associated with dissatisfaction with the mission experience. Those missionaries with negative or mixed feelings were about average on the Compulsive scale at a mean percentile of 53. Those with positive feelings were significantly higher at the 77th percentile. With regard to the Submissive scale, there was a significant negative correlation ($-.26$) with missionaries' willingness to question mission policies. Essentially, those who questioned policy were more aggressive.

These special scales seem to work well when MCMIs are behaving poorly in multivariate work and when researchers wish to measure more narrow or more global variables associated with the psychopathology tapped by the MCMI.

CLINICAL USE OF THE SPECIAL SCALES

The clinical utility of these special scales can be gleaned both by looking at their development and through their direct use.

Often special additional scales are used without much understanding of their development and what that says about the manner in which a test, as well as the special scales, behave. The MCMI is a strong test due to its domains and development, and as such it is highly reflective of clinical pathology. It can tell a great deal about the manner in which psychopathology behaves. Note the recurring theme in which Schizoid and Avoidant scales covary. The nonoverlapping scales failed to reveal an avoidant factor in the face of the Schizoid scale. As well, in both sets of the factor based scales Schizoid and Avoidant load on the same factors and scales. In the case of the personality factor scales, those two domains define the high end of the aloof factor. Further, Histrionic loads the bottom end of that factor.

Applying these analyses to profile interpretation, allows the clinician to understand the profile patterns in light of the underlying scale covariances. In the above case, one should expect Schizoid and Avoidant to either both be high or both be low. Indeed fleshing out the rest of the aloof factor, if a patient displays primary aloof tendencies, one should normally see Schizoid, Avoidant, and Schizotypal all high and Histrionic should be low. That one factor drives at least four scales. This makes a great deal of clinical sense and is an accurate representation of psychopathology.

The overall Submissive factor is somewhat more narrow. In essence, Dependence and Antisocial strongly negatively covary. As such, in a patient with a submissive tendency, Dependent should be high and Antisocial as well as Narcissistic should be low. Conversely, profiles that display high Antisocial and Narcissistic scales will very rarely have high Dependence scales. Again, clinical reality is well measured.

The last personality factor, Labile, shows a strong dimension with Passive-aggressive and Avoidant at one end with Compulsive at the other. In this case, the profile that is high on Compulsive will rarely have high scores on Avoidant or Passive-aggressive. A look at the correlation table with the regular MCMI scales will also show that high compulsive scales will also drive down Borderline, Anxiety, Dysthymia, and Psychotic Depression. Clinicians should expect these profiles and deviations from the expected often point to fairly serious yet narrow conflicts.

The clinical convergence scales, similarly, quantify underlying profile factors across the entire test. The best factor for demonstration purposes is in some ways similar to the labile personality factor covary. The Distress clinical convergence factor is a global response to the test that is often situational, showing pan disturbance. This "fake bad" or "cry for help" factor is usually an overreport of symptomotology. Convergently, it is also often highly associated with high weight/disclosure scores which at times suggest invalid profiles. This profile includes high Avoidance, Passive-aggressive, Borderline, Anxiety, Dysthymia, and Psychotic Depression. This factor scale score and profile are common and should be interpreted with the above in mind. Perhaps more interesting is what this tells us about the scales not driven up by this factor. Dependence, Histrionic, Antisocial, Paranoid, Hypomania, and Drug Abuse are particularly resistant to this factor. It seems logical then, that perhaps even in the face of a technically invalid profile, that these scales may still be interpretable. Traditionally, an invalid profile implies that all scales are invalid but this does not appear to be the case. Obviously, more work is necessary in this area. Understanding what these special scales operationalize in terms of the MCMI regular scales and profiles is an indirect use of these scales.

The direct use of these scales is more straightforward. The nonoverlapping personality and clinical special scales are probably at their best in teasing apart conflicting regular MCMI scales. Again, several MCMI scales can be high because a patient is endorsing primary symptoms of a pathology on one scale which are secondary symptoms on another. The nonoverlapping scales, when compared to the regular scales, can clarify the scores.

The factor based scales are highly reliable measures of global pathology which are well accepted in one form or another in most theories of personality. As such they allow for an understanding of a patient at a higher level than the very specific MCMI scales. A high Submissive score implies cognitions, affect, and behavior across a wide range of situations.

In short, the use of special additional scales for the MCMI allow clinicians and researchers additional information. These special scales are well built psychometrically and should stand the test of cross validation.

REFERENCES

Adams, W., & Clopton, J. (1990). Personality and dissonance among Mormon missionaries. *Journal of Personality Assessment, 54*, 684–693.

Butters, M., & Retzlaff, P., & Gibertini, M. (1986). Non-adaptability to basic training and the Millon Clinical Multiaxial Inventory. *Military Medicine, 151*, 574–576.

Gibertini, M., Baile, W., Scott, L., Endicott, J., & Ross, E. (in press). Personality traits of patients undergoing evaluation for head and neck cancer. *Journal of Personality Assessment*.

Gibertini, M., Brandenburg, N., & Retzlaff, P. (1986). The operating characteristics of the Millon Clinical Multiaxial Inventory. *Journal of Personality Assessment, 50*(4), 554–567.

Gibertini, M., & Retzlaff, P. (1988). Factor invariance of the Millon Clinical Multiaxial Inventory. *Journal of Psychopathology and Behavioral Assessment, 10*(1), 65–74.

Millon, T. (1969). *Modern psychopathology*. Philadelphia: Saunders.

Millon, T. (1981). *Disorders of Personality: DSM-III, Axis II*. New York: Wiley.

Millon, T. (1983). *Millon Clinical Multiaxial Inventory Manual*. Minneapolis, MN: National Computer Systems.

Millon, T. (1987). *Manual for the MCMI-II*. Minneapolis, MN: National Computer Systems.

Nunnally, J. (1978). *Psychometric theory*. New York: McGraw-Hill.

Retzlaff, P., & Gibertini, M. (1987). Factor structure of the MCMI basic personality scales and common item artifact. *Journal of Personality Assessment, 51*(4), 588–594.

Widiger, T. A., Frances, A., Spitzer, R. L., & Williams, J. B. W. (1988). The DSM-III-R personality disorders: An overview. *American Journal of Psychiatry, 145*(7), 786–795.

15

Measuring Millon's Personality Styles in Normal Adults

Stephen Strack, Ph.D.

With the increasing interest in personality pathology that was ushered in by the inclusion of Axis II in the *Diagnostic and Statistical Manual of Mental Disorders* (DSM-III; American Psychiatric Association [APA], 1980) there has come an understanding that we must examine not only disturbance of character but also the nature of normal personality (e.g., Costa & McCrae, 1990; Grove & Tellegen, 1991; Sabshin, 1989; Strack, 1987). Although diagnosis of personality disorders remains a categorical distinction in DSM-III-R (APA, 1987), the belief that normal and abnormal personality are dimensional in nature has become increasingly prevalent in the psychiatric community (e.g., Frances, 1982; Livesley, 1991). This shift in thinking poses a number of important questions: What makes a personality normal or disordered? How are normal and abnormal personalities of the same type similar and different? Which traits are shared by normals and patients and which are unique to each population? Questions such as these challenge clinicians and researchers alike to re-examine current conceptions of normality and pathology.

This chapter addresses Millon's (1969/1983b, 1981, 1986a, 1986b, 1990) model of personality as it applies to normals and focuses on measurement of his styles in nonpatient populations. Major elements of the model that distinguish normal and pathological character are presented along with a review of *Millon Clinical Multiaxial Inventory-I* (MCMI-I; Millon, 1983a) and *Millon Clinical Multiaxial Inventory-II* (MCMI-II; Millon, 1987) studies that examined personality in normal adults. This leads to an item analysis of MCMI-I and MCMI-II personality scales for the purpose of evaluating their usefulness in nonpatient samples. Next, a detailed presentation is made of the *Personality Adjective Check List* (PACL; Strack, 1987, 1990), a measure developed specifically to assess Millon's personalities in normal form. Finishing the chapter are conclusions and recommendations for future research.

NORMALITY AND PATHOLOGY IN MILLON'S MODEL

Although centered on disorders, Millon's (1969/1983b, 1981, 1986a, 1986b, 1990) model of personality can serve as a useful guide in the search for knowledge about normal character, and the interface between normality and pathology. An integral feature of this model is the assumption that normal and abnormal personality lie along a continuum, with disordered character representing an exaggeration or distortion of normal traits. Normal and abnormal persons are viewed by Millon as sharing the same basic styles. Disordered persons are depicted as a small subset of the pool of all persons who, for various biological, psychological, environmental, and social reasons, have developed traits that are rigid and maladaptive.

In deriving his personalities, Millon (1981, 1990) distinguished four points along the normal-abnormal continuum, that is, normal character, and styles exhibiting mild, moderate, and severe pathology. Ten personality types, that is, asocial, avoidant, submissive, gregarious, narcissistic, antisocial, aggressive, conforming, negativistic, and self-defeating, are considered to exist in normal form as well as in mild or moderate pathological form (Millon, 1986a, 1986b). Three severe styles—schizoid, cycloid, and paranoid—are thought to be variants of the mildly and moderately pathological personalities and not to have direct counterparts in the normal domain.

Two sets of concepts were outlined by Millon to distinguish his personalities at the various continuum points. One set of concepts defines the relative position of normal and pathological individuals on his three evolutionary polarities, that is, self-other, active-passive, and pleasure-pain (Millon, 1990). Normal individuals are thought to be balanced in each of these areas, for example, possessing both moderate self-esteem and empathic regard for others. Mild or moderate pathology would be apparent among persons showing excesses or deficits in self- or other-regard, active or passive coping, and/or pleasure-pain orientation. Severe pathology would be marked by extremes or distortions on these polarities.

A second set of ideas used by Millon to distinguish normal and abnormal personality focuses on interpersonal functioning, namely, an individual's level of flexibility, stability, and tendency to foster "vicious cycles" (1969/1983b, 1986a). Healthy persons are viewed as interpersonally flexible, adaptive in coping, ego-resilient, and able to avoid, escape from, or move beyond pathogenic

attitudes, behaviors, or situations. In contrast, mildly and moderately pathological persons exhibit rigidity in interpersonal relations, nonadaptive coping, low
ego-strength, and a tendency to become mired in dysfunctional schemas or
transactions with others and the environment. More severely disturbed individuals are viewed as strongly rigid and inflexible, lacking in adaptive coping
skills, possessing extreme ego deficits, and unable to avoid, escape, or move
through pathological thought processes and relationships.

MCMI-I AND MCMI-II

While his model is attentive to issues of normality, Millon's empirical work has
almost exclusively been geared toward further explication of personality disorders. As such, his clinical assessment instruments, including the MCMI-I (Millon, 1983a) and MCMI-II (Millon, 1987), were developed and normed for use in
patient populations. Items for MCMI-I and MCMI-II personality scales were
written to measure prototypes of his styles as they appear in mildly to severely
disturbed form. Scales were developed based on endorsement frequencies and
item-scale correlations obtained exclusively from patient samples. Essentially all
validation data for both instruments were obtained on patients. Additionally, the
normative data used to create base rate (BR) scores were also derived from
patients.

The MCMI-I and MCMI-II have proven themselves to be quite useful in
clinical populations. However, Millon's extensive use of patients in developing,
validating, and norming scales for these instruments poses problems for their use
with normal adults. While many of the personality items appear to measure
normal traits (e.g., from MCMI-II, "I am content to be a follower of others" and
"I think I am a very sociable and outgoing person"), scales contain varying
numbers of items likely to be endorsed only by patients (e.g., from MCMI-II,
"Most people think that I'm a worthless nothing" and "I hate or fear most
people"). Furthermore, MCMI-I and MCMI-II BR scores are essentially unus-
able with normals since they are geared to prevalence rates for the various
disorders as found in clinical populations (Millon, 1983a, 1987).

Studies with Normal Adults

In spite of potential shortcomings, a number of investigators have employed the
MCMI-I (Auerbach, 1984; Emmons, 1987; Holliman & Guthrie, 1989; Lemkau,
Purdy, Rafferty, & Rudisill, 1988; Montag & Comrey, 1987; Piersma, 1987;
Retzlaff & Gibertini, 1987a, 1987b, 1988; Tango & Dziuban, 1984; Wheeler &
Schwarz, 1989) and MCMI-II (Costa & McCrae, 1990; Retzlaff, Lorr, Hyer, &
Ofman, in press; Retzlaff, Sheehan, & Fiel, 1991; Retzlaff, Sheehan, & Lorr,

1990; Strack, 1991b; Strack, Lorr, & Campbell, 1989) personality scales in research on normal adults.[1] Essentially all of these studies were descriptive or correlational in nature, and examined personality trait levels, factor structure, or relationships with other tests. Most were conducted on college undergraduates although samples of seminary students, Air Force pilot trainees, family practice residents, and Israeli driver license applicants were also utilized. Major findings are summarized next.

MCMI-I studies reporting means for the personality scales consistently showed high-points for normals on the Histrionic, Narcissistic, Antisocial, and Compulsive scales (Holliman & Guthrie, 1989; Lemkau et al., 1988; Montag & Comrey, 1987; Piersma, 1987; Retzlaff & Gibertini, 1987a, 1988; Wheeler & Schwarz, 1989). Both MCMI-II studies reporting means noted the Histrionic, Narcissistic, and Aggressive scales as being among the profile high-points, although not the Antisocial or Compulsive scales (Retzlaff, Sheehan, & Fiel, 1991; Strack, Lorr, & Campbell, 1989).

Retzlaff and Gibertini (1987b) factor analyzed MCMI-I basic personality scales in two samples of normal adults and three patient samples. They found the same three bipolar factors among normals and patients, namely, Aloof-Social, Aggressive-Submissive, and Lability-Restraint. A recent factor analysis of MCMI-II basic personality measures in normals that also included PACL scales (Strack, 1991b) revealed three bipolar factors among weighted raw residual scores that were very similar to those noted by Retzlaff and Gibertini.

In various forms, MCMI-I personality scale data have been correlated with the *Beck Depression Inventory* (Holliman & Guthrie, 1989), *California Psychological Inventory* (CPI; Holliman & Guthrie, 1989), *Comrey Personality Scales* (CPS; Montag & Comrey, 1987), *Maslach Burnout Inventory* (Lemkau et al., 1988), *Minnesota Multiphasic Personality Inventory* (MMPI; Montag & Comrey, 1987), *Narcissistic Personality Inventory* (Auerbach, 1984; Emmons, 1987), *NEO Personality Inventory* (NEO-PI; Costa & McCrae, 1990), *Strong Vocational Interest Blank* (SVIB; Tango & Dziuban, 1984), and to clusters derived from the *Personality Research Form* (Retzlaff & Gibertini, 1987a). Thus far, MCMI-II scales have been correlated with the NEO-PI (Costa & McCrae, 1990) and PACL (Strack, 1991b; Strack, Lorr, & Campbell, 1989).

Most of the extratest correlational findings indicated that MCMI-I and MCMI-II personality scales behaved relatively well with normal subjects. For example, Holliman and Guthrie (1989) noted that the MCMI-I Schizoid and Avoidant scales, and to a lesser extent the Dependent and Passive-Aggressive scales, were negatively associated with the six CPI Class I scales measuring interpersonal involvement, social dominance, and well-being. They also found that dysphoric subjects (as measured by the BDI) obtained their highest MCMI-I scores on the

---

[1]Excluded from this review were a small number of clinical studies that used normals for comparison purposes only.

Passive-Aggressive and Avoidant scales. In a study of occupational interests, Tango and Dziuban (1984) noted that subjects with elevated MCMI-I Aggressive and Narcissistic scales (canonical variate II) favored occupations involving athletics, management, and public speaking. Among their findings for the MCMI-II, Costa and McCrae (1990) reported that Compulsive was the only personality scale positively linked to the NEO-PI Conscientiousness factor, and Dependent the only scale positively associated with the NEO-PI Agreeableness dimension (Costa & McCrae, 1990).

Psychometric problems were noted in some of the studies. Auerbach (1984) found low internal reliability for the MCMI-I Narcissistic scale in his sample of 148 undergraduates (coefficient alpha = .66). Costa and McCrae (1990) found low correlations for the MCMI-II Paranoid scale on NEO-PI factors and surmised that low endorsement rates for scale items might be at fault. Canonical correlation analyses performed by Montag and Comrey (1987) on MCMI-I, MMPI, and CPS scales yielded first canonical variates that loaded most of the MCMI-I measures. A similar finding was reported by Tango and Dziuban (1984) in their analysis of the MCMI-I basic scales and SVIB. Undifferentiated variates such as these suggest the presence of an acquiescence response bias, a problem noted in factor results for the MCMI-II personality scales among both normals and patients (Strack, 1991b; Strack, Lorr, & Campbell, 1989, 1990).

Only one of the published MCMI-I studies, and none of the MCMI-II reports, addressed reliability of the personality scales among normals. Wheeler and Schwarz (1989) obtained 3-year test-retest data on MCMI-I scales from 225 college undergraduates who were participants in a longitudinal study of family dynamics and college adjustment. They also secured ratings of subjects on the MCMI-I from roommates and friends. Three-year stability coefficients for the personality scales ranged from .37 for Paranoid to .66 for Dependent. The basic eight personality scales were found to be more stable (Median r = .58) than those measuring the three severe styles (Median r = .42). Nevertheless, most of the correlations were lower than would be anticipated given the relatively high coefficients found among patients across 1 to 6-week intervals (Range = .77–.91, Millon, 1983a, p. 47; there are no published data for more extended periods of time).

MCMI-I ratings obtained from roommates and friends were correlated with subject self-reports to yield coefficients of self-other agreement. Values ranged from a low of .18 for Borderline to a high of .55 for Histrionic. Again, correlations were higher for the basic eight scales (Median r = .40) than for the three severe personality scales (Median r = .23).

Evaluating their results, Wheeler and Schwarz (1989) surmised that at least some of the low test-retest correlations were due to restrictions in the range of scores, especially for the severe disorder scales. Their conclusion was supported by the finding that self-other agreement coefficients were strongly related to the proportion of items endorsed for each scale, with greatest self-other agreement obtained for scales having the highest item endorsement rates. Scales with lower endorsement rates (e.g., the severe disorder scales) had the lowest self-other agreement.

Item Endorsement Rates and Internal Consistency Estimates for MCMI-I and MCMI-II Personality Scales in Normal Samples

The findings of Wheeler and Schwarz (1989) and others (Costa & McCrae, 1990) highlight significant problems in using the MCMI-I and MCMI-II with normals, namely, that temporal stability of the personality scales, self-other agreement, and extratest correlations may be lower for normals than patients because of poor endorsement rates for items on some scales. Auerbach's (1984) finding of a low alpha coefficient for the MCMI-II Narcissistic scale raises questions about internal consistency of the other measures. If scale reliability is lower among normals than patients, this would serve to further attenuate most types of correlations. Unfortunately, Wheeler and Schwarz did not report internal consistency estimates for the MCMI-I personality scales and none of the other published MCMI-I and MCMI-II studies provides this information.

To further evaluate the problem of low endorsement rates for scale items and to provide internal consistency estimates for the personality scales in normals, item-scale analyses were conducted on MCMI-I and MCMI-II personality scales. Two samples for each test were obtained for analysis from previously published data: *MCMI-I Sample 1* consisted of the responses of 295 male Air Force pilot trainees used by Retzlaff and Gibertini (1987a, 1988). Subjects were between 22 and 27 years-of-age and were given the MCMI-I during class training. *MCMI-I Sample 2* was comprised of data from 109 male and 132 female college students employed by Wheeler and Schwarz (1989; Time 2 data were used). Subjects were between 22 and 29 years-of-age and were paid for their participation in the study. *MCMI-II Sample 1* consisted of data from 159 male and 281 female college students used in an item factor analysis conducted by Retzlaff et al. (1991). Subjects came from two universities and were between 19 and 21 years-of-age. *MCMI-II Sample 2* contained item responses from 65 male and 75 female college students collected by Strack (1991b). Subjects ranged in age from 17 to 27 years and received course credit for completing the test.

Data were analyzed by me using the SPSS/PC+ (Norusis & SPSS Inc., 1990) statistical package, except for those of MCMI-I Sample 2, which were analyzed by David Wheeler using SAS (SAS Institute, Inc., 1990). By sample, item endorsement frequencies, corrected item-total correlations, and alpha coefficients (Cronbach, 1951) were calculated for the personality scales. False-keyed items were reversed prior to analysis. Since Millon (1987) apparently did not weight MCMI-II items before estimating internal consistency of the scales, they were not weighted here.[2]

Rates of Extreme Item Endorsement. Millon (1987) selected items for MCMI-I and MCMI-II scales that were endorsed by at least 15% and no more than 85% of his patients. Millon surmised that items with more extreme endorsement frequencies would not be good at making discriminations among people, and would be strongly influenced by social desirability (p. 41). Table 15.1 presents the percentages of MCMI-I and MCMI-II personality scale items endorsed by less than 15% or more than 85% of normal subjects. As can be seen in the table, virtually all MCMI-I and MCMI-II personality measures had significant numbers of items with endorsement frequencies lying outside the range that Millon used for scale development. Endorsement extremes were more common for MCMI-I than MCMI-II scale items. Nevertheless, all of the MCMI-II scales had 10% or more of their items in the extreme endorsement range.[3] The Avoidant, Schizotypal, and Borderline scales appeared most susceptible to endorsement bias on both instruments. Histrionic and Compulsive were least effected by this bias on MCMI-I, while Compulsive, Histrionic, and Narcissistic were least effected on MCMI-II. Surprisingly, the Paranoid scale was impacted much less by endorsement bias than the other two severe disorder scales.

Item-Scale Correlations. To ensure high internal consistency for MCMI-I and MCMI-II scales among patients, Millon (1983a, 1987) eliminated items that had corrected item-scale correlations of less than .30. For MCMI-I, the median item-scale correlation was .58 (Millon, 1983a, p. 38). Millon did not report comparable information for the MCMI-II; however, item selection criteria were essentially the same as those employed for MCMI-I.

Table 15.2 presents median item-scale correlations (corrected for overlap) for MCMI-I and MCMI-II personality scales among normals. As noted in the table, each of the scales for the two tests exhibited relatively low correlations. The highest median for both measures was found on the Borderline scale (.35 for both MCMI-I and MCMI-II). Recognizing that fully half the items had item-scale correlations *less* than the values listed in the table (some were negative), it can be concluded that large numbers of items are not strongly linked to the scales on which they are scored.

---

[2]Item weighting should not appreciably effect item-scale correlations or internal reliability estimates. To test this assumption, I recalculated the MCMI-II item-scale correlations and alpha coefficients presented in Tables 2 and 3 using weighted items. Values were practically identical to those reported in the tables. They differed by only ±.04 points and did not effect overall findings or conclusions.

[3]Some test developers, including myself, have successfully used less stringent criteria for selecting personality scale items. Applying a more lenient 5%–95% endorsement range, I still found that 9 of 11 MCMI-I scales and 5 of 13 MCMI-II scales had at least 10% of their items outside these limits.

TABLE 15.1
Percentages of MCMI-I and MCMI-II Scale Items With Extreme Endorsement Frequencies in
Normal Samples

Endorsement Rate and Scale	MCMI-I		MCMI-II	
	Sample 1 (295)	Sample 2 (241)	Sample 1 (440)	Sample 2 (140)
Less than 15%				
Schizoid	54.1	54.1	31.4	25.7
Avoidant	85.4	68.3	46.3	41.5
Dependent	42.4	24.2	13.5	16.2
Histrionic	0	0	12.5	7.5
Narcissistic	11.6	11.6	10.2	2.0
Antisocial	18.8	12.5	35.6	26.7
Aggressive	–	–	22.2	22.2
Compulsive	0	2.4	5.3	5.3
Passive-Aggressive	69.4	66.7	19.5	22.0
Self-Defeating	–	–	42.5	42.5
Schizotypal	81.8	68.2	54.5	52.3
Borderline	93.2	77.3	50.0	46.8
Paranoid	38.9	38.9	18.2	11.4
Greater than 85%				
Schizoid	0	0	0	0
Avoidant	0	0	0	0
Dependent	3.0	0	16.2	13.5
Histrionic	23.3	20.0	2.5	5.0
Narcissistic	30.2	20.9	2.0	2.0
Antisocial	25.0	9.4	2.2	4.4
Aggressive	–	–	0	2.2
Compulsive	35.7	28.6	5.3	5.3
Passive-Aggressive	0	2.8	0	0
Self-Defeating	–	–	0	0
Schizotypal	0	0	0	0
Borderline	0	0	0	0
Paranoid	0	0	2.3	0

Note. Numbers in parentheses are Ns. MCMI-I Sample 1 was made up of Air Force pilot trainees (Retzlaff & Gibertini, 1987a, 1988). Subjects in MCMI-I Sample 2 were college students from Wheeler and Schwarz's (1987) Time 2 follow-up. MCMI-II Sample 1 (Retzlaff, Lorr, Hyer, & Ofman, 1991) and MCMI-II Sample 2 (Strack, 1991) contained college student subjects.

Alpha Coefficients.   Millon (1983a) presented internal consistency estimates for MCMI-I personality scales among patients that ranged from .73 for Schizoid to .95 for Borderline (Median = .82; p. 47). MCMI-II internal consistency estimates among patients were reported to range from .86 to .93 (Median = .90; Millon, 1987, p. 129). Table 15.3 presents alpha coefficients for the scales in normal samples. Comparisons of table values with those presented by Millon for patients revealed lower reliability for all scales among normals than patients. Significantly, 9 of 11 MCMI-I scales and 5 of 13 MCMI-II scales had alpha coefficients below .70 on at least one sample (.70 is often considered a lower limit for acceptable internal consistency in measures of personality). Median alpha for MCMI-I across samples was .69, while for MCMI-II it was .76.

TABLE 15.2
Median Item-Scale Correlations for MCMI-I and MCMI-II Personality Scales in Normal Samples

Scale	MCMI-I		MCMI-II	
	Sample 1	Sample 2	Sample 1	Sample 2
Schizoid	.09	.15	.18	.22
Avoidant	.21	.27	.32	.31
Dependent	.18	.24	.18	.19
Histrionic	.26	.21	.17	.22
Narcissistic	.19	.19	.16	.20
Antisocial	.17	.20	.26	.25
Aggressive	–	–	.21	.31
Compulsive	.19	.18	.12	.15
Passive-Aggressive	.20	.32	.30	.31
Self-Defeating	–	–	.32	.28
Schizotypal	.22	.26	.27	.29
Borderline	.29	.35	.30	.35
Paranoid	.22	.19	.22	.29

Implications for Use of the MCMI-I and MCMI-II With Normals. The extreme endorsement frequencies, low item-scale correlations, and low internal consistency estimates found here point to significant limiting factors for use of MCMI-I and MCMI-II personality scales in normal samples. Perhaps most important is that each of these elements reduce reliability of the scale scores. They result in attenuated correlations in most applications, for example, in evaluations of scale stability over time, self-other agreement, and relationships with other tests. Additionally, it is plausible to assume that the items with poor endorsement properties decrease the scales' overall ability to discriminate, and increase the likelihood that social desirability will confound the scores.

The presence of poor item-scale correlations calls into question the integrity

TABLE 15.3
Alpha Coefficients for MCMI-I and MCMI-II Personality Scales in Normal Samples

Scale	MCMI-I		MCMI-II	
	Sample 1	Sample 2	Sample 1	Sample 2
Schizoid	.50	.59	.62	.68
Avoidant	.73	.69	.80	.78
Dependent	.58	.69	.66	.65
Histrionic	.70	.66	.61	.71
Narcissistic	.67	.69	.69	.73
Antisocial	.61	.68	.75	.80
Aggressive	–	–	.74	.81
Compulsive	.69	.68	.50	.61
Passive-Aggressive	.70	.78	.81	.84
Self-Defeating	–	–	.81	.77
Schizotypal	.74	.69	.80	.80
Borderline	.79	.87	.88	.88
Paranoid	.67	.67	.74	.82

of the scales as measures of Millon's styles in normal form. Findings indicate that many items selected to measure the personalities as disorders do not belong on scales measuring the personalities among normals. This is not surprising, but it does imply that MCMI-I and MCMI-II scales do not adequately measure the constellation of traits that represent Millon's personalities in normal form.

PACL

The only assessment device currently available that was designed specifically to measure Millon's personalities in a normal population is the PACL (Strack, 1987, 1990).[4] The check list originated at the University of Miami in the early 1980s in a research group led by Theodore Millon, Catherine Green, and Robert Meagher, Jr.[5] At the time, very little empirical work had been done on Millon's model and it seemed that advances could be made through development of an interpersonally-oriented measure of his styles that could be used with normal adults. In the tradition of LaForge and Suzek's (1955) *Interpersonal Check List,* and Gough's (Gough & Heilbrun, 1983) *Adjective Check List,* we decided to create an adjective measure that would allow for observer ratings as well as self-reports. Following Millon's (1983a) strategy for MCMI-I, Loevinger's (1957) three-stage model of test development was employed.

In its initial, experimental form, the PACL was composed of 405 theory-derived adjectives keyed to measure normal versions of Millon's (1969/1983b) eight basic and three severe personality styles. Items were culled from numerous sources, including *Modern Psychopathology* (MP; Millon, 1969/1983b), and were selected based on rater judgments that each item had a clear best-fit for one style.

Scale development and validation took place using the responses of over 2000 normal adults from numerous samples across the United States (Strack, 1987, 1990). Adjectives for the refined scales were selected from among items endorsed by at least 5% and no more than 80% of subjects.[6] Additional standards included minimum item-scale correlations of .25, and maximum within-scale item-item correlations of .49 (to prevent redundancy; Strack, 1987, p. 577).

---

[4]Although the *Millon Behavioral Health Inventory* (Millon, Green, & Meagher, 1982b) and *Millon Adolescent Personality Inventory* (Millon, Green, & Meagher, 1982a) measure non-disordered forms of Millon's basic eight personality styles, they were developed and normed on patient samples and emphasize maladaptive traits.

[5]Other members of the research group were Leonard Bard, Nancy Firestone, Richard Garvine, and Steven Hentoff.

[6]Item selection standards were different for the PACL than MCMI-I and MCMI-II because people respond differently to check lists than statement-based measures, and because normals respond differently than patients (e.g., normals endorse fewer negative items).

Using these criteria, scales with satisfactory internal consistency and temporal reliability were created for each of Millon's eight basic styles. Alpha coefficients for the scales ranged from .76 to .89 (new sample Median = .83; Strack, 1987, p. 578), while test-retest correlations over a 3-month period ranged from .60 to .85 (Median = .72 across sexes; Strack, 1987, p. 578). Scales could not be developed to measure the three severe personalities because of extremely low endorsement rates (<5%) for most keyed items. Rather than throw away the handful of good items that remained for these measures, they were combined into an experimental problem indicator scale, PI, which we thought might be useful in identifying persons with personality disorders.

In addition to the personality and experimental scales, I developed three response bias indices to aid in the detection of faked protocols (Strack, 1990), namely, Random (R), Favorable (F), and Unfavorable (UF). Separate groups of college students were asked to complete the PACL randomly, or with intent to give an overly favorable or overly unfavorable self-report. Discriminant function analyses were used to distinguish the faked tests from PACLs completed under the normal instructional set. Equations were derived from these analyses (separately for men and women) and were cross-validated with independent samples. The equations were able to correctly identify a large majority of faked (75%–91%) and normal tests (60%–94%).

Extensive validity data have been reported for PACL scales in the form of correlations with other tests of personality, mood, and dispositional variables, and reports from subjects about current and past behavior (Horton & Retzlaff, 1991; Pincus & Wiggins, 1990; Strack, 1987, 1990, 1991b; Strack & Lorr, 1990; Strack, Lorr, & Campbell, 1989; Wiggins & Pincus, 1989). My own research has noted that each PACL scale is in line with theoretical expectations and measures milder versions of Millon's (1969/1983b) pathological styles. For example, the scale measuring the avoidant personality (Inhibited) was positively associated with measures of shyness, submissiveness, and social anxiety, and negatively associated with measures of sociability, dominance, and emotional well-being (Strack, 1990). The scale measuring aggressive traits (Forceful) was positively linked to measures of arrogance, dominance, assertiveness, and autonomy, and negatively linked to measures of deference, submissiveness, and conscientiousness (Strack, 1990). In a study comparing the PI scores of psychiatric patients ($n = 124$) and normal adults ($n = 140$), I (Strack, 1991a) found that 84% of PI scales with scores of 60 or above were obtained by patients. Only 16% of the normals had scores over 59.

Other investigators have reported expected relationships between PACL scales and other measures. Horton and Retzlaff (1991) correlated the PACL with Moos' *Family Environment Scale* in a sample of 65 undergraduates. They found that family cohesion and expressiveness were strongly associated with cooperative and sociable personality styles, while conflict was most prevalent in the families of sensitive and forceful persons. High scores on the Respectful scale were linked to family environments in which cohesion, organization, and religiosity were salient features.

Wiggins and Pincus (1989; Pincus & Wiggins, 1990) examined the PACL in the context of MMPI personality disorder scales, Big Five *Interpersonal Adjective Scales* (IAS-B5), the NEO-PI, and a circumplex version of Horowitz's *Inventory of Interpersonal Problems*. PACL scales exhibited anticipated relationships with each of the tests in correlational, canonical, and factor analyses. For example, PACL Introversive and Sociable were loaded (in opposite directions) on a factor that included the MMPI Schizoid and Histrionic scales, NEO-PI Extraversion, and IAS-B5 Dominance. PACL Forceful was correlated .59 with interpersonal problems associated with dominance behavior, while PACL Cooperative was correlated .48 with problems involving exploitation by others.

In keeping with the emphasis on normality, PACL scales were normed as *T* scores rather than BR scores. Normative data (Strack, 1990) were obtained from 2507 normal adults between the ages of 16 and 72. Subjects were sampled between 1980–1986 with 90% coming from colleges and 10% from businesses. Men comprised 47.4% of sample and women 52.6%. Ethnic make-up was 65.2% non-Hispanic White, 17.3% Hispanic, 9.1% Black, 7.6% Asian, and 0.8% Native American Indian or Eskimo.

The PACL is currently available as a paper-and-pencil measure that can be hand-scored. A full-color, computerized version of the check list, called AUTO-PACL (Robbins, 1991), is also available for IBM-compatible computers that permits computer administration of test, automatic scoring, and printing of profile plots of scores as well as narrative interpretations. The program allows for unlimited uses on a single computer and, as an aid to researchers, can produce exportable files containing test data for multiple subjects. The narrative interpretations were written by me for use in counseling and personnel settings, and were based on Millon's (e.g., 1969/1983b) writings, empirical information obtained during test construction and validation (e.g., Strack, 1990), and clinical experience with the test. A sample print-out from AUTOPACL, including a narrative interpretation of results, is presented in Fig. 15.1. PACL items are given on the last page of the print-out. Endorsed adjectives are identified with asterisks (e.g., **self-satisfied**).

Comparison With MCMI-I and MCMI-II.   The PACL was designed exclusively on the basis of Millon's (1969/1983b) model as presented in MP. This is in contrast to the MCMI-I and MCMI-II which were designed to match DSM-III (APA, 1980) and DSM-III-R (APA, 1987) Axis II criteria for personality disorders. The MP model also differs slightly from that found in Millon's (1986a, 1986b, 1990) more recent writings where he expanded his detached-dependent-independent-ambivalent axis to include a fifth branch, *discordant*, to encompass the two provisional personality disorders found in DSM-III-R (i.e., aggressive/sadistic and self-defeating/masochistic).

----------------------- IDENTIFYING INFORMATION -----------------------

```
ID: 999999999        TEST DATE: 01/15/92    REPORT DATE: 01/26/92
NAME: Eric S                SEX: Male    AGE: 41
RESEARCH CODE: 00000        EDUCATION: 16
ETHNIC: Non-Hispanic White  MARITAL: Divorced
RELIGION: Protestant
```

-------------------------- VALIDITY INDICES --------------------------

```
                  UNLIKELY              :CONSIDER:      LIKELY
    BIAS                                 \       /
        -30  -25  -20  -15  -10   -5    0    5   10   15   20   25   30
        +----+----+----+----+----+----+----:----:----+----+----+----+
 R   -7.65 |RRRRRRRRRRRRRRRRRRRRRRR        :    :                    |
 F   -4.95 |FFFFFFFFFFFFFFFFFFFFFFFFFF     :    :                    |
 UF -15.71 |UUUUUUUUUUUUUUUU               :    :                    |
        +----+----+----+----+----+----+---:+----+----+----+----+----+
        -30  -25  -20  -15  -10   -5    0    4   10   15   20   25   30
    BIAS                                 /   \
                  UNLIKELY              :CONSIDER:      LIKELY
```

```
        NUMBER OF ADJECTIVES CHECKED = 62   NUMBER CHECKED IS OK
                        R   SCORE IS OK
                        F   SCORE IS OK
                        UF  SCORE IS OK
        Note: Validity indices should be interpreted with care - see Manual
```

-------------------------- PACL SCALES --------------------------

```
              T SCORE-> 10   20   30   40   50   60   70   80   90  100  110
      SCALE     raw  ----+----+----:----+----|----+----:----+----+----+----+
1 INTROVERSIVE    1  |XXXXXXXXXXXXXX:XXXX 39           :
2 INHIBITED       6  |XXXXXXXXXXXXXX:XXXXXXX   |44     :
3 COOPERATIVE    14  |XXXXXXXXXXXXXX:XXXXXXX   |47     :
4 SOCIABLE       10  |XXXXXXXXXXXXXX:XXXXXXXXX |49     :
5 CONFIDENT      12  |XXXXXXXXXXXXXX:XXXXXXXXX |XXXX 58 :
6 FORCEFUL       17  |XXXXXXXXXXXXXX:XXXXXXXXX |XXXXXX 62:
7 RESPECTFUL     10  |XXXXXXXXXXXXXX:XXXXX 43  :
8 SENSITIVE       7  |XXXXXXXXXXXXXX:XXXXXXXXX |46     :
9 PI              1  |*************:**** 38    :
      SCALE     raw  ----+----+----:----+----|----+----:----+----+----+----+
              T SCORE-> 10   20   30   40   50   60   70   80   90  100  110
```

INTRODUCTION

The Personality Adjective Check List (PACL) is a comprehensive, objective measure of eight basic personality styles outlined by Theodore Millon. A ninth PI scale measures aspects of three more severe personality styles and may be used as an indicator of personality disturbance. This test was designed for use with normal adults who read at minimally the eighth grade level. The PACL was developed, validated, and normed using the responses of over 2500 men and women from across the United States. All of the people measured in the course of test development were presumed to have normal personalities. Therefore, even extreme elevations on PACL scales should not be interpreted as indicating disordered personality.

FIG. 15.1. Measuring Millon's personality styles in normal adults. PACL and narrative interpretation. Copyright (1986, 1990) Stephen Strack, AUTOPACL V1.1. Copyright (1991) Brian Robbins. Published by 21st Century Assessment, South Pasadena, California.

Computer-generated PACL test reports are intended for use by qualified professionals only. Interpretive statements made in the test reports are based on empirical data and theoretical inference. They are probabilistic in nature and cannot be considered definitive. The report should be evaluated along with other information available about the respondent, for example, background characteristics and other test and interview data, before conclusions are made. Users of the test reports should be familiar with the PACL's assets and limitations as described in the test manual.

RESPONDENT CHARACTERISTICS AND TEST VALIDITY

This 41 year old, Non-Hispanic White, Protestant, divorced, male respondent, with 16 years of education, completed the PACL on 01/15/92. He marked 62 adjectives as self-descriptive, which is within the valid range of 20-110 items checked. Response style indices indicate no unusual test-taking biases.

NARRATIVE DESCRIPTION

This person is characteristically aggressive, hardheaded, and ascendant. Ambitious and competitive, he can be overbearing and gruff. While he sees the world as a harsh place where he must be on guard at all times, this person is also confident of his ability to attain his wishes. He frequently bullies his way to success but can be refined, engaging, and even charming in order to achieved desired ends. This person tends to feel privileged and superior and may expect others to cater to him. Viewing himself as exempt from social responsibilities, he is often self-centered, exploitive, and unwilling to reciprocate favors or kindness. He may have a low tolerance for frustration. When crossed, pushed on personal matters, or faced with embarrassment, this person may respond quickly and become angry, revengeful, and vindictive. Beneath his rugged exterior, this person may be afraid of letting down his guard. Because he fears that others will use his sensitivities to humiliate or exploit him, expressions of emotion and vulnerability are usually short-lived.

This person is likely to enjoy challenging, competitive work settings which allow him independence and control. Although he can tolerate group work environments, his single-mindedness, gruff style, and insensitivity may be hard on others. Not only is he able to work alone or in situations involving some difficulty, he may even excel in these circumstances. In general, he is a dedicated worker who won't let obstacles get in his way. Others typically see him as aggressive, undaunted, and achievement-minded.

When troubled, this person may exaggerate his usual coping strategies, becoming excessively angry, tyrannical, and reckless. He is unlikely to seek help on his own, even when in significant distress. His defensiveness and fear of being viewed as weak make it difficult for him to trust anyone or to admit shortcomings. He is likely to experience discomfort in a therapy client role and will probably find it difficult to explore personal issues which impact his problems. He may view therapists as threatening or in competition with him. Taking a firm but nonthreatening approach which enables this person to feel more like a collaborator than a patient is best. A nondirective, supportive style aimed at restoring lost self-esteem and bolstering current coping strategies may prove useful. If amenable to more probing forms of therapy, this person may benefit from reassessing his attitudes toward self and others, developing interpersonal sensitivities, increasing self-control, and learning new, prosocial behaviors for obtaining desired ends.

FIG. 15.1
(*Continued*)

```
---------------------------- ITEM ENDORSEMENTS ----------Total endorsed: 62
```

1. PLAYFUL	52.**ANNOYED**	103. SELF-ADMIRING
2.**SELF-SATISFIED**	53.**LIVELY**	104.**GENTLE**
3. RESERVED	54. RIGID	105. THEATRICAL
4.**CONSENTING**	55. NAIVE	106.**SWEET**
5. IGNORED	56. IRRITABLE	107. FORMAL
6.**INSECURE**	57. SHY	108. GROUCHY
7. BOASTFUL	58. DISCIPLINED	109. OVERLOOKED
8.**STRICT**	59. UNINSPIRED	110.**SELF-CONTENTED**
9. EXTRAVAGANT	60. EXCLUDED	111.**BOSSY**
10. OVERSENSITIVE	61.**FEARLESS**	112. SUSPICIOUS
11. APPREHENSIVE	62.**BAFFLING**	113.**EFFICIENT**
12.**CAREFUL**	63. NEAT	114.**SELF-CONSCIOUS**
13.**INTIMIDATING**	64. SOLITARY	115.**EGOISTIC**
14. BUBBLY	65. TOUCHY	116. CONFUSING
15. EDGY	66. SECRETIVE	117. MEAN
16. REMOTE	67.**OUTGOING**	118. MORALISTIC
17.**COURAGEOUS**	68. TRADITIONAL	119. CONCEITED
18. TIMID	69. SUBDUED	120. DISAGREEABLE
19. ERRATIC	70. FICKLE	121.**POWERFUL**
20. INNOCENT	71.**ANIMATED**	122.**HELPFUL**
21.**COMPETITIVE**	72. MOODY	123. DEPENDENT
22.**INDUSTRIOUS**	73.**TALKATIVE**	124.**ORGANIZED**
23. UNEASY	74. NAGGING	125. SELF-IMPORTANT
24. CHAOTIC	75.**DECENT**	126.**DOMINEERING**
25.**GREGARIOUS**	76. EXPRESSIONLESS	127. REVENGEFUL
26. ARROGANT	77. CONFORMING	128. RIGHTEOUS
27. FRAGMENTED	78. COY	129. ILL-AT-EASE
28. AFRAID	79. DRAMATIC	130.**REJECTED**
29.**YIELDING**	80.**MILITANT**	131. UNAFRAID
30. VIRTUOUS	81.**BLUNT**	132. SERIOUS
31. SLUGGISH	82.**ADVENTUROUS**	133.**COOPERATIVE**
32. UPRIGHT	83. HESITANT	134.**IMMODEST**
33.**SELFISH**	84. INDIFFERENT	135.**FORCEFUL**
34.**WORRIED**	85. PROPER	136.**TRUSTFUL**
35.**STRAIGHT-LACED**	86.**COMMANDING**	137.**TOUGH**
36. AGGRAVATED	87. NERVOUS	138.**RESPECTFUL**
37. PRECISE	88. CARE-FREE	139.**FLIRTATIOUS**
38.**COOL**	89. UNNOTICED	140. DISINTERESTED
39. VIVACIOUS	90.**ORDERLY**	141. IMPERSONAL
40.**DARING**	91. DOCILE	142. INEXPRESSIVE
41. APATHETIC	92.**LONELY**	143. SWEET-TEMPERED
42. FLUCTUATING	93.**SOCIABLE**	144.**VAIN**
43.**AGREEABLE**	94.**OBEDIENT**	145.**HARD-HEADED**
44. PEPPY	95. ANXIOUS	146. PESSIMISTIC
45.**TEMPERAMENTAL**	96. COMBATIVE	147.**WARM-HEARTED**
46.**SELF-CENTERED**	97.**COMPLAINING**	148.**HARD-WORKING**
47. TESTY	98. DESPONDENT	149. MERRY
48. DEPRESSED	99. DETACHED	150. DISTANT
49. UNEMOTIONAL	100. APOLOGETIC	151.**UNDERSTANDING**
50. FEARFUL	101.**SEDUCTIVE**	152.**AGGRESSIVE**
51. OVERCONFIDENT	102. UNCOMFORTABLE	153. HOSTILE

FIG. 15.1

In accord with Millon's (1969/1983b, 1987) model and akin to MCMI-I and MCMI-II, PACL personality scales contain varying numbers of overlapping items, ranging from one for the Respectful scale to nine for the Sensitive scale. The percentage of overlapping items on PACL scales is substantially lower than that for MCMI-I (1983a) and MCMI-II (1987) scales, and ranges from 5% to 35%. As a result, scale intercorrelations for the PACL are somewhat lower than those for MCMI-I and MCMI-II (Median $r = |.35|$ across sexes; Strack, 1987, p. 579). Also as a result, PACL scales containing only nonoverlapping items have

TABLE 15.4
Corresponding Scales for the PACL, MCMI-I, and MCMI-II

PACL	MCMI-I	MCMI-II
Introversive	Schizoid	Schizoid
Inhibited	Avoidant	Avoidant
Cooperative	Dependent	Dependent
Sociable	Histrionic	Histrionic
Confident	Narcissistic	Narcissistic
Forceful	Antisocial	Antisocial
		Aggressive
Respectful	Compulsive	Compulsive
Sensitive	Passive-Aggressive	Passive-Aggressive
		Self-Defeating

Note. The PACL PI scale measures aspects of the schizotypal, borderline, and paranoid styles, but does not directly assess these personalities.

been found to be quite reliable on their own, and to yield essentially the same factors as the overlapping scales (Pincus & Wiggins, 1990; Wiggins & Pincus, 1989; Strack, 1990).

Table 15.4 lists corresponding personality measures for the PACL, MCMI-I, and MCMI-II. Two MCMI-II scales are listed for both PACL Forceful and Sensitive. This is because Millon's (1986a) new model divides his original (1969/1983b) aggressive (Forceful) style into Antisocial and Aggressive, and his original negativistic (Sensitive) style into Passive-Aggressive and Self-Defeating. An examination of items for these scales suggested that MCMI-II Aggressive and Passive-Aggressive may be closer to the PACL Forceful and Sensitive scales, respectively, than MCMI-II Antisocial and Self-Defeating, although research is needed to verify this impression.

In practice, correspondence between the PACL and MCMI-I and MCMI-II is reduced by the dissimilar test formats (adjectives versus statements), models used, and focus on normality versus pathology. In spite of these differences, I (Strack, 1991b) found the eight PACL and ten MCMI-II basic personality scales to be correlated between .39 and .67 (Median = .52, using MCMI-II weighted raw scores) in a sample of 65 male and 75 female college students. The lowest values were found for PACL Sensitive/MCMI-II Self-Defeating (.39) and PACL Forceful/MCMI-II Antisocial (.41), suggesting that these MCMI-II scales are not strongly aligned with Millon's original (1969/1983b) MP model. By comparison, the MCMI-II Aggressive scale was correlated .53 with PACL Forceful and the MCMI-II Passive-Aggressive scale was correlated .51 with PACL Sensitive.

Factor analyses of PACL, MCMI-I, and MCMI-II personality scales have revealed very similar results. The three higher-order dimensions found in the PACL (Strack, 1987), that is, Neuroticism, Assertiveness-Aggressiveness, and Social Extraversion-Introversion, correspond to the three factors found by Retzlaff and Gibertini (1987b) for MCMI-I basic eight scales among psychiatric patients and normal adults, and by Strack, Lorr, Campbell, and Lamnin (1992) for the 13 MCMI-II personality scales with patients. A joint factor analysis of PACL and MCMI-II basic personality scales among college students also yielded three factors (using residual scores), with corresponding PACL and MCMI-II scales loading on the same dimensions (Strack, 1991b).

Strack, Lorr, and Campbell (1990) examined the circular ordering of MCMI-II personality disorder scales in a mixed group of psychiatric patients and compared results with those from the PACL in normals. Plotted against the orthogonally-rotated first two principal components, they found a reasonably good circle for MCMI-II scales (using residual scores) that, for the most part, followed Millon's (1987, p. 20) predictions. Ordering for the PACL scales was similar, although a less complete circle was noted for PACL than MCMI-II.

Millon's Personalities as Measured by the PACL.   The correlational evidence presented earlier indicated that normal versions of Millon's basic styles are milder variants of the personalities as disorders. Unfortunately, behavioral studies and side-by-side comparisons of matched groups of normals and patients on the PACL, MCMI-I, and MCMI-II have not been carried out. As a result, data are not available to address the important questions posed at the beginning of the chapter concerning the precise nature of similarities and differences between normal and disordered forms of character.

With regard to the appearance of Millon's personalities in normal form, what can be offered at this point is a summary of empirical findings from studies associating PACL scales with other measures of personality, mood, and dispositional variables. Presented below are listings of the most frequently endorsed adjectives for PACL personality scales and statements from correlated tests (*rs* > |.40|). All statements describe those who obtain high scale scores and were summarized from data presented in the PACL test manual (Strack, 1990). The descriptions are a first step toward the development of normal prototypes and will hopefully serve to flesh-out aspects of the normal types not readily grasped by extrapolations from Millon's (e.g., 1981) writings on pathological personalities. Especially noteworthy among the normals are their positive dispositional features and interpersonal attitudes. Even less desirable traits are placed within a normal frame of reference.

Introversive   (Millon's asocial, passive-detached style). PACL items: Serious, reserved, yielding, solitary, remote.

1. Avoids social interactions and rebuffs the friendly overtures of others; is introverted, distant, aloof; friendly interactions are avoided by restricting social life, refusing invitations, and not taking the time or making the effort to interact with others (*Interpersonal Adjective Scales-Revised,* IAS-R, Aloof-Introverted).

2. Shy, withdrawing, cautious, retiring, a "wallflower"; has inferiority feelings; is slow and impeded in speech and self-expression; dislikes occupations with personal contacts; prefers one or two close friends to large groups (*Sixteen Personality Factors Questionnaire*, 16PF, Shy).

3. Methodical, conservative, dependable, conventional, easygoing, quiet; is self-abasing and given to feelings of guilt and self-blame; passive in action; narrow in interest (CPI, Self-acceptance).

4. Socially anxious; resentful (IAS-R, Gregarious-Extraverted).

5. Restrained, reticent, introspective; dour, pessimistic, unduly deliberate; often considered smug and primly correct by observers; tends to be sober and dependable (16PF, Sober).

6. Detached; seeks privacy; likes being alone (*Interpersonal Style Inventory*, ISI, Sociable).

7. Cautious, holds back, avoids conflict; gives in so as to escape interpersonal stress or controversy; tends to shrink from encounters in which they will be visible or "on stage" (*Adjective Check List*, ACL, Exhibition).

Inhibited (Millon's avoidant, active-detached personality). PACL items: Self-conscious, shy, moody, anxious, oversensitive.

1. Shy, withdrawing, cautious, retiring, a "wallflower;" has inferiority feelings; is slow in speech and self-expression; dislikes occupations with personal contacts; prefers one or two close friends to large groups (16PF, Shy).

2. Lacks self-confidence; prefers to be on the periphery of group enterprise; shuns situations calling for competition or self-assertion (ACL, Dominance).

3. Has difficulty mobilizing resources and taking action; viewed by others as inhibited and withdrawn (ACL, Self-confidence).

4. Tends to ask little of others; tends to submit to others' wishes and demands; avoids conflict at all costs; the interpersonal world is viewed with worry and foreboding; others are seen as stronger, more effective, and more deserving (ACL, Abasement).

5. Awkward, conventional, quiet, and unassuming; detached and passive in attitude; suggestible and overly influenced by others' reactions and opinions (CPI, Sociability).

6. Clever, enthusiastic, imaginative; quick, informal, spontaneous, talkative; active and vigorous; has an expressive, ebullient nature (CPI, Social-presence).

7. Socially anxious; is uncomfortable in the presence of others; is sensitive to the evaluation of others; attempts to escape from social situations; avoids eye contact; inhibits speech or other social behavior; may stammer, stutter, or appear clumsy with others (*Self-consciousness Scale*, Social Anxiety).

8. Timid, fearful, and submissive in social transactions; low self-confidence

and self-esteem; is meek and self-doubting; evades situations involving social challenge, power over others, and being the center of attention (IAS-R, Lazy-Submissive).

Cooperative (Millon's submissive, passive-dependent type). PACL items: Understanding, helpful, agreeable, trustful, respectful.

1. Unassuming, patient, conscientious; defers to others without loss of self-respect; prefers anonymity and freedom from conflict (ACL, Deference).

2. Makes few if any demands on others; is forbearing and conciliatory (ACL, Aggression).

3. Likes people; is cooperative and unaffected; has a tactful social manner; is sympathetic and supportive (ACL, Nurturance).

4. Conventional; seeks security in the tried and true; avoids risks; welcomes direction from trusted superiors (ACL, Autonomy).

5. Tends to ask little of others; tends to submit to others' wishes and demands; avoids conflict at all costs; the interpersonal world is viewed with worry and foreboding; others are seen as stronger, more effective, and more deserving (ACL, Abasement).

6. Is warm, nurturant, sympathetic, and caring in social transactions; sympathetic, forgiving, kind, and soft-hearted; provides material or emotional benefits to others who are in trouble, need help, are ill, or otherwise in need of care and support (IAS-R, Warm-Agreeable).

7. Reliable; considerate of others; free of pretense; comfortable in interpersonal relationships (CPI, Communality).

Sociable (Millon's gregarious, active-dependent style). PACL items: Playful, sociable, adventurous, lively, outgoing.

1. Sociable, bold, and ready to try new things; spontaneous; abundant in emotional responsiveness; "thick skinned"; is able to face wear and tear in dealing with people and grueling emotional situations without fatigue; careless to detail; ignores danger signals; talkative; pushy; actively interested in the opposite sex (16PF, Venturesome).

2. Forceful, obtrusive, bombastic; insists on winning attention; impatient with opposition and delay; willing to coerce or manipulate someone whose acquiescence is desired (ACL, Exhibition).

3. Cheerful, active, talkative, frank, expressive, effervescent, and care-free; frequently chosen as leader; impulsive and mercurial (16PF, Happy-go-lucky).

4. Outgoing and vivacious in social transactions, and actively seeks out settings and situations that will permit harmonious interactions with others;

friendly; looks for jobs, social events, organized activities, hobbies, parties, and social clubs that will provide settings for maximal social interaction (IAS-R Gregarious-Extraverted).

5. Plunges into life with gusto; responds warmly to interpersonal encounters; has vigorous erotic drives; appears to be blessed by good health and abundant vitality (ACL, Heterosexuality).

6. Intelligent, outspoken, sharp-witted; demanding, aggressive, and self-centered; persuasive and verbally fluent; self-confident and self-assured (CPI, Self-acceptance).

7. Clever, enthusiastic, imaginative; quick, informal, spontaneous, talkative; active and vigorous; expressive, ebullient nature (CPI, Social-presence).

Confident (Millon's narcissistic, passive-independent personality). PACL items: Self-satisfied, cool, daring, extravagant, care-free.

1. Assertively self-confident; responds quickly; insist on obtaining what they judge to be their just rewards (ACL, Abasement).

2. Self-assured and independent-minded; austere; a law to themselves; hostile and extrapunitive; authoritarian; disregards authority (16PF, Assertive).

3. Independent, autonomous, and self-willed; indifferent to the feelings of others; viewed as egotistical and domineering by others (ACL, Autonomy).

4. Delights in competition, taking risks, and defeating rivals; headstrong and impulsive behavior frequently leads to conflict with others (ACL, Deference).

5. Forceful, obtrusive, bombastic; insists on winning attention; impatient with opposition and delay; willing to coerce or manipulate someone whose acquiescence is desired (ACL, Exhibition).

6. Clever, enthusiastic, imaginative; quick, informal, spontaneous, talkative; active and vigorous; has an expressive, ebullient nature (CPI, Social-presence).

7. Sociable, bold, and ready to try new things; spontaneous; abundant in emotional responsiveness; "thick skinned"; is able to face wear and tear in dealing with people and grueling emotional situations without fatigue; careless to detail; ignores danger signals; talkative; pushy; actively interested in the opposite sex (16PF, Venturesome).

Forceful (Millon's aggressive, active-independent type). PACL items: Competitive, adventurous, cool, daring, courageous.

1. Expresses anger and irritation toward others in the form of humiliation and exploitation; egotistical, arrogant, cunning, and exploitive; puts others in their place, proves them wrong, and criticizes them publicly; has a cynical world view; competition and exploitation are viewed as means for survival (IAS-R, Arrogant-Calculating).

2. Ambitious, assertive; impatient when blocked or frustrated; quick to take the initiative and get things moving; stubbornly insistent on attaining their goals (ACL, Masculinity).

3. Competitive and aggressive; others are viewed as rivals to be vanquished; strong impulses are often undercontrolled and tend to be expressed with little regard for the courtesies of conventional society (ACL, Aggression).

4. Strong-willed, determined, forceful; free of self-doubt in the pursuit of goals; little if at all inhibited by the disapproval or opposition of others; affiliative and adroit in directing group actions toward the attainment of socially worthy objectives (ACL, Dominance).

5. Assertively self-confident; responds quickly; insist on obtaining what they judge to be their just rewards (ACL, Abasement).

6. Self-assured and independent-minded; austere; a law to themselves; hostile and extrapunitive; authoritarian; disregards authority (16PF, Assertive).

7. Expedient; takes advantage of people for own ends; undependable (ISI, Conscientious).

Respectful (Millon's conforming, passive-ambivalent style). PACL items: Careful, respectful, serious, disciplined, organized.

1. Seeks objectivity and rationality; firm in controlling impulses; unswerving in the pursuit of goals; setbacks and distractions are not easily endured, nor are change and variety welcomed (ACL, Orderly).

2. Conscientious; eschews frivolity and the nonessential; conservation of the tried and true is deemed more important than the discovery of the new and different (ACL, Endurance).

3. Seeks stability and continuity in the environment; avoids ill-defined and risky situations; tends to lack verve and imagination (ACL, Change).

4. Exacting in character; responsible, planful; moralistic; prefers hard-working people to witty companions; strong superego (16PF, Conscientious).

5. Oriented toward duties and obligations; holds fast to an agreed-upon line of action; works hard to see that consensual goals are attained; exerts a steadying influence on others; values good organization and careful planning; not at all temperamental or high-strung (ACL, Military Leadership).

6. Orderly, organized; lives and works by systematic plan in an orderly fashion (ISI, Orderly).

7. Persistent; persists at tasks or goals until they are completed, despite difficulty or the amount of time required (ISI, Persistent).

8. Deliberate; stops and thinks before acting; is able to resist and delay gratification of impulses (ISI, Deliberate).

Sensitive (Millon's negativistic, active-ambivalent personality). PACL: Moody, anxious, temperamental, apprehensive, fluctuating.

1. High-strung and moody; avoids close relationships with others; worries about ability to deal with the stresses and strains of life; viewed by others as defensive, preoccupied, and easily distracted (ACL, Personal Adjustment).

2. Poor morale; tends to feel defeated by life; finds it difficult to set and attain goals; kind, modest, and considerate of the rights and wishes of others (ACL, Ideal Self).

3. Generally anxious and dysphoric (*Multiple Affect Adjective Check List-General Form,* Anxiety and Depression).

4. Tends to agonize over the meaning of relationships, complicates them, and fears involvement; self-preoccupation and an underlying current of anxiety make wholehearted participation in social interactions difficult if not impossible (ACL, Affiliation).

5. Pessimistic; tends to expect negative outcomes (*Life Orientation Test,* Pessimism).

6. Inhibited, cautious, shrewd, wary, aloof, and resentful; is cool and distant in relationships with others; is self-centered and little concerned with the needs and wants of others (CPI, Good Impression).

7. Feels inadequate in coping with stress and crises; tends to retreat into fantasy (ACL, Succorance).

CONCLUSIONS AND FUTURE DIRECTIONS

Millon's normal personality styles, and the relationship between healthy and pathological variants of the same types, are topics of scientific inquiry with considerable promise that have only recently begun to garner the attention of researchers. This chapter highlighted some of Millon's (1969/1983b, 1986a) theoretical assumptions in these areas and offered empirical evidence for the existence of normal versions of his styles that appear strongly linked to their pathological counterparts.

Concerning measurement of Millon's personalities among normal adults, it was noted that summary MCMI-I and MCMI-II scale scores are problematic. Although the scales behaved reasonably well in some studies with normals, their low item endorsement rates, internal reliability, and test-retest stability greatly reduce their effectiveness as measures of normal personality. Findings for the summary scale scores should not, however, discourage research focusing on MCMI-I and MCMI-II scale items. Studies comparing item response patterns of matched groups of normals and patients may shed light on important similarities and differences between these populations. Such studies might also lead to the development of scales for these instruments that are reliable and valid among patients and normals alike.

Existing data indicated that the PACL is a satisfactory measure of Millon's basic eight personality patterns among normal adults. Data also showed that while there are a number of similarities between PACL and MCMI-I and MCMI-II scales, there are a number of differences as well. As such, PACL scales should not be viewed as being identical to MCMI-I and MCMI-II personality measures (or DSM-III-R Axis II disorder constructs).

The PACL can be fruitfully employed in studies that further describe Millon's personalities in normal form, and examine major premises of his model thought to differentiate normal and abnormal persons. For experimental purposes, there may be some value in using the PACL with patient samples and/or combining the PACL with the MCMI-I or MCMI-II. PACL item responses may provide information about the normal characteristics of patients not tapped by MCMI-II, and the scale scores can show how subjects deviate from a normal mean, something MCMI-I and MCMI-II BR scores cannot do.

Concerning future directions for research, there is still much to be learned about the appearance of Millon's personalities in normal form. Empirical evidence in this realm will further explicate the normal prototypes presented earlier and, in the process, should provide clearer avenues for research relating normal and abnormal styles. Millon's ideas about the differences between normal and abnormal personalities are also important targets for research. At this point, we simply don't know whether disordered styles are less interpersonally flexible and stable, and more pathogenic, than normal types. Likewise, there is no research information available concerning the relative position of normal and abnormal types on Millon's self-other, active-passive, and pleasure-pain polarities.

In describing personality development, Millon (1969/1983b, 1981, 1990) emphasized a number of individual difference and process elements thought to be influential in creating either normal or dysfunctional character, for example, biological predispositions (including temperament), early learning experiences, and parent-child relations. Many of these elements are central to his model and deserve careful scrutiny in both retrospective and longitudinal investigations.

A large body of research now supports a five-factor model of normal personality (for a review, see Digman, 1990). Studies relating the five-factor model to Millon's derivation of pathological styles should illuminate significant features of both approaches and, as a byproduct, may provide a bridge between the separate normal and clinical traditions in personality research (Costa & McCrae, 1990). A marriage of resources from these traditions promises to give us a more complete picture of the meaning and function of those enduring human characteristics we experience as personality in all individuals.

ACKNOWLEDGMENTS

This chapter is dedicated to the memory of Robert B. Meagher, Jr.

Preparation of this manuscript was facilitated by a U. S. Department of Veterans Affairs grant.

Data from Wheeler and Schwartz (1989) were collected and analyzed with the support of PHS grant R01 MH31750-01-6 and 5R01 AA06754-01-03, and funds from the University of Connecticut Research Foundation and Computer Center. Data from Retzlaff, Lorr, Hyer, and Offman (1991) were collected with the help of U. S. Department of Veterans Affairs Research funds.

I thank Paul Retzlaff, David Wheeler, and J. Conrad Schwarz for their generosity in providing data for the MCMI-I and MCMI-II item analysis.

Requests for reprints should be directed to Stephen Strack, Psychology Service 116B, Veterans Affairs Outpatient Clinic, 425 South Hill Street, Los Angeles, CA 90013.

REFERENCES

American Psychiatric Association. (1980). *Diagnostic and statistical manual of mental disorders* (3rd ed.). Washington, DC: Author.

American Psychiatric Association. (1987). *Diagnostic and statistical manual of mental disorders* (3rd ed., rev.). Washington, DC: Author.

Auerbach, J. S. (1984). Validation of two scales for narcissistic personality disorder. *Journal of Personality Assessment, 48,* 649–653.

Costa, P. T., & McCrae, R. R. (1990). Personality disorders and the five-factor model of personality. *Journal of Personality Disorders, 4,* 362–371.

Cronbach, L. J. (1951). Alpha coefficient and the internal structure of tests. *Psychometrika, 16,* 542–548.

Digman, J. M. (1990). Personality structure: Emergence of the five-factor model. *Annual Review of Psychology, 41,* 417–440.

Emmons, R. A. (1987). Narcissism: Theory and measurement. *Journal of Personality and Social Psychology, 52,* 11–17.

Frances, A. J. (1982). Categorical and dimensional systems of personality disorder. *Comprehensive Psychiatry, 23,* 516–527.

Gough, H. G., & Heilbrun, A. B. (1983). *The Adjective Check List manual* (1983 edition). Palo Alto, CA: Consulting Psychologists Press.

Grove, W. M., & Tellegen, A. (1991). Problems in the classification of personality disorders. *Journal of Personality Disorders, 5,* 31–41.

Holliman, N. B., & Guthrie, P. C. (1989). A comparison of the Millon Clinical Multiaxial Inventory and the California Psychological Inventory in assessment of a nonclinical population. *Journal of Clinical Psychology, 45,* 373–382.

Horton, A. D., & Retzlaff, P. D. (1991). Family assessment: Toward DSM-III-R relevancy. *Journal of Clinical Psychology, 47,* 94–100.

LaForge, R., & Suczek, R. F. (1955). The interpersonal dimensions of personality: III. An interpersonal check list. *Journal of Personality, 24,* 94–112.

Lemkau, J. P., Purdy, R. R., Rafferty, J. P., & Rudisill, J. R. (1988). Correlates of burnout among family practice residents. *Journal of Medical Education, 63,* 682–691.

Livesley, W. J. (1991). Classifying personality disorders: Ideal types, prototypes, or dimensions? *Journal of Personality Disorders, 5,* 52–59.

Loevinger, J. (1957). Objective tests as instruments of psychological theory. *Psychological Reports, 3,* 635–694.

Millon, T. (1981). *Disorders of personality.* New York: Wiley.

Millon, T. (1983a). *Millon clinical multiaxial inventory manual* (3rd ed.). Minneapolis, MN: National Computer Systems.

Millon, T. (1983b). *Modern psychopathology.* Prospect Heights, IL: Waveland Press. (Original work published 1969)

Millon, T. (1986a). A theoretical derivation of pathological personalities. In T. Millon & G. L. Klerman (Eds.), *Contemporary directions in psychopathology: Toward the DSM-IV* (pp. 639–670). New York: Guilford.

Millon, T. (1986b). Personality prototypes and their diagnostic criteria. In T. Millon & G. L. Klerman (Eds.), *Contemporary directions in psychopathology: Toward the DSM-IV* (pp. 639–670). New York: Guilford.

Millon, T. (1987). *Manual for the MCMI-II* (2nd ed.). Minneapolis, MN: National Computer Systems.

Millon, T. (1990). *Toward a new personology.* New York: Wiley.

Millon, T., Green, C., & Meagher, R. B. (1982a). *Millon Adolescent Personality Inventory manual.* Minneapolis, MN: National Computer Systems.

Millon, T., Green, C., & Meagher, R. B. (1982b). *Millon Behavioral Health Inventory manual.* Minneapolis, MN: National Computer Systems.

Montag, I., & Comrey, A. L. (1987). Millon MCMI scales factor analyzed and correlated with MMPI and CPS scales. *Multivariate Behavioral Research, 22,* 401–413.

Norusis, M. J., & SPSS Inc. (1990). *SPSS/PC+ Statistics* (Version 4.0). Chicago: SPSS Inc.

Piersma, H. L. (1987). The use of the Millon Clinical Multiaxial Inventory in the evaluation of seminary students. *Journal of Psychology and Theology, 15,* 227–233.

Pincus, A. L., & Wiggins, J. S. (1990). Interpersonal problems and conceptions of personality disorders. *Journal of Personality Disorders, 4,* 342–352.

Retzlaff, P. D., & Gibertini, M. (1987a). Air force pilot personality: Hard data on the "right stuff." *Multivariate Behavioral Research, 22,* 383–399.

Retzlaff, P. D., & Gibertini, M. (1987b). Factor structure of the MCMI basic personality scales and common-item artifact. *Journal of Personality Assessment, 51,* 588–594.

Retzlaff, P. D., & Gibertini, M. (1988). Objective psychological testing of U.S. Air Force officers in pilot training. *Aviation, Space, and Environmental Medicine, 59,* 661–663.

Retzlaff, P. D., Lorr, M., Hyer, L., & Ofman, P. (1991). An MCMI-II item-level component analysis: personality and clinical factors. *Journal of Personality Assessment, 57,* 323–334.

Retzlaff, P. D., Sheehan, E., & Fiel, A. (1991). MCMI-II report style and bias: Profile and validity scales analyses. *Journal of Personality Assessment, 56,* 466–477.

Retzlaff, P. D., Sheehan, E., & Lorr, M. (1990). MCMI-II scoring: Weighted and unweighted algorithms. *Journal of Personality Assessment, 55,* 219–223.

Robbins, B. (1991). *AUTOPACL user's guide.* South Pasadena, CA: 21st Century Assessment.

Sabshin, M. (1989). Normality and the boundaries of psychopathology. *Journal of Personality Disorders, 3,* 259–273.

SAS Institute, Inc. (1990). *SAS/STAT user's guide. Version 6.* (Vol. 1, 4th ed.). Cary, NC: Author.

Strack, S. (1987). Development and validation of an adjective check list to assess the Millon personality types in a normal population. *Journal of Personality Assessment, 51,* 572–587.

Strack, S. (1990). *Manual for the Personality Adjective Check List (PACL) (Rev.).* South Pasadena, CA: 21st. Century Assessment.

Strack, S. (1991a). *Comparison of PACL PI scale elevations in samples of psychiatric patients and normal adults.* Unpublished manuscript.

Strack, S. (1991b). Factor analysis of MCMI-II and PACL basic personality scales in a college sample. *Journal of Personality Assessment, 57,* 345–355.

Strack, S., & Lorr, M. (1990). Three approaches to interpersonal behavior and their common factors. *Journal of Personality Assessment, 54,* 782–790.

Strack, S., Lorr, M., & Campbell, L. (1989, August). *Similarities in Millon personality styles among normals and psychiatric patients.* Paper presented at the annual convention of the American Psychological Association, New Orleans, LA.

Strack, S., Lorr, M., & Campbell, L. (1990). An evaluation of Millon's circular model of personality disorders. *Journal of Personality Disorders, 4,* 353–361.

Strack, S., Lorr, M., Campbell, L., & Lamnin, A. (1992). Personality and clinical syndrome factors of MCMI-II scales. *Journal of Personality Disorders, 6,* 40–52.

Tango, R. A., & Dziuban, C. D. (1984). The use of personality components in the interpretation of career indecision. *Journal of College Student Personnel, 25,* 509–512.

Wheeler, D. S., & Schwarz, J. C. (1989). Millon Clinical Multiaxial Inventory (MCMI) scores with a collegiate sample: Long-term stability and self-other agreement. *Journal of Psychopathology and Behavioral Assessment, 11,* 339–352.

Wiggins, J. S., & Pincus, A. L. (1989). Conceptions of personality disorders and dimensions of personality. *JCCP: Psychological Assessment, 1,* 305–316.

16 The Combined Use of the MCMI and MMPI

Michael Antoni, Ph.D.

Until the official publication of the DSM-III (American Psychiatric Association, 1980), distinctions between what are termed clinical syndromes (Axis I) and personality disorders (Axis II) were not made, although it had long been recognized as a useful distinction. The DSM-III made explicit the practice of differentiating longstanding, deep-seated patterns of behavior, affect, cognition, and interpersonal style (personality) from more transitory, time-limited, and obvious deviations from characteristic behaviors (clinical syndromes). This approach reflects an evolution in the understanding of psychopathological processes, namely, that the picture a patient presents will depend on his/her characteristic, longstanding perceptual and behavioral tendencies, as well as the more transitory stressors of everyday life.

As prescribed by DSM-III-R (American Psychiatric Association) comprehensive clinical diagnostics involve a multidimensional assessment featuring at least two major sets of variables. On the one hand, there are "process variables," including perceptions of self–others and environmental demands, and there are reactions to these, which occur on the behavioral, interpersonal, and emotional level. These reactions may vary in terms of the severity and direction (inward vs. outward) in which they are expressed. These process or personality variables tend to perpetuate one another, thereby creating a "loop," manifest as a pervasive and lifelong pattern or style. The DSM-III Axis II categories comprise this realm of functioning.

On the other hand, clinical syndromes can be seen as "output" variables in reference to their genesis from the personality loop. These output variables tend to encompass static, point-in-time outcomes, manifest in overt behaviors and phenomenological reports. From this standpoint, a clinical syndrome (Axis I)

279

may result from several different loops (Axis II), or it may be one of several syndromes output from the same loop. Consideration of both the process variables and outcome variables is critical to a comprehensive diagnostic assessment.

The Millon Clinical Multiaxial Inventory (MCMI) was designed to assess personality disorders, specifically as established in the DSM-III. At the present time, the MCMI is the only objective, self-report inventory explicitly created to elucidate this realm of psychopathology. Some have gone so far as to proclaim the MCMI as the prime competitor of the MMPI (Butcher & Owen, 1978; Korchin & Schuldberg, 1981). The MMPI is the best documented instrument designed to assess the presence of specific clinical syndromes (Axis I), whereas the MCMI provides an in-depth view of the personality pattern (Axis II). The MCMI also assesses levels of personality disorder severity or "organization" (i.e., borderline). Together, the MMPI and MCMI provide data on different domains of psychological functioning, both of which are essential to the elucidation of a complete clinical picture.

Although the combination of multiple assessment instruments (e.g., TAT and Rorschach) is a common practice, little research has tested the utility of integrating two or more "objective" inventories. Our work has shown that the combination of MMPI and MCMI data might be useful in two ways. This procedure could, on the one hand, identify the relationship between Axis I (MMPI) and Axis II (MCMI) syndromes. On the other hand, each test might enrich and refine data obtained from one instrument alone (Antoni, Tischer, Levine, Green, & Millon, 1985; Millon, 1984).

MMPI 2-point codes often suggest multiple interpretations, some of which contain contradictory "within code" descriptors. We reasoned that the addition of MCMI data may help to confirm MMPI hypotheses in some cases and resolve MMPI descriptive contradictions in others. We now present some well-accepted descriptions of commonly observed MMPI 2-point codes. As will be evident, these are wrought with discrepancies.

CONTRADICTORY DESCRIPTORS FOR MMPI TWO-POINT CODES

MMPI 28/82

Individuals with the MMPI 28/82 code type are basically dependent and submissive with difficulties in being assertive. They appear irritable and resentful, fear losing control, deny undesirable impulses, occasionally act-out and express guilt afterwards. Seen by some as stubborn and moody at times, they are considered peaceable and docile to others. These people are judged by some to be in a state of profound inner turmoil over highly conflictual, insoluble problems; others view them as somehow "resigned" to their psychosis. In some cases anxious, agitated depression may be seen while in others soft, reduced speech and retarded stream of thought are noted. Individuals with the 28/82 MMPI code appear most likely to receive a diagnosis of either manic-depressive psychosis or schizophrenia, schizoaffective type. A significant segment of 28/82 individuals exhibit psychotic upsets, often preceded by hypochondriacal and hysterical episodes. Psychotic symptomatology may include bizarre mentation, delusions, hallucinations, social alienation, sleep disturbance, poor family relationships, and difficulties in impulse control. Unusual thoughts may take a specific form (hallucinations and suicidal ideation) or more diffuse symptomology (general confusion, disorganization, and disorientation) (Dahlstrom, Welsh, & Dahlstrom, 1972; Graham, 1977). Overall, the 28/82 type appears to suffer from a heterogeneous group of disorders and syndromes characterized by disturbances of thinking, mood, and behavior. (Antoni, Levine, Tischer et al., 1985, pp. 393).

This collection of descriptors presents an assortment of behavioral, interpersonal, and affective components that at times seem to contradict one another, making clear hypothesis formation difficult. These contradictions appear at the *behavioral* level (denial of undesirable impulses vs. acting-out behaviors), the *interpersonal* level (withdrawn vs. hysterical), and at the *emotional* level (stubborn and moody vs. peaceable and docile). While some descriptors reflect an outwardly directed response style (hostility and aggression), others portray a more inwardly directed mode (retreat into fantasy via hallucinations). Diagnostic disparities also seem to be prevalent with the 28/82 type including hysterical and manic syndromes on the one hand and schizoidal and schizophrenic symptoms on the other.

MMPI 24/42

The 24/42 type, often referred to as "psychopaths in trouble," are known for their recurrent acting-out and subsequent periods of guilt and depression. They are noted as impulsive, unable to delay gratification and to have little respect for societal standards. Frustrated by their own limited achievements, resentful of the demands and expectations of others, they often experience a mixture of anger and guilt that manifests itself in agitated depression. Some are overcontrolled, avoid confrontations, and express feelings of inadequacy and self-punitive rumination. Many also engage in asocial or antisocial behaviors, such as stealing, sexual acting-out, and drug or alcohol abuse. Often described as immature and narcissistic, they appear unable to maintain deep relationships. Beneath the carefree and confident facade of many will often reside either worry and dissatisfaction, or an absence of any emotional response. Their failure to achieve life satisfactions results either in self-blame and depression or in a projection of blame and paranoid ideation. In some cases, prepsychotic behavior and suicide attempts may be seen (Dahlstrom et al., 1972; Graham, 1977). (Antoni, Tischer, Levine et al., 1985, p. 509).

Some of these statements appear to be contradictory at the *behavioral* (asocial vs. antisocial), and *emotional* levels (worry and anger vs. absence of emotional response). As noted previously, while some descriptors reflect an outwardly directed response (extrapunitive, projected blame), others indicate a more inwardly directed response (self-blame, depression).

MMPI 89/98.

Individuals with the 89/98 code type have been described as being self-centered and infantile in their expectations of others, demanding a great deal of attention, and responding with resentment and hostility when demands are not met. Fearing emotional involvement they avoid close relationships and tend to be socially withdrawn and isolated. Characterized as hyperactive, emotionally labile and unrealistic in self-appraisal, these individuals may impress others as grandiose, boastful and fickle. Their feelings of inadequacy and low self-esteem tend to limit the extent to which they involve themselves in competitive and achievement-oriented activities. However, these individuals usually emphasize achievement as a means of gaining status and recognition. Their affect is characterized by some as inappropriate, unmodulated, irritable and hostile, yet they may also tend to be ruminative, over-ideational and withdrawn, fearing any type of outward communication with others. Highly suspicious and distrustful of others, these individuals may display unusual and unconventional thought processes including delusions of a religious nature, feelings of grandiosity, hallucinations, poor concentration and negativism. These individuals may receive a diagnosis of either schizophrenia, stressing an interpersonal element, or manic depression, manic type, stressing the emotional features. Drug abuse is a common accompanying symptom. (Dahlstrom et al., 1972; Graham, 1977). (Antoni, Levine, Tischer et al., 1986, pp. 66–67).

These features, taken as a whole, seem to contradict one another at the *behavioral* level (avoidance of achievement-oriented activities vs. emphasis on achievement as a means of gaining status and recognition), the *interpersonal* level (socially withdrawn and inadequate vs. grandiose and boastful) and at the *emotional* level (ruminative and fearful of emotional involvement vs. overt hostility and emotional lability). Diagnostic disparities also appear in the 89/98 MMPI type including schizophrenia, on the one hand, and manic-depressive syndromes on the other.

MMPI 78/87

Individuals with the 78/87 code type are often described as experiencing a good deal of psychic turmoil. Usually introspective and obsessional, they spend much of their time being worried, tense, and depressed. Often indecisive, these individuals usually show poor judgment when they do act and may appear to others as jumpy and socially inept. In interpersonal situations, the 78/87 type comes across as shy and hard to get to know at times, yet sentimental, sensitive, and softhearted on other occasions. These individuals characteristically maintain a rigid hold on affect, yet may be prone to displays of immaturity and emotionality. These people tend to deal with their psychic and social discomfort by withdrawal into a rich fantasy experience, often of a sexual nature (Dahlstrom et al., 1972; Graham, 1977). (Antoni, Levine, Tischer et al., 1987, p. 377).

DSM-III diagnoses for this 2-point code range from the neurotic to psychotic level, with primary emphasis being placed on Axis I in some cases and Axis II in others. In terms of Axis II diagnoses, these range from passive dependent and schizoid to schizotypal and borderline. Several inconsistencies and ambiguities occur across interpersonal, behavioral, and emotional spheres of functioning. Within the *interpersonal* realm, these individuals have been characterized as introverted, and hard to get to know on the one hand, yet sentimental, sensitive, and softhearted on the other (Dahlstrom et al., 1972). Thus these descriptors appear to present a simultaneous "moving away from" and "moving toward" others. In the *behavioral* domain, the 78/87 type has been described with terms that emphasize both compulsivity and impulsivity (Dahlstrom et al., 1972; Graham, 1977). Finally, on the *emotional* level of functioning, the 78/87 type has been presented by some as rigid, affectively restrained, and introspective, yet by others as immature and emotional (Dahlstrom et al., 1972). The DSM-III diagnoses often associated with this code type also vary in terms of the degree to which they emphasize behavioral (compulsive behaviors), interpersonal (schizoid, passive-dependent), and affective (depression) features. Some have utilized the relative elevations of Scales 7 and 8 for differentiating neurotic from psychotic or schizoid disorders (Graham, 1977).

A MODEL FOR PREDICTING RESPONSES TO STRESSORS

Many tenable hypotheses may be generated for each of the 2-point codes presented. These hypotheses, when taken together, may cloud necessary diagnostic and therapeutic decision-making processes. Our previous work has suggested that by combining information from the MCMI and MMPI, many of these contradictions can be sorted out into consistent subtypes of each MMPI 2-point code, each representing different coping styles. One way to summarize the large collection of subtypes that we have identified is to view them within the framework of a stress-coping model. One of the most valuable benefits of personality diagnosis is the ability to predict future behaviors across a wide range of settings. Although many different personality styles present on the surface as similar at regular samplings, it is likely that during periods of acute stress or throughout periods of unremitting and severe burden that the pathognomonic signs of each personality style will present themselves. Whereas reactions to acute, short-lived stressors may reach extreme levels (manifest as clinical syndromes) these episodes may be as short-lived as their associated stimuli. More long-term, uncontrollable and unremitting stressors can be associated with more chronic changes in physical (e.g., immune system changes; Antoni, Schneiderman, Fletcher et al., 1990; McKinnon et al., 1989) and psychiatric (e.g., decompensation to a borderline level of psychopathology, Millon, 1981) status. A model that we have used to guide our empirical investigations is one derived from the personality theory of Millon (1981). This model views reactions to acute stressors along two dimensions: reactive *currency* and *direction*. We have proposed that one pervasive stressor, loss or threatened loss of reinforcement, can lead to responses comprised of interpersonal or emotional *currencies,* which are expressed in an outward or inward *direction*. Together these dimensions would make up the individual's coping style—a "program" that sets into motion several strategies that are employed in demanding situations. When individuals experience chronic unremitting periods of burden, especially to the extent that such burdens are perceived as uncontrollable, their coping style will be ineffective in regaining reinforcements and support. According to Millon (1981) the stressed individual's reactions to this loss expressed in distinct currencies and in a characteristic direction may spiral him/her into a state of self and/or social alienation followed by decompensation to a more severe variant of personality pathology. Millon has defined these decompensated patterns as schizotypal, borderline, and paranoid (Millon, 1981; see Table 16.1). We have used this model to interpret the findings of our research with the MCMI–MMPI battery.

One way that the MMPI and MCMI can offer clinical utility when combined as a battery, is in their ability to generate testable predictions of short-term responses to acute stressors as well as the more decompensatory sequelae of chronic stressors. In this chapter we present a summary of our previous work with such an "objective test battery" and how these findings might be useful in making predictions concerning such stress response/outcomes. Moreover, we demonstrate how such a battery can be used to clarify some of the previously

TABLE 16.1
A Model for Predicting Responses to Acute and Chronic,Severe Stressors

I. *Reactions to Acute Stressors*

    A. *Level*
       Emotional
       Interpersonal
    B. *Direction*
       Inward action
       Outward action

II. *Sequelae of Severe, Chronic Stressors*

    A. *Schizotypal pattern*
    B. *Borderline pattern*
    C. *Paranoid pattern*

TABLE 16.2
Demographic Characteristics of the Sample

Patients	Proportion of Sample
Status	
Outpatients	76.4%
Inpatients	21.3%
Not specified	2.3%
Gender	
Male	50.8%
Female	45.5%
Not specified	3.7%
Age (years)[a]	
20-34	31.4%
35-44	29.1%
45-54	19.2%
55-64	15.9%
65+	4.4%

[a]Percentages are based on that 90% of the sample for which demographic information was supplied. From Antoni, Levine, Tischer, Green, and Millon (1987). Reproduced by permission of Lawrence Erlbaum Associates.

presented contradictory descriptions that can result from relying on MMPI two-point codes alone.

Research Strategy

Sampling. Approximately 175 clinicians, all frequent users of both the MMPI and MCMI, were contacted and asked to participate in a study involving the administration of these two instruments to their patients. Data were collected over a 16-month period from a total of 46 clinicians in various geographical regions and professional settings resulting in a total return of 3283 sets of MMPI and MCMI batteries. Twenty-four of the clinicians responding were in private practice; 15 worked in community mental health centers, shared practices, clinics or other group settings; 3 were in Veterans Administration Medical Centers; and 4 worked in other hospital settings.

Exact figures on sample age and sex were unavailable owing to the failure of several participants to supply this information. Estimates drawn from samples of the data indicate slightly more female than male subjects. The age of the samples was widely distributed with no systematic bias. Approximately 85% of the subjects were outpatients and 15% were inpatients. The demographic characteristics of the overall sample are displayed in Table 16.2. In order to characterize the diagnostic spectrum making up the sample the proportion of primary DSM-III Axis I and II diagnoses was computed (see Table 16.3). Affective and anxiety

TABLE 16.3
Primary Diagnoses of the Sample

Primary Diagnosis	Proportion of Sample
No diagnosis provided	27%
Diagnosis	73%
Among Axis I	
Affective disorders	19%
Anxiety disorders	18%
Schizophrenic disorders	14%
Adjustment disorders	9%
Alcohol abuse disorders	9%
Drug abuse disorders	8%
Disorders with incidence <5%	23%
Among Axis II	
Dependent	24%
Avoidant	18%
Atypical/Mixed	11%
Passive-Aggressive	10%
Borderline	10%
Schizotypal	9%
Schizoid	7%
Compulsive	5%
Disorders with incidence <5%	5%

disorders were predominant along Axis I whereas Axis II primary diagnoses included a large number of dependent and borderline classifications.

Procedure.   Raw score data were reduced to the two highest scores for each instrument, provided that at least two scale scores were above a K-corrected T-score of 70 for the MMPI and a base rate (BR) score of 65 for the first eight or "basic" personality scales of the MCMI. If no MMPI scales were elevated then the profile was listed as flat. For MCMI data it was also noted whether any of the three severe personality disturbance scales (Schizotypal, Borderline, and Paranoid) was elevated. High point codes for each subject on the MCMI were tallied and percentages of the largest and most theoretically relevant code types were computed. Code types were included only when a minimum of 10 cases were used. This cut-off point is somewhat more stringent than those employed in other research designs examining MMPI overlap with measures of psychopathology (Gilberstadt & Duker, 1965; Kelly & King, 1977; Vincent et al., 1983). It was judged that this rule would reduce the possibility of subtypes emerging by chance.

Summary of Previously Published Findings

From the 3,283 MCMI–MMPI batteries, we anticipated that Ns of 200–300 would be available for each of the more commonly observed MMPI 2-point codes. To date we have published the results of six of the most prevalent MMPI 2-point codes. The sample sizes, and the relative proportion of the 3,283 cases

TABLE 16.4
Sample Sizes for Each of the Most Prevalent MMPI Two-Point Codes Studies

MMPI Code	N	% of Overall	Publication
28/82	353	10.8%	Antoni, Tischer, Levine et al., 1985a
24/42	318	9.7%	Antoni, Tischer, Levine et al., 1985b
49/94	305	9.3%	Levine, Antoni, Tischer et al., 1986
78/87	272	8.3%	Antoni, Levine, Tischer et al., 1987
98/89	228	6.9%	Antoni, Levine, Tischer et al., 1986
27/72	228	6.9%	Levine, Tischer, Antoni et al., 1985

collected for each of these six are displayed in Table 16.4. It is beyond the scope of this chapter to provide a detailed "cookbook" for every subtype of each MMPI 2-point code that we have studied. Rather we have summarized the findings from four commonly encountered, though somewhat disparate, 2-point code types with an emphasis placed on stress response predictions that can be made on the basis of MCMI–MMPI covariations. These four MMPI 2-point codes are those that were presented previously in the section on contradictory descriptors thus providing a demonstration of how such contradictions may be resolved with the "objective test battery" approach. For detailed descriptions of the results of each study the reader is referred to the primary reference.

MMPI 28/82

The results of our first MCMI–MMPI study indicated that covariations between the MMPI 28/82 type and MCMI high-point scales could enable the clinician to locate three distinct groups of individuals differing across dimensions. To reiterate some of the aspects of the model proposed previously, the interpersonal style can take the form of a detached or ambivalent one; and the reaction to loss of reinforcement is manifested in reactive currency (behavioral, interpersonal, or emotional) and direction (inward or outward). Each group represented a unique constellation of these dimensions. The first group (MCMI 12, 21), *the interpersonally acting-in group,* anticipates no reinforcement and therefore employs an interpersonal style of detachment or withdrawal. These individuals tend to react to stress with inwardly directed self-punitive responses on the behavioral and interpersonal level. The second group (MCMI 8, 82, 28), the *emotionally acting-out group,* seeks reinforcement from external sources, displays an ambivalent interpersonal style, and reacts to loss of support with outwardly directed unpredictable and dramatic emotional responses. The third group (MCMI 23, 32), the *emotionally acting-in group,* seeks reinforcements from external sources, moves between ambivalent and withdrawn interpersonal styles, and may react to loss of support with inwardly directed negative emotional experiences.

If stress should become excessive in any of these groups, thereby "overwhelming" their interpersonal style, they may become ineffective in securing reinforcements and support. The reactions to this loss expressed in their distinct currencies and in a characteristic direction (inward, outward) could spiral such individuals into a state of alienation followed by decompensation. In the emotional acting-out group, this alienation is likely to precipitate as self-alienation and identity problems. Our data suggested that decompensation appears to follow into a borderline pattern in this group. The interpersonally acting-in group may experience total alienation with decompensation to a schizotypal pattern when under unremitting stress. Finally, the emotionally acting-in group, possessing traits of both of the other two groups, may display borderline and schizotypal patterns of decompensation.

In sum, it appears that the primary sources of ambiguity in the MMPI 28/82 code description—the level (emotional vs. interpersonal) and direction (inward vs. outward) on which these individuals react to stress—may have been clarified by the use of MMPI-MCMI clusters into subtypes, named according to the configuration of these two dimensions.

MMPI 24/42

Analysis of the MCMI-MMPI battery for subjects classified as MMPI 24/42 produced three subtypes with at least one of these appearing to break into two variants. For this reason, we discuss our findings for this MMPI code type in somewhat more detail with an emphasis on stress responses within each subtype.

Interpersonally Acting-Out Group

We designated one subtype as the interpersonally acting-out group to describe their tendency to react to stress on the behavioral and interpersonal level through impulsive, outwardly directed, and projected responses. For these individuals it is likely that MMPI scale 4 elevations approximate their personality core and scale 2 elevations reflect a failure clinical outcome, when they are unable to acquire the reinforcements they need. Individuals comprising this group (MCMI scale 6, 65, 67, 5) are related in their arrogance, aggressiveness, and self-centeredness. When criticized, these individuals may become explosive and display overtly antisocial behaviors, such as brutality, alcoholism, drug addiction, and other forms of acting-out.

Acute Stress Response.   The first variant of this subtype (MCMI scale 6, primary elevation) appears driven by fear and a mistrust of others, resulting in hostile acting-out, angry rejection of social norms, and an undercurrent of inadequacy and self-dissatisfaction. This "desire to provoke fear and intimidate others" may stem either from a need to compensate for a sense of inner weakness or from a wish to vindicate past injustices (Millon, 1969, 1981).

The second variant (primary elevations on MCMI scale 5) appear guided by their high self-esteem, leading to arrogance and a disregard for social constraints. They may come across as charming and exhibitionistic, yet manipulative. The individual in this subgroup is rarely likely to experience self-doubt, although psychosocial stress may bring about unpredictable acting-out behaviors (addictions, sexual excesses) as a means of restoring equilibrium.

Chronic Stress Sequelae. Should these individuals meet with repeated failure in their attempt to secure support and reinforcement, paranoid-like behaviors may become evident. In support of this hypothesis, we found that over half of the interpersonally acting-out group (primary elevations on MCMI scale 6) also showed high elevations on the MCMI Paranoid scale—a scale measuring symptoms such as ideas of reference, vigilant mistrust and grandiose self-image. It is noteworthy also that those with primary elevations on MCMI scale 5 showed no elevations on the three, more severe personality scales.

Interpersonally Acting-In Group

Acute stress response. A second subtype composes a more unitary group and was referred to as an interpersonally acting-in group to emphasize their tendency to react to stressors on the behavioral and interpersonal levels through withdrawal, self-depreciation, and self-punitive responses. Individuals in this group (MCMI 1, 13–8) may be self-belittling, and possess a self-image of being weak and ineffectual. The intrapunitive nature of the interpersonally acting-in group seems the polar opposite of the extrapunitive and blaming nature of the acting-out group. According to Millon (1981) this group may comprise individuals who have neither internal nor external sources of reinforcement and therefore turn neither inward nor outward to acquire psychic pleasure or support. These individuals exhibit a deflated sense of self-esteem and experience a pan-social isolation, both of which would contribute to their high endorsement of MMPI scale 2 items. Importantly, isolation for this group is likely to reflect an indifference to social interaction rather than an active disdain or rejection of others, which is more characteristic of the interpersonally acting-out group.

Chronic Stress Sequelae. Should these individuals continue to experience both self and social alienation, they may decompensate into a pattern marked by behavioral eccentricities, ideas of reference, cognitive slippage, magical thinking, and depersonalization anxieties. These symptoms characterize a Schizotypal personality pattern. We found that a large proportion of patients in this interpersonally acting-in group showed distinct and frequent elevations on the Schizotypal scale of the MCMI.

Emotionally Acting-Out Group

Acute Stress Response.   The two subtypes discussed thus far, both representing variations of the MMPI 24/42 type, differ in both the "direction" of their expressive functioning (acting-out vs. acting-in), as well as in their likely course of decompensation. A third MMPI 24/42 group, referred to as the *emotionally acting-out* group, is best characterized by their tendency to exhibit demodulated, labile, and outwardly expressed affect employed to gain attention and support. Their coping pattern may volley between the traits of MMPI scales 2 and 4. In their case, the contradictory nature of the MMPI 24/42 code type descriptors portray, at least to some extent, the intrinsically contradictory nature of ambivalent interpersonal styles (Millon, 1969, 1981). Individuals included in this group (MCMI 34/43, 83, 84) may vacillate between irritably depressive moods and manic-like euphoric or hostile episodes. The unifying element in these emotional expressions appears to be their dramatic nature. According to Millon (1981) these displays might be designed to regain a "lost" source of reinforcement or support. Actively seeking reinforcement from external sources, these individuals are characterized both by an extreme dependency and a self-alienation. Central to these behaviors is a resentful ambivalence, possibly generated by conflict between dependency needs and a desire to be autonomous.

Chronic Stress Sequelae.   We hypothesized that when these individuals fail to gain and sustain attention and support, a mixed and conflicting set of emotions such as rage, guilt, and love may surge to the surface. These periods may be characterized by cognitive confusions over goals and identity, as well as desultory energy levels, and irregularities in the sleep–wake cycle. Supportive of this notion is the fact that a significant proportion of those in the emotionally acting-out group showed marked elevations on the MCMI Borderline personality scale, a scale reflecting such traits as identity confusion and sleep irregularity.

Resolution of Contradictions

Based on the results of the MCMI-MMPI analysis just summarized, it appears that the MMPI 24/42 code represents in the *interpersonally acting-out group,* an acting-out type in which scale 4 relates to the personality, whereas scale 2 reflects a more transient clinical outcome occurring when these individuals are unable to acquire reinforcements. High scale 2 in the *interpersonally acting-in group* seems to reflect the personality style, whereas scale 4 represents the clinical outcome of withdrawal via asocial behaviors and interpersonal indifference. The contradictory descriptors of the MMPI 24/42 code appear to accurately reflect the essential ambivalent nature of the third, or *emotionally acting-out group,* whose coping style waffles between the aspects of the MMPI scale 2 and 4.

MMPI 89/98

As noted previously, traditional descriptions of individuals revealing the 89/98 MMPI code type contain apparent contradictions at the behavioral, interpersonal, and emotional levels. We identified three subtypes that begin to explain the roots of these discrepancies.

Interpersonally Acting-Out Group

The largest subtype, comprised of individuals with elevations on MCMI scale 6 (antisocial) was referred to as the *interpersonally acting-out* group to portray their tendency to respond to stressors with impulsive outwardly-directed and projected responses. Criticism and assaults on their self-image may result in explosive antisocial behaviors such as substance abuse and frank brutality. The behaviors of this subtype may be "driven" by a fear and mistrust of others, resulting in hostile acting-out, rejection of social norms and an avoidance of close relationships stemming from a need to compensate for an inner sense of weakness or from a wish to vindicate past injustices (Millon, 1969, 1981).

Interpersonally Grandiose Group

Individuals with this subtype (with primary elevations on MCMI scale 5) are believed to be motivated by high self-esteem, feelings of grandiosity, disregard for social constraints, and interpersonal arrogance. These individuals, though charming and exhibitionistic during periods of low stress, may be prone to periods of acting-out (e.g., substance abuse, sexual excesses) when experiencing mounting stressors.

Chronic Stress Sequelae.   Should either of the two subtypes just discussed encounter periods of unremitting stress in which they meet with repeated failures to secure support and reinforcement, they may evince paranoid-like changes (e.g., magnifying the incidental remarks of others). This hypothesis was supported by our observation that a large proportion of individuals in both groups showed clear elevations on the MCMI Paranoid scale. This scale measures symptoms such as ideas of reference, vigilant mistrust, and grandiose self-image.

Emotionally Acting-Out Group

Acute Stress Responses.   The third subtype, made up of individuals with primary elevations on MCMI scale 8 (passive-aggressive) and scale 3 (dependent) are referred to as the *emotionally acting-out group* to describe their tendency to react to stressors with demodulated, labile, unpredictable, and intense affective responses. Because these individuals actively seek reinforcers from external sources they are susceptible to periods of extreme dependency and self-alienation. These individuals are also untrusting, fear domination, and are suspiciously alert to efforts to undermine their ambivalent and veiled movements toward closeness and intimacy. As such their coping style for dealing with interpersonal stressors is marked by ambivalence.

Chronic Stress Sequelae.   When these individuals' attempts at securing social support and attention fail, conflicting emotions of guilt, rage, and love may emerge. We hypothesized that such periods may be characterized by cognitive confusions over identity, extreme suspiciousness, and unpredictable succession of moods. In support of this notion was our observation that a substantial proportion of those people in the *emotionally acting-out group* showed elevations on both the MCMI Borderline and Paranoid Scales.

MMPI 78/87

Interpersonally Acting-In Group

Acute Stress Responses.   One subtype of the MMPI 78/87, comprised of individuals with elevations on MCMI scale 1 (schizoid) and 2 (avoidant) was termed the *interpersonally acting-in group* to describe their predicted tendency to react to stressors on the interpersonal level with indecision, withdrawal, pervasive anxiety, and obsessional thoughts. Millon (1969, 1981) states that the withdrawal and acting-in quality of this group may result from an inability to experience pleasure. This subtype can be seen as a group of individuals who are often socially alienated and self-alienated, and who experience a chronic state of psychic turmoil. Because such individuals are unsuccessful in reducing this chronic turmoil through interpersonal channels, they may engage in repetitive and ritualistic behaviors. Indeed, this subtype may be comprised of those MMPI 78/87 patients who receive obsessive-compulsive diagnoses.

Chronic Stress Sequelae.   Because these individuals are isolated from social feedback they may under periods of persistent and severe stress, decompensate into a pattern of behavioral eccentricities, ideas of reference, depersonalization anxieties, cognitive slippage, and magical thinking (i.e., schizotypal pattern). This hypothesis is supported by our observation that a large proportion of individuals in the *interpersonally acting-in group* also showed elevations on the MCMI Schizotypal scale.

Emotionally Acting-Out Group

Acute Stress Responses.   Other MMPI 78/87 descriptions focus on a more agitated clinical picture featuring outwardly expressed affect. These features mirror a second subtype which we termed the *emotionally acting-out group* to capture their tendency to react to stressors with labile emotional responses that volley between angry defiance and sullen moodiness. As opposed to the former MMPI 78/87 subtype these individuals actively seek reinforcement from others and are best characterized by extreme dependency, self-alienation, and interpersonal ambivalence. Their ambivalence over relationships can be manifest as hostility and demonstrative emotional displays which act to repel the significant others that they desperately need. As such this subtype fits the MMPI 78/87 descriptors that pertain to high affect and immaturity.

Chronic Stress Sequelae.   When under periods of chronic, uncontrollable demands, these individuals may become frustrated in their attempts to secure support and attention from others, especially to the extent that they have rebuffed members of their social network in the past. During such periods they may experience conflicting emotions related to others (e.g., guilt, love, rage), identity confusion, and physiological changes such as sleep irregularities. These predictions are supported by our observations that individuals in the *emotionally acting-out group* obtain elevations on the MCMI Borderline scale.

Emotionally Acting-In Group

Acute Stress Response.   A final subtype with the MMPI 78/87 code includes individuals with primary elevations on MCMI scale 2 (avoidant) and 3 (dependent) who we have designated as the *emotionally acting-in group.* This group of individuals is likely to respond to stress with inwardly directed anger and frustration, which Millon (1981) has hypothesized results from an intense conflict between opposing sources of reinforcement (other, self, none) and alternating approaches to securing that support (active, passive). Out of a fear of rejection by others, they may withdraw from their only source of reinforcement resulting in loneliness, social isolation, and mixed feelings of anxiety, sadness, anger, and guilt.

Chronic Stress Sequelae.   If reinforcers are unavailable for extended periods these individuals may become emotionally drained and may translate anger at others into self-degradation and feelings of unworthiness. Because of this relentless, downwardly spiralling conflict they may decompensate to either a schizotypal pattern, a borderline pattern, or some mixture of both. Associated symptoms would include acute emotional turmoil, irrational thinking, and periods of despondency. In support of these predictions we noted that a large proportion of individuals with this subtype also obtained elevations on both the MCMI Borderline and Schizotypal scales.

Summary

The results of our subtype analyses are summarized in Table 16.5. We believe that conceptualizing the various MMPI 2-point codes as distinct subtypes will

TABLE 16.5

Subtypes of Some Common MMPI Two-Point Codes Derived From the MCMI-MMPI Battery

MMPI 2-Point Codes and Subtypes	Key MCMI Elevations	Predicted Response to Stressors	Predominant Severe Variants
28/82			
Interpersonally acting-in	1, 2, 21	withdrawal, self-depreciation and self-punitive responses	schizotypal
Emotionally acting-out	8, 82, 28	labile, polar, and intense outwardly expressed affect	borderline
Emotionally acting-in	23, 32	anger, frustration, and restraint	schizotypal, borderline, or mixed
24/42			
Interpersonally acting-out	6, 65, 67, 5	antisocial behaviors (brutality substance abuse)	paranoid
Interpersonally acting-in	1, 13-8	self and social alienation, asocial behaviors	schizotypal
Emotionally acting-out	34/43, 83, 84	intense outwardly expressed affect, interpersonal ambivalence	borderline
89/98			
Interpersonally acting-out	65/56, 61, 6, 67	impulsive, outwardly-directed and projected responses	paranoid
Interpersonally grandiose	5	substance abuse, sexual excesses	paranoid
Emotionally acting-out	85, 86, 35, 34/43, 83	unpredictable intense impulsive angry outbursts	borderline, paranoid
78/87			
Interpersonally acting-in	12, 21	withdrawal, indecision, pervasive anxiety, obsessional thoughts	schizotypal
Emotionally acting-out	28, 82, 84, 83	outwardly expressed affect with vacillation between angry defiance, manic-like episodes and sullen moodiness	borderline
Emotionally acting-in	23, 32	inward-directed anger and frustration, social isolation	schizotypal:. borderline, or mixed

Included are predicted responses to acute stressors and severe personality variants potentially reflecting sequelae of more severe and chronic stressors.

facilitate making predictions concerning the coping responses that these individuals will employ in periods of acute stress and the route of decompensation that they will take should stressors persist and coping resources become insufficient. The discriminations that become available with this test battery may be useful in cases where the clinician needs to determine the salience and centrality of behavioral, interpersonal, and affective issues and observations.

Previously Unpublished Findings

For the purpose of illustrating our research strategy in greater detail as well as providing information that is not available in published form elsewhere this section provides a step-by-step analysis of the MCMI-MMPI covariation for the MMPI 48/84 2-point code. We also examine differences in cognitive style in this study.

Background

Primary elevations of MMPI scales 4 (psychopathic deviate) and 8 (schizophrenia) are relatively common among clinical populations, accounting for approximately 5.2% of inpatients and 6.0% of outpatients (Dahlstrom et al., 1972). The practice of treating the 48 and 84 patterns as equivalent is supported by research that failed to differentiate between the two patterns across most dimensions (Dahlstrom et al., 1972; Graham, 1977). Individuals receiving the 48/84 code type are often described as odd and peculiar, and not fitting in well with their environments. They are nonconforming and resentful of authority and have problems with impulse control. They tend to be angry and irritable, often behaving in erratic and unpredictable ways, while harboring deep feelings of insecurity along with exaggerated needs for attention and affection. They have poor self-concepts, and often set themselves up for rejection and failure. They are impaired empathically and usually maintain a socially isolated existence. Seeing the world as a hostile and rejecting place they may try to manipulate others to meet their needs and often accept little responsibility for their own behavior, which is often angry and threatening (preceding taken from Graham, 1977). Marks, Seeman, and Haller (1974) describe the features of the 48/84 pattern, which they refer to as "paranoid," as characterized by hostile and moody tendencies, inappropriate emotionality, and ideas of reference. Some are routinely diagnosed as paranoid schizophrenics, although many professionals prefer to label them "paranoid personalities" (Gilberstadt & Duker, 1965). Indeed, Marks and his colleagues (1974) state that 48/84 individuals show less of the florid thought disorders characteristic of other profiles with marked scale 8 elevations (e.g., MMPI 38/83, 68/86, 89/98).

The preceding descriptive review presents several plausible but often conflicting portrayals. For some the 48/84 MMPI code suggests a longstanding paranoid personality pattern, distinguishing such individuals from those with more acute schizophrenic or paranoid disorders. Other MMPI 48/84 descriptive differences are found in the representation of their interpersonal qualities (manipulation of others vs. withdrawal), emotional functioning (empathically impaired vs. angry and impulsive) and cognitive style (accepting little responsibility vs. self-doubt and insecurity). Taken together, these descriptors would make individual predictions highly unreliable, or ambiguous at best.

We investigated the clinical utility of employing an MCMI–MMPI battery with this code type. The first step in this procedure was to determine the pattern of covariations that would be found between MMPI 48/84 code types and MCMI high point profiles. Based on these covariations, the clinical significance of MCMI elevations was useful in refining some of the diverse descriptions usually assigned this code type in the MMPI literature. Of the total 3,283 cases collected, 6.2% (N = 202) were found to have MMPI scales 4 and 8 as their primary elevations. These were the subjects used for the present analysis.

RESULTS

The results of the covariation analysis between the MMPI 48/84 code type and the MCMI high-point types are depicted in Fig. 16.1. The covariation analysis yielded seven MCMI profiles that accounted for a significant segment of the MMPI 48/84 code type. These MCMI profiles are listed along the horizontal axis of Fig. 16.1. The vertical axis represents the percentage of patients receiving each MCMI type who also received elevations on the MMPI 48/84 (for example,

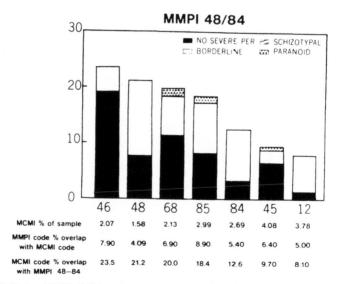

FIG. 16.1.   MMPI 48/84 code % overlap with MCMI high point codes.

20.0% of all patients with an MCMI 68 profile also obtained the 48/84 MMPI code).

Also represented on the bar graphs in Fig. 16.1 is the percent of each MCMI profile that also showed elevations on the severe personality disorder scales (Schizotypal, Borderline, and Paranoid). For example, of those receiving an MMPI code type of 48/84 and MCMI profile *48*, 63.6% also showed an elevation on the Borderline scale. The percentages for all the MCMI profiles were as follows: MCMI 46/64, 18.8% Borderline; MCMI *48*, 63.6% Borderline; MCMI *68*, 35.7% Borderline, 7.1% Paranoid; MCMI *85–86*, 50.0% Borderline, 5.6% Paranoid; MCMI *84*, 72.7% Borderline; MCMI *45*, 23.1% Borderline, 7.7% Paranoid; and MCMI *12*, 80.0% Borderline.

The MCMI profile data from this study established several distinctions among respondents obtaining the MMPI 48/84 code type. These results and their interpretation would appear to provide a basis for gauging severity of disturbance, as well as differentiating among seemingly contradictory descriptors generated by the MMPI high point code alone. As noted previously, analyses of the overlap between the MMPI and the MCMI yielded three distinct groups. These included one group, with a primary elevation on MCMI scale 8, a second group of patients with primary elevations on scale 6 of the MCMI, and a third, smaller group, marked by elevations on MCMI scales 1 or 2. The first two groups mentioned often present similar clinical pictures, thus leading to frequent confusions between them. Both are marked by a high degree of interpersonal manipulativeness, hostility, and aggressive behavior, traits often noted in MMPI 48/84 descriptions. However, important differences between these two groups exist, most notably in their emotional and cognitive styles. The smaller group, characterized by a detached, avoidant interpersonal style, is also worthy of note. Thus, MMPI 48/84 descriptors, often contain adjectives such as isolated and avoidant, a portrayal that conflicts with the hostile and manipulative pattern of the two larger groups. The following analyses should help illuminate and refine these clinical subtypes.

The Emotionally Acting-In/Out Group:
The Ambivalent Pattern

This first group, composed of those with elevations on MCMI scale 8 (passive aggressive) is referred to as the *emotionally acting in/out group* to represent the central role that ambivalence plays in their interpersonal, affective and cognitive styles. Deeply conflicted over their dependency needs, these patients often alternate between an angry manipulativeness and a dependent acquiescence (Millon, 1969, 1981). This pattern is captured well by most MMPI 48/84 descriptors, which note tendencies toward both manipulation and dependency. These patients tend also to be self-disparaging, and their cognitive style is characterized by self-doubt and insecurity. The dynamic struggle of need for support versus fear of being hurt is constantly being played out resulting in frequent or repeated alienations from those with whom they wish to be close.

The degree of internal conflict experienced by these individuals is evidenced also in the high percentage of MCMI Borderline personality scale elevations among these patients. Although the emotional lability and dysregulation indicated by the MCMI Borderline scale are not uncommon in the other subgroups, they are notably prevalent among this group. This ambivalence, expressed alternately in hostile manipulativeness, acquiescent dependency, and self-disparaging cognitions, may be observed at varying levels of severity, with concomitant disturbances in their ability to cope. In the following section, we distinguish between those whose manipulative hostility stems from emotional ambivalence and those who evidence these behaviors for other less conflictual reasons.

The Emotionally Acting-Out Group: The Contemptuous Pattern

This large group, distinguished by marked MCMI scale 6 (Antisocial–Aggressive) elevations, often appears similar clinically to the previous subtype. These individuals are also angry and frequently aggressive, as well as interpersonally manipulative. They are much less conflicted, however, appreciably less concerned than the emotionally ambivalent with issues of dependency or the securing of support and nurturance from others. Rather, their manipulativeness stems from an uncomplicated disregard, if not contempt for others, often displayed in scornful derogation typically rationalized by a "get them before they get you" attitude. Cognitively, this group fits well those MMPI descriptors that stress impaired empathy and a tendency to assume little or no responsibility for the consequence of their actions.

Further distinctions within this group may be made also on the basis of severity of disturbance. Elevations on the MCMI Borderline personality scale, emotional lability and dyscontrol, are present here in significant numbers. A small but meaningful number of patients in this group also show elevations on the MCMI Paranoid scale. Those whose disturbance is manifested primarily in paranoid ideation are likely to receive the clinical label of paranoid personality or even paranoid schizophrenia, although the actual incidence of these disorders is somewhat low. Emotional dyscontrol and lability are fairly common, however, and it is also clear that this group will respond differently to therapeutic attempts at rapport and empathy at least as compared to the emotionally ambivalent group.

The Interpersonally Acting-In Group: The Detached Pattern

A small proportion of patients receiving MMPI 48/84 elevations showed their primary elevations on MCMI scales 1 (schizoid) and/or 2 (avoidant). The resulting subtype is characterized by significant degrees of social isolation owing

either to affective deficits or protective withdrawal behaviors. Among those in the latter variant (high MCMI scale 2), the individual may have isolated himself in response to perceiving the world as a hostile, threatening place where relationships with others bring only pain (Millon, 1969, 1981). MMPI 48/84 descriptors include this pattern of isolation with the more common 48/84 picture of interpersonal manipulativeness and belligerence.

Many respondents in this detached group also show elevations on the MCMI Borderline scale, indicating a significant degree of psychic turmoil, emotional lability, and cognitive diffusion. The dimensions of interpersonal relationships and emotional regulation appear diagnostically important among these patients, especially if they are to be distinguished from the prior two MMPI 48/84 subtypes. Further, it would appear that patients falling in this group may be comprised of those respondents who are likely to decompensate toward schizophrenic processes in light of their tendencies toward withdrawal and isolation.

Summary

In this study, three subtypes within the MMPI 48/84 pattern were differentiated: an Ambivalent pattern, a Contemptuous pattern, and a Detached pattern. The Ambivalent and the Contemptuous groups often present features in common, notably that of hostile and manipulative interpersonal style. Important differences between the two groups were outlined as well, specifically, the need for support and nurturance from others. It is plausible further that attitudes and behaviors associated with each of these groups may appear in one individual, especially when followed over a period of time.

The results of this study further show that only a small percentage of those with the MMPI 48/84 pattern obtain elevations on the Paranoid scale of the MCMI, in contrast to what one might have expected based on the MMPI literature. In fact, half or more of those receiving elevations on the basic MCMI clinical scales showed no elevations on the more severe scales. Interestingly, the elevations of greatest frequency and severity were on the Borderline scale. This suggests that the MMPI 48/84 may be tapping more into emotional dysregulation, and not into blatant schizophrenic withdrawal or paranoid ideation. It suggests further that although the MMPI 48/84 pattern is indicative of emotional turmoil, it by no means indicates the presence of severe Axis I disorders such as paranoid schizophrenia. Differentiating between individuals whose primary difficulties lie in the paranoid or borderline realm, in addition to those with no severe personality pathology, may become possible when MCMI and MMPI data are combined. The data obtained in this study provide further support for the practice of combining different "objective" assessment instruments in a battery approach. Both the MMPI and the MCMI sampled from a wide range of personality variables-behavior, affect, cognition, interpersonal style, and probable mechanisms of defense. The MMPI high point code alone did not appear sufficient to discriminate among subtypes in as refined a manner as would be desirable.

Conclusion

The goal of our work was not only to demonstrate the utility of an MMPI–MCMI "battery" in terms of the refinement of personality diagnosis, but to lay the groundwork for empirical tests of diagnostic categories assessed by this battery. The descriptive stage in this process was the aim of our previous studies. The second step (empirical stage) necessarily involves external criteria against which these categories can be compared (e.g., clinical observations). This latter stage is the focus of other research in our laboratory in which clinicians' ratings, DSM-III diagnoses, and MCMI high-point codes are compared (Antoni, Green, Sandberg, & Millon, 1987).

Other gains may be derived from these studies aside from the clarification and refinement of MMPI interpretations. Supplementary elements of a taxonomic system include (a) a listing of central and salient clinical criteria, (b) separation and specification of clinical syndromes (Axis I) from personality disorders (Axis II), and (c) a variety of therapeutic implications. As we have already pointed out in this and prior studies, the individuals comprising a given MMPI code type display heterogeneity across many spheres of functioning (Antoni, Levine, Tischer et al., 1985; Antoni, Tischer, Levine, et al., 1985). The variability described for these groups may be found across behavioral, interpersonal, and affective realms and is manifest in specific "styles" of reinforcement acquisition, and decompensation. This variance describes the configurations of assorted clinical features, some describing a core issue and others representing more or less "spinoffs" of this central feature. We have demonstrated a format that gives a focus to the clinical picture by specifying particular spheres of psychosocial functioning and impairment (behavioral, cognitive, interpersonal, emotional), thereby establishing subtypes with distinct clusters of clinical symptoms.

Does one assign primacy to Axis I or Axis II in the DSM-III multidimensional schema? It is often uncertain, according to the set of descriptions provided for MMPI 2-point code types, which axis should be considered primary and which secondary in arriving at a diagnosis. It is equally unclear as to which Axis II disorder is most likely to "coexist" with an accompanying Axis I syndrome. Admittedly, the approach of our work has been to assign primacy to Axis II; hence, all the subgroups identified and described had a primary label along this axis. However, this formulation did allow for the explanation of clinical syndromes that would very likely be present in each subtype and, in so doing, united the most likely Axis I-Axis II combinations. The elucidation of these combinations is essential for accurate and comprehensive diagnosis and can help predict probable clinical course and treatment prognosis.

A third contribution of this test battery approach involves the therapeutic arena. With an understanding of the central clinical features, along with a clear picture of the primacy of syndrome and disorder in a given case, the clinician may be better prepared to decide on a treatment approach based on the efficacy of one intervention modality over another. Also, the identification of the spheres of functioning (e.g., interpersonal vs. emotional) may help clinicians with general "rapport" and communication ·... ·s, allowing them to work more efficiently with patients in familiar ways.

REFERENCES

American Psychiatric Association (1980). *Diagnostic and Statistical Manual of Mental Disorders.* American Psychiatric Association.

Antoni, M., Green, C., Sandberg, M., & Millon, T. (1987). *On the relationship between the DSM-III and the Millon Clinical Multiaxial Inventory.* Unpublished manuscript. University of Miami.

Antoni, M. H., Levine, J., Tischer, P., Green, C., & Millon, T. (1987). Refining personality assessments by combining MCMI high point profiles and MMPI codes, part V: MMPI code 78/87. *Journal of Personality Assessment, 51*(3), 375–387.

Antoni, M. H., Levine, J., Tischer, P., Green, C., & Millon, T. (1986). Refining personality assessments by combining MCMI high point profiles and MMPI codes, part IV: MMPI code 89/98. *Journal of Personality Assessment, 50*(1), 65–72.

Antoni, M. H., Levine, J., Tischer, P., Green, C., & Millon, T. (1985). Refining MMPI code interpretations by reference to MCMI scale data, part I: MMPI Code 28/82 *Journal of Personality Assessment, 49*(4), 392–398.

Antoni, M. H., Schneiderman, N., Fletcher, M. A., Goldstein, D., Ironson, G., & LaPerriere, A. (1990). Psychoneuroimmunology and HIV-1. *Journal of Consulting and Clinical Psychology, 58*(1), 38–49.

Antoni, M. H., Tischer, P., Levine, J., Green, C., & Millon, T. (1985). Refining personality assessments by combining MCMI high point profiles and MMPI codes, Part III: MMPI Code 24/42, *Journal of Personality Assessment, 49*(5), 508–515.

Butcher, J. N., & Owen, P. L. (1978). Objective personality inventories: Recent research and some contemporary issues. In B. B. Wolman (Ed.), *Clinical diagnosis of mental disorders: A handbook.* New York: Plenum Press.

Dahstrom, W. G., Welsh, G. S., & Dahlstrom, L. E. (1972). *An MMPI Handbook, Volume I: Clinical Interpretation.* Minneapolis: University of Minnesota Press.

Gilberstadt, H., & Duker, J. (1965). *A handbook for clinical and actuarial MMPI interpretation.* Philadelphia: W. B. Saunders.

Graham, J. R. (1977). *The MMPI: A practical guide.* New York: Oxford University Press.

Kelly, C., & King, G. D. (1977). MMPI behavioral correlates of spike 5 and two-point code types with scale 5 as one elevation. *Journal of Clinical Psychology, 33,* 180–185.

Korchin, S. J., & Schuldberg, D. (1981). The future of clinical assessment. *American Psychologist, 36,* 1147–1148.

Levine, J., Antoni, M. H., Tischer, P., Green, C., & Millon, T. (1985). Refining MMPI code interpretations by reference to MCMI scale data, part II: MMPI Code 27/72. *Journal of Personality Assessment, 49*(5), 501–507.

Levine, J., Tischer, P., Antoni, M. H., Green, C., & Millon, T. (1986). Refining personality assessments by combining MCMI high point profiles and MMPI codes, part VI: MMPI code 49/94. *Journal of Personality Assessment, 51.*

Marks, P., Seeman, W., & Haller, D. (1974). *The actuarial use of the MMPI with adolescents and adults.* Baltimore, MD: Williams and Wilkins.

McKinnon, W., Weisse, C., Reynolds, C., Bowles, C., & Baum, A. (1989). Chronic stress, leukocyte subpopulations, and humoral responses to latent viruses. *Health Psychology, 8*(4), 389–402.

Millon, T. (1969). *Modern Psychopathology. A biosocial approach to maladaptive learning and functioning.* Philadelphia: W. B. Saunders.

Millon, T. (1981). *Disorders of personality: DSM-III: Axis II.* New York: Wiley Interscience.

Millon, T. (1984). An interpretive guide to the Millon Clinical Multiaxial Inventory. In P. McReynolds & G. Chelune (Eds.), *Advances in psychological assessment* (Vol. 6). San Francisco: Jossey-Bass.

Vincent, K. R., Castillo, I., Hauser, R. I., Stuart, H. J., Zapata, J. A., Cohn, C. K., & O'Shanick, G. J. (1983). MMPI code type and DSM-III diagnoses. *Journal of Clinical Psychology, 39*(6), 829–842.

Author Index

Subject Index